Health and Disease
A READER

This reader is one part of an Open University integrated teaching system and the selection is therefore related to other material available to students. It is designed to evoke the critical understanding of students. Opinions expressed in it are not necessarily those of the course team or of the University.

Health and Disease

A READER

Edited by
Nick Black, David Boswell, Alastair Gray, Sean Murphy and Jennie Popay
at the Open University

Open University Press

Milton Keynes · Philadelphia

Open University Press,
12 Cofferidge Close, Stony Stratford,
Milton Keynes MK11 1BY, England
and
242 Cherry Street,
Philadelphia PA 19106, U.S.A.

First published 1984
Reprinted 1986, 1988, 1989

British Library Cataloguing in Publication Data

Health and disease.
  1. Health
  I. Black, Nick
  613   RA776

  ISBN 0–335–15017–9
  ISBN 0–335–10593–9 Pbk

Library of Congress Cataloguing in Publication Data

Health and disease
  Bibliography: p.
  Includes index.
  1. Public health—Social aspects—Addresses, essays, lectures.   2. Medical
care—Social aspects—Addresses, essays, lectures.   I. Black, Nick. [DNLM:
1. Health—collected works. 2. Disease—collected works. 3. Medicine—
collected works. 4. Delivery of Health Care—collected works. 5. Sociology,
Medical—collected works. WA 31 H434]
RA436.H43 1984   362.1   84–18913

  ISBN 0–335–15017–9
  ISBN 0–335–10593–9 (pbk.)

Text design by Clark Williams
Typesetting by S & S Press, Abingdon, Oxfordshire
Printed in Great Britain by
M. & A. Thomson Litho Limited,
East Kilbride, Glasgow,
Scotland

Contents

Part 6 Experiencing health and disease

Part 7 Prospects and speculations

Acknowledgements

During the planning phase of this Reader we were pleased to receive many suggestions from members of the U205 Course Team and help with editing, particularly Steven Rose, Phil Strong, Basiro Davey and Liz Lane. In many cases the authors of the articles contained in this Reader made useful suggestions as to their editing and we thank them and the publishers for their cooperation.

Finally, we were maintained through our task by Sylvia Bentley who, in addition to her extensive involvement in preparing the associated Open University course, prepared much of the final manuscript.

Copyright Permissions

1.1 Abridged selections (pp. 2–232) from *Mirage of Health: Utopias, Progress and Biological Change* by René Dubos, Vol. 22 in *World Perspectives* planned and edited by Ruth Nanda Anshen, © 1959 René Dubos, reprinted by permission of Harper & Row Publishers Inc.

1.2 Reprinted from *Culture, Medicine and Psychiatry* 2, 1978, 107–37, copyright © 1978 by D. Reidel Publishing Company, Dordrecht, Holland, by permission of D. Reidel Co., and from *New Society*, 5 November 1981, by permission of *New Society*.

1.3 Reprinted from D. Pillsbury, 'Doing the month' in *Social Science and Medicine* Vol. 12, 11–22, by permission of Pergamon Press.

1.4 Reprinted from C. Smith-Rosenberg, 'the hysterical woman' in *Social Research* Vol. 39 No. 4 (1972) by permission of *Social Research*.

1.5 Reprinted from M. Blaxter, 'The courses of disease' in *Social Science and Medicine* Vol. 17, 59–69, by permission of Pergamon Press.

1.6 Original article by I. Loudon © The Open University 1984, by permission of the Open University.

1.7 Reprinted from T. Posner, 'Magical Elements in Orthodox Medicine' in Dingwall et al. (eds), *Health Care and Health Knowledge,* Croom Helm 1977, by permission of Croom Helm Ltd.

2.1 Reprinted from F. Engels, *The Condition of the Working Class in England,* translated by the Institute of Marxism-Leninism, Moscow, Panther Books 1969, by permission of Panther Books and Lawrence and Wishart.

2.2 Reprinted from P. Harrison, *Inside the Inner City,* Pelican Books 1983, 21–44, 253–9, © Paul Harrison 1983, by permission of Penguin Books Ltd. and Paul Harrison.

2.3 Reprinted from R. Titmuss, *Essays on the Welfare State,* Allen & Unwin 1958, by permission of George Allen & Unwin (Publishers) Ltd.

2.4 Reprinted from O. Tuckett and J. M. Kaufert (eds), *Basic Readings in Medical Sociology,* Tavistock 1978, by permission of Associated Book Publishers Ltd.

2.5 Reprinted from A. Sen, *Poverty and Famines,* ILO 1981, 154–66, © 1981 International Labour Office, Geneva, by permission of the ILO.

2.6 Reprinted from Sir MacFarlane Burnet, 'Biomedical research' in *Perspectives in Biology and Medicine,* Vol. 24, No. 4, 511–24, by permission of the University of Chicago Press.

2.7   Reprinted from the Royal College of Physicians Medical Services Study Group, 'Deaths Under 50' in *British Medical Journal* 2, 1061–2, by permission of the *British Medical Journal*.

2.8   Reprinted from R. Asher, *Talking Sense*, Pitman 1972 by permission of Pitman Publishing Ltd.

3.1   Reprinted from T. McKeown, *The Modern Rise of Population*, Edward Arnold, 1976, by permission of Edward Arnold Publishers Ltd.

3.2   Reprinted from A. L. Cochrane, *Effectiveness and Efficiency: Random Reflections on Health Services*, Nuffield Provincial Hospitals Trust, 1971, © A. L. Cochrane, by permission of the author.

3.3   Reprinted from P. Beeson, 'Changes in medical therapy', *Medicine*, 1980, 59, 79–84, © 1980 The Williams and Wilkins Co, Baltimore, by permission.

3.4   Reprinted from J. T. Hart, 'A new kind of doctor' in the *Journal of the Royal Society of Medicine* 74, 1981, 871–83, by permission of the *J.R.S.M.*

3.5   Reprinted from D. Piachaud and J. Weddell, 'The economics of treating varicose veins' in the *International Journal of Epidemiology*, 387–93, by permission of the I.J.E.

3.6   Reprinted from *The Lancet, The Guardian* and the *British Medical Journal* by permission.

3.7   Reprinted from I. Illich, *Limits to Medicine*, Marion Boyars, 1976, by permission of Marion Boyars Publishers Ltd.

3.8   Reprinted from V. Navarro, *Medicine under Capitalism*, Prodist, 1976, by permission of the author.

3.9   Reprinted from A. Oakley, Women Confined, Martin Robertson 1980, by permission of Basil Blackwell Ltd.

3.10 Reprinted from D. Werner, 'The Village Health Worker' in Skeet & Elliott (eds), *Health Auxiliaries and the Health Team*, Croom Helm 1978, by permission of Croom Helm Ltd.

4.1   Reprinted from R. Stevens, 'The Evolution of the Health-Care Systems in the US and the UK', by permission of the author.

4.2   Original article by G. Bevan © The Open University 1984, by permission of the Open University.

4.3   Reprinted from A. Ramesh and B. Hyma, 'Traditional Indian Medicine in practice in an Indian metropolitan city' in *Social Science and Medicine* Vol. 15, 69–81, by permission of Pergamon Press Ltd.

4.4   Reprinted from T. Bossert, 'Health policy-making in a revolutionary context' in *Social Science and Medicine* Vol. 15, 225–31, by permission of Pergamon Press Ltd.

4.5   Reprinted from M. Strassburg, 'The global eradication of smallpox' in the *American Journal of Infection Control* Vol. 19, 53–9, by permission of the C. V. Mosby Company.

4.6   Reprinted from *Drug Problems in the Sociocultural Context*, World Health Organization 1980, by permission of the WHO.

5.1   Reprinted from E. Goffman, 'The Insanity of Place', *Psychiatry*, 1969, 32. 357–88, © 1969 by the William Alanson White Psychiatric Foundation, Inc., by special permission of The William Alanson White Psychiatric Foundation, Inc. and from *Relations in Public*, Allen Lane, 1971, 335–90, by permission of Penguin Books Ltd.

5.2   Reprinted from E. Paterson, 'Food-work' in P. Atkinson and C. Heath (eds), *Medical Work*, Gower, 1981, by permission of Gower Publishing Co. Ltd.

5.3   Reprinted from R. Jeffrey, 'Normal rubbish' in *Sociology of Health and Illness* Vol. I, No. 1, 1979, by permission of Routledge and Kegan Paul plc.

5.4   Reprinted from the *Report of the Committee on Nursing (Chairman Professor Asa Briggs)*, 1972, Her Majesty's Stationery Office, 1972, by permission of HMSO.

6.1   Reprinted from J. Van den Berg, *The Psychology of the Sickbed*, Humanities Press, 1981, by permission of Humanities Press Inc., Atlantic Highlands, N.J. 07716.

6.2   Reprinted from S. Macintyre and D. Oldham, 'Coping with Migraine' in Davis and Horobin (eds), *Medical Encounters*, Croom Helm 1977, by permission of the authors.

6.3   Reprinted from A. Shearer, *Disability: Whose Handicap?*, Basil Blackwell, 1981, by permission of Basil Blackwell.

6.4   Reprinted from Ellen Newton, *This Bed My Centre*, Virago Press 1980, by permission of Virago Press.

6.5   Reprinted from A. Bowling and A. Cartwright, *Life After Death: A study of elderly widowed*, Tavistock, 1982, by permission of Associated Book Publishers Ltd.

6.6   Reprinted from R. Littlewood and M. Lipsedge, *Aliens and Alienists*, Pelican Books 1982, 25–8 and 65–7, by permission of Penguin Books Ltd.

6.7   Reprinted from B. Earthrowl and M. Stacey 'Social class and children in hospital' in *Social Science and Medicine* Vol. 11, 83–8, by permission of Pergamon Press Ltd.

7.1   Reprinted from J. D. Bernal, *The World, The Flesh and the Devil*, Jonathan Cape, 1929, by permission of Routledge and Kegan Paul plc.

7.2   Original article by B. Durie © The Open University 1984, by permission of the Open University.

7.3   Reprinted from E. Frei, 'The National Cancer Chemotherapy Program' *Science* 217, 1982, 600–6, by permission of *Science*.

7.4   Edited material from *Inequalities in Health* (Chairman Sir Douglas Black), Her Majesty's Stationery Office, 1980, by permission of HMSO; extracts from Introduction to P. Townsend and N. Davidson, *Inequalities in Health*, Pelican Books, 1982, 16–24, by permission of Penguin Books Ltd.; material from *Lancet* and *British Medical Journal* by permission.

7.5   Original article © Alain C. Enthoven 1984, by permission of the author.

7.6   Original article by R. West © The Open University 1984, by permission of the Open University.

7.7   Reprinted from *Disease: Cancer; Cause: Work; Task: Prove It*, by permission of the General Municipal Boilermakers and Allied Trades Union.

7.8   Excerpt from A. Huxley, *Brave New World*, © 1932 by Aldous Huxley, renewed 1960 by Aldous Huxley. Reprinted by permission of Mrs Laura Huxley and Chatto & Windus, and by permission of Harper & Row, Publishers, Inc.

General Introduction

Although there has been a great expansion of interest, research and publishing related to health and disease in recent years, much of it has made little attempt to acknowledge, far less surmount, the constraints imposed by different disciplinary boundaries. In particular, there has been a general failure of biological science, of medicine and of social science to speak to one another. This Reader is committed to the view that neither health nor disease are straightforward matters, and that they can only be fully understood by adopting an interdisciplinary stance.

The frequent failure to take such a stance is exemplified in the UK by the strong bias towards pure clinical research exhibited by the Medical Research Council; by the small numbers of social scientists willing to engage in collaborative research on health and disease topics; and by the low status often ascribed to such research. And yet there are many examples of the benefits which can result from adopting an interdisciplinary approach to questions of health and disease. A contemporary instance might be the development of a method of preventing neural-tube defects (spina bifida): biological science has provided a simple screening test which can identify pregnancies at risk. The spreading medical application of the screening procedure has not only posed a number of epidemiological questions concerning the distribution of defects, but has created ethical and psychological difficulties for providers and recipients, raised economic questions concerning the relative benefits and costs of the procedure, and even spilled over into legal aspects when screening fails to detect an affected foetus. The perspective of individual disciplines in such cases is somewhat blinkered, while the great majority of people quite correctly perceive that to understand the full implication of such a development it is necessary and indeed natural to move between the biological, the medical and the social.

The material collected into this Reader is drawn mainly from the biological, medical and social sciences. The intention is to advertise the advantages of a broader perspective, by drawing attention to the handicaps which disciplinary boundaries can impose.

In all, fifty articles have been included, of which five have not previously been published and the remainder have been drawn from a wide variety of sources. The articles differ greatly in style, content, focus and perspective. Given this diversity, and the broad reach of the collection, it is worth stating briefly the principles and objectives underlying the arrangements of the book's contents and the selection of the articles included.

The readings have been grouped around seven headings: concepts of health and disease; factors influencing patterns of health and disease; the role of medicine; aspects of health care systems; organisations and occupations within health care; the experience of health care; and prospects and speculations. These topics have been chosen because they seem to be areas of enquiry that have been given some priority by several disciplines. Within each topic the emphasis has been on maintaining representation, rather than equality, of biological, medical and social sciences. Each part of this book has a short introductory text prepared by the editors, as a guide to the readings and their authors.

In selecting material for inclusion, the editors decided to opt for the policy of a larger number of edited articles rather than a much smaller number in unabridged form. Nevertheless, many difficult decisions had to be made on what to include or exclude. Apart from maintaining the overall thematic and disciplinary balance of the readings, decisions on what to include could not be reduced to any neat set of criteria: some readings have been included because of their 'classic' status, some as participants in key controversies or debates. Others were included because they are difficult or had been unjustifiably neglected. The editors sought, and are pleased to acknowledge, the co-operation of authors or trustees in reducing the length of the original texts and we hope that the substance and style have been largely retained. Where substantial and significant parts of the text have been removed, this has been indicated in the source note at the end of the article, where short descriptions of the authors are appended, together with the full original reference of that material previously published.

The Reader has been devised to accompany an Open University second-level course— *U205 Health and Disease*. The major aim of this course is 'to educate the student concerning those factors physical, biological, and social, which are responsible for the state of our own health and the health of the society and world in which we live'.

This course has been able to explore in depth the possibilities of an interdisciplinary approach to a whole range of health and disease topics by combining this Reader with extensive and specially prepared teaching texts and audiovisual materials. For students taking the course, this Reader is indispensable, but the collection has also been designed to stand as a coherent and self-contained entity, accessible to the wider reading public. Among this wider audience, the editors hope that doctors, nurses and others involved in the health and welfare services will find this collection of readings to be of particular value. It will also be relevant to the undergraduate studies of medical and social science students, as well as being of interest to the general public.

Part 1

Concepts of health, disease and illness

Introduction

Concepts have their own history, and should be seen within a framework of related ideas and beliefs. This is as true of science and medicine as it is of theology and politics. The articles selected for this part exemplify some of the approaches needed to understand the meaning and significance of both popular and professional conceptions of health, disease and illness.

Most societies maintain some myth of a Golden Age which, while usually set in the past, may be considered to be attainable in the future if the appropriate policies and practices are adopted. René Dubos, who was a microbiologist, argued that health is such a concept, with the difference that it is considered to be attainable now, not only by individuals but also collectively by society. The notion of the 'noble savage' corrupted by civilisation, or the rural community disturbed by urbanisation, has a direct parallel in holistic conceptions of health as a state of harmony with nature.

Such a view of health is mirrored by one of illness and disease as disharmony. Cecil Helman, a general practitioner and social anthropologist, demonstrates how fundamental this is for understanding popular explanations of ill-health in the UK. He shows how ways of dealing with colds and fevers are influenced by the classical tradition of 'medical' natural philosophy that was expounded by the Greeks and codified by the Roman physician, Galen. Similarly, Barbara Pillsbury shows that this is also a potent force in the behaviour of other cultures. In China, 'doing the month' after childbirth involves mothers in restoring their equilibrium. It is intended both to be physically therapeutic and to prevent misfortune falling on other people. It therefore provides a way for women to regain a safe place in society.

Women's bodily functions have been closely linked with expectations of their roles in society as mothers, home keepers and definers of morality. Yet, at the same time, women have occupied socially inferior positions and been dependent on men. Against such a background, Carroll Smith-Rosenberg argues that the way hysteria was diagnosed and treated by physicians in the nineteenth century may have resulted not only from such conflicting demands made of women, but also from the reactions of physicians as men. Although blame for hysteria was often laid on the indolence and self-pitying indulgence of middle-class urban women and the fecklessness and sexual indulgence of working-class women, there is powerful evidence to suggest that hysteria may have been women's only possible 'escape', given their subordinate position in society.

The subject of blame and responsibility for the causes of ill health has always been part of the popular conception of disease. Helman argues that the attractiveness of the germ theory of disease, with its notion of external agents, may lie in the fact that it relieves those afflicted of responsibility (provided they have taken normal precautions). This can be seen in the work of Mildred Blaxter, a British sociologist, who found that Aberdonian working-class grandmothers believed that a variety of environmental factors—stress, trauma and poverty, as well as the natural process of ageing—also contributed to the relief of responsibility. Individuals had no more control over these factors than they did over a body which, once weakened, was liable to suffer further complications as diseases developed.

Where, then, does modern scientific medicine fit into the picture? Is it some separate force with its own model of causation and treatment? The answer, as can be seen in these articles, is a complicated one. Professionalised medicine may, as Smith-Rosenberg argues, largely reflect general social roles and values; for example, the reaction of male doctors to isolated, lonely and depressed women and the labelling of these women as hysterical. Professionalised medicine may also strike a bargain with patients by putting across modern medical ideas and explanations that meet the expectations of well-established popular images of disease. Helman suggests that this is the situation in the NHS and may account for its overprescription of medicines. And Blaxter describes how women's notions of the causation of disease arise from information received, not only from doctors but also from their own parents, ideas current in their community, and what is put across in advertising and on television.

Whatever their interrelationship, the potentially fundamental difference between scientific and popular conceptions of the causation of disease and appropriate treatment cannot be ignored. Pillsbury indicates through her Chinese examples that, while some Western-trained health staff look for analogies between these traditional beliefs and practices and those in their own societies, some reject them, and yet others merely select the parts that seem to work.

The case for medical intervention, though sometimes based on incomplete rather than comprehensive understanding of causation, is made by Irvine Loudon, a retired general practitioner and medical historian. His article analyses the progress made towards success in treating pernicious anaemia in the absence of a full explanation of its cause. However, there are many examples of treatments which failed as a consequence of inappropriate theories of causation and which sometimes resulted in mistreatment, even to the extent of harming patients. This is the basis for Tina Posner's discussion of the treatment of diabetes. She argues that, because reducing the level of blood sugar to that normally found in the general population is an accepted medical treatment, one of the most common problems for people with diabetes is hypoglycaemic coma, which is a direct result of insulin therapy. She goes on to argue that the desire to control the level of blood sugar is, in any case, largely an act of faith on the part of doctors, many of whom are well aware that they are in the dark as to whether such control confers any long-term benefit. Posner suggests that such behaviour is not unlike that of magical practitioners in other societies who feel they have to do something in critical and desperate circumstances, are uncertain what to do, and hold fast to a fixed belief in traditional practices. In this context Loudon also draws parallels with the situation that lasted for many years in the treatment of pernicious anaemia.

This poses the question as to whether there is a difference between belief in witchcraft and belief in these therapies? When witchcraft fails, it is the method of applying it which is questioned by the believers rather than the whole system. Similarly, the very doubts that doctors have about treating diabetes should make them susceptible to change their practices if better evidence comes their way. In the meantime, they pin their faith on the belief that long-term benefits ought to accrue from controlling blood sugar levels, despite no demonstration of this effect.

The association between popular images of health and disease, patterns of belief and of social behaviour, and the development and practice of scientific medicine is intricate and problematic. These articles exemplify the wide range of approaches to these matters and the different observations and conclusions to which investigators have been drawn.

1.1

Mirage of Health

René Dubos

The Gardens of Eden

The illusion that perfect health and happiness are within man's possibilities has flourished in many different forms throughout history. Primitive religions and folklores are wont to place in the remote past this idyllic state of paradise on earth. In the Old Testament the Patriarchs are said to have lived hundreds of years, while their descendants can hardly aspire to more than threescore and ten. The ancient Greeks believed in the existence of happy races, vigorous and virtuous, in inaccessible parts of the earth. According to their legends, the Hyperboreans and the Scythians in the north, the Ethiopians in the south, lived exempt from toil and warfare, from disease and old age, in everlasting bliss like the dwellers in the Isles of the Blest at the edge of the Western Sea.

The Return to Nature

Like primitive peoples, men in civilized societies commonly believe in the possibility of an ideal state of health and happiness. But, instead of expressing this belief through legends and folklore, they are apt to rationalize it in the form of philosophical theories and to assert that a healthy mind in a healthy body can be achieved only by harmonizing life with the ways of nature. The latter part of the eighteenth century proved particularly receptive—in theory at least—to the gospel that all human problems could be solved by returning to the ways of nature. Jean Jacques Rousseau asserted that man in his original state was good, healthy, and happy and that all his troubles came from the fact that civilization had spoiled him physically and corrupted him mentally. 'Hygiene,' Rousseau claimed, 'is less a science than a virtue.' Sickness being the result of straying away from the natural environment, the blessed original state of health and happiness could be recaptured only through abiding by the simple order and purity of nature—or, as Voltaire said in maliciously paraphrasing Rousseau, through learning again to walk on all fours.

Since very ancient times the theory that most of the ills of mankind arise from failure to follow the laws of nature has been endlessly reformulated in every possible form and mood, in technical and poetical language, in ponderous treatises and witty epigrams. In particular, the Taoist philosophy which has so profoundly influenced Chinese life and art is pervaded by reverence for nature. Lao-tzu, the Jean Jacques Rousseau of ancient China, was followed by many translators and imitators. Chuang-tzu wrote of the time when 'the ancient men lived in a world of primitive simplicity. . . . That was the time when the *yin* and the *yang* worked harmoniously, and the spirits of men and beasts did not interfere with the life of the people, when the four seasons were in order and all creation was unharmed, and the people did not die young.'

Modern man has done many odd things to display his faith in the fundamental goodness of nature. Following in the steps of Rousseau, one hundred million Central Europeans went botanizing in the hope of discovering among lowly flowers both the soul of the universe and natural remedies for chest troubles. More prosaic twentieth-century man tries to re-establish contact with this forgotten biological past in countless country clubs, hunting or ski lodges and beach bungalows, through clambakes in the moonlight and barbecue parties in suburban gardens and picnic groves. Whatever his inhibitions and tastes, Western man believes in the natural holiness of seminudism and raw vegetable juice, because these have become for him symbols of unadulterated nature.

The Concept of Nature

It is probable that a few people now and then in limited periods of history have enjoyed relative peace in a fairly constant physical and social environment. But the state of equilibrium never lasts long and its characteristics are at best elusive, because the word 'nature' does not designate a definable and constant entity. With reference to life there is not one *nature*; there are only associations of states and circumstances, varying from place to place and from time to time.

Living things can survive and function effectively only if they adapt themselves to the peculiarities of each individual situation. For some sulphur bacteria, nature is a Mexican spring with extremely acid water at very high temperature; for the reindeer moss, it is a rock surface in the frozen atmosphere of the arctic. The word 'nature' also means very different things to different men. Man, by manipulating the external world, renders 'natural' for his individual taste many kinds of environments which display an astonishingly wide range of moods.

Harmonious equilibrium with nature is an abstract concept with a Platonic beauty but lacking the flesh and blood of life. It fails, in particular, to convey the creative emergent quality of human existence. [For man] the seasons and the soil, the plants and the beasts, the permanent dwellers and the distant visitors with which he came into contact during his long journey, all the factors of his total environment, differed from one place to another, from one period to another, and their temporary association constituted the 'nature' to which he had to adapt in each situation and at each moment.

The Doctrine of Specific Etiology

Until late in the nineteenth century disease had been regarded as resulting from a lack of harmony between the sick person and his environment. Louis Pasteur, Robert Koch, and their followers took a far simpler and more direct view of the problem. They showed by laboratory experiments that disease could be produced at will by the mere artifice of introducing a single specific factor—a virulent microorganism—into a healthy animal.

From the field of infection the doctrine of specific etiology spread rapidly to other areas of medicine; a large variety of well-defined disease states could be produced experimentally by creating in the body specific biochemical or physiological lesions. Microbial agents, disturbances in essential metabolic processes, deficiencies in growth factors or in hormones, and physiological stresses are now regarded as specific causes of disease. The ancient concept of disharmony between the sick person and his environment seems very primitive and obscure indeed when compared with the precise terminology and explanations of modern medical science.

Unquestionably the doctrine of specific etiology has been the most constructive force in medical research for almost a century and the theoretical and practical achievements to which it has led constitute the bulk of modern medicine. Yet few are the cases in which it has provided a complete account of the causation of disease. Despite frantic efforts, the causes of cancer, of arteriosclerosis, of mental disorders, and of the great medical problems of our times remain undiscovered. It is generally assumed that these failures are due to technical difficulties and that the cause of all diseases can and will be found in due time by bringing the big guns of science to bear on the problems. In reality, however, search for *the* cause may be a hopeless pursuit because most disease states are the indirect outcome of a constellation of circumstances rather than the direct result of single determinant factors.

It is true that in a few cases—far less common than usually believed—the search for *the* cause has led to effective measures of control. But it does not follow that these measures provide information as to the nature of the trouble that they correct. While drenching with water may help in putting out a blaze, few are the cases in which fire has its origin in a lack of water. Effective therapies do not constitute evidence for the doctrine of specific etiology.

Darwin and Bernard

By equating disease with the effect of a precise cause—microbial invader, biochemical lesion, or mental stress—the doctrine of specific etiology had appeared to negate the philosophical view of health as equilibrium and to render obsolete the traditional art of medicine. Oddly enough, however, the vague and abstract concepts symbolized by the Hippocratic doctrine of harmony are now re-entering the scientific arena. Hippocratic medicine has acquired a more profound significance from the implications of the discoveries that Darwin and Claude Bernard were making around 1850—even before Pasteur and Koch had made their contributions to the etiology of disease. Darwinism implies that the individual and species which survive and multiply selectively are those best adapted to the external environment. Claude Bernard supplemented the doctrine of evolutionary adaptation by his visionary guess that fitness depends upon a constant interplay between the internal and the external environment of the individual. He emphasized that at all levels of biological organization, in plants as well as in animals, survival and fitness are conditioned by the ability of the organism to resist the impact of the outside world and maintain constant within narrow limits the physicochemical characteristics of its internal environment. In other words, life depends not only upon the reactions through which the individual manages to grow and to reproduce itself but also upon the operation of the control mechanisms which permit the maintenance of individuality. The dual concept of fitness to the external environment and fixity of the internal environment is the modern expression of the Hippocratic dictum that health is universal sympathy.

The Gods of Health

The word 'hygiene' now conjures up smells of chlorine and phenol, pasteurized foodstuffs and beverages in cellophane wrappers, a way of life in which the search for pleasurable sensations must yield to practices that are assumed to be sanitary. Its etymology, however, bears no relation to this pedestrian concept. Hygiene is the modern ersatz for the cult of Hygeia, the lovely goddess who once watched over the health of Athens. She was the guardian of health and symbolized the belief that men could remain well if they lived according to reason.

Throughout the classical world Hygeia continued to symbolize the virtues of a sane life in a pleasant environment, the ideal of *mens sana in corpore sano*. Hygeia was not an earthbound goddess of ancient origin. Her name derives from an abstract word meaning health. For the Greeks she was a concept rather than a historical person remembered from the myths of their past. She was not a compelling Jeanne d'Arc but only an allegorical goddess Liberty and she never truly touched the hearts of the people. From the fifth century BC on, her cult progressively gave way to that of the healing god, Asclepius.

To ward off disease or recover health, men as a rule find it easier to depend on healers than to attempt the more difficult task of living wisely. Asclepius, the first physician according to Greek legend, achieved fame not by teaching wisdom but by mastering the use of the knife and the knowledge of the curative virtues of plants. In contrast to Hygeia, the name Asclepius is of very ancient origin. Apparently Asclepius lived as a physician around the twelfth century BC. He was already known as a hero during Homeric times and was created a god in Epidaurus around the fifth or sixth century BC. His popularity spread far and wide, even beyond the boundaries of Greece. Soon Hygeia was relegated to the role of a member of his retinue, usually as his daughter, sometimes as his sister or wife, but always subservient to him. In most of the ancient iconography from the third century on, as well as in all subsequent representation, Asclepius appears as a handsome, self-assured young god, accompanied by two maidens: on his right Hygeia and on his left Panakeia. Unlike Hygeia, her sister, Panakeia became omnipotent as a healing goddess through knowledge of drugs either from plants or from the earth. Her cult is alive today in the universal search for a panacea.

The myths of Hygeia and Asclepius symbolize the never-ending oscillation between two different points of view in medicine. For the worshippers of Hygeia, health is the natural order of things, a positive attribute to which men are entitled if they govern their lives wisely. According to them, the most important function of medicine is to discover and teach the natural laws which will ensure to man a healthy mind in a healthy body. More skeptical or wiser in the ways of the world, the followers of Asclepius believe that the chief role of the physician is to treat disease, to restore health by correcting any imperfection caused by the accidents of birth or of life.

Hippocratic Wisdom

Hippocratic writings occupy a place in medicine corresponding to that of the Bible in the literature and ethics of Western peoples. Just as everyone quotes from the Bible, it is the universal practice to look to Hippocrates for statements that give the sanction of authority and of time to almost any kind of medical views, profound or banal. For twenty-five centuries Hippocrates has personified in the Western world the rational outlook of the philosopher, the objective attitude of the scientist, the practical approach of Asclepius, and the human traditions of Hygeia.

It is implicit in the Hippocratic teachings that both health and disease are under the control of natural laws and reflect the influence exerted by the environment and the way of life. Accordingly, health depends upon a state of equilibrium among the various internal factors which govern the operations of the body and the mind; this equilibrium in turn is reached only when man lives in harmony with his external environment. [Hippocrates'] writings are pervaded with the concept that the life of the patient as a whole is implicated in the disease process and that the cause is to be found in a concatenation of circumstances rather than in the simple direct effect of some external agency.

The Modern Public Health Movement

Rudolf Virchow deserves special mention at this point because of his immense prestige as experimenter, scientist, and writer in several medical and other biological fields. During his student days, Virchow had been influenced by the political philosophy of the German Social Democratic Party. At the age of twenty-six in 1847, he was appointed member of a commission organized by the Prussian government to study the epidemic which was then raging in the industrial districts of Upper Silesia. In a minority report Virchow traced the origin of the epidemic to unfavourable meteorological conditions. Heavy rains had ruined the year's crops and this had resulted in famine. Furthermore, the winter following had been extremely severe, forcing the poor people to huddle together in their homes, cold and hungry. It was then that typhus had broken out, first spreading rapidly through the poor population and eventually reaching the wealthier classes. His experience in Silesia led Virchow to start in 1848 the new journal, *Medizinische Reform*. In it he professed, as did his French predecessors inspired by the philosophers of the Enlightenment, that poverty was the breeder of disease and that it was the responsibility of physicians to support social reforms that would reconstruct society according to a pattern favourable to the health of man. Thus, according to Virchow, the treatment of individual cases is only a small aspect of medicine. More important is the control of crowd diseases which demand social and, if need be, political action. In this light medicine is a social science.

Despite its vigorous intellectual and social basis, the early nineteenth-century health movement in France and Germany was rather ineffective in the way of practical reforms. The goals of the French and German philosophers and physicians were to a large extent political and therefore difficult to reach except by revolutionary action. Furthermore, their doctrines were presented to the public in somewhat abstract terms. In England, by contrast, the leadership was taken by practical men who succeeded in finding a formula that appealed to elementary emotions and was meaningful to everyone. To a group of public-minded citizens guided by the physician Southwood Smith and the engineer Edwin Chadwick it appeared that, since disease always accompanied want, dirt, and pollution, health could be restored only by bringing back to the multitudes pure air, pure water, pure food, and pleasant surroundings.

This simple concept was synthesized in the movement 'The Health of Towns Association', the prototype of the present-day voluntary health associations throughout the world. Its aim was to 'substitute health for disease, cleanliness for filth, order for disorder ... prevention for palliation ... enlightened self-interest for ignorant selfishness and bring home to the poorest ... in purity and abundance, the simple blessings which ignorance and negligence have long combined to limit or to spoil: *Air, Water, Light.*'

Faith in the healing power of pure air, with much contempt for the germ theory of disease, was also the basis of Florence Nightingale's reforms of hospital sanitation during the Crimean War. 'There are no specific diseases,' she wrote. 'There are specific disease conditions.'

The conquest of epidemic diseases was in large part the result of the campaign for pure food, pure water, and pure air based not on a scientific doctrine but on philosophical faith. It was through the humanitarian movements dedicated to the eradication of the social evils of the Industrial Revolution, and the attempt to recapture the goodness of life in harmony with the ways of nature, that Western man succeeded in controlling some of the disease problems generated by the undisciplined ruthlessness of industrialization in its early phase.

Defining Health

Health and disease cannot be defined merely in terms of anatomical, physiological, or mental attributes. Their real measure is the ability of the individual to function in a manner acceptable to himself and to the group of which he is part.

For several centuries the Western world has pretended to find a unifying concept of health in the Greek ideal of a proper balance between body and mind. But in reality this ideal is more and more difficult to convert into practice. Poets, philosophers, and creative scientists are rarely found among Olympic laureates. It is not easy to discover a formula of health broad enough to fit Voltaire and Jack Dempsey, to encompass the requirements of a stevedore, a New York City bus driver, and a contemplative monk.

Among other living things, it is man's dignity to value certain ideals above comfort, and even above life. This human trait makes of medicine a philosophy that goes beyond exact medical sciences, because it must encompass not only man as a living machine but also the collective aspirations of mankind. A perfect policy of public health could be conceived for colonies of social ants or bees whose habits have become stabilized by instincts. Likewise it would be possible to devise for a herd of cows an ideal system of husbandry with the proper combination of stables and pastures. But, unless men become robots, no formula can ever give them permanently the health and happiness symbolized by the contented cow, nor can their societies achieve a structure that will last for millennia. As long as mankind is made up of independent individuals with free will, there cannot be any social status quo. Men will develop new urges, and these will give rise to new problems, which will require ever new solutions. Human life implies adventure, and there is no adventure without struggles and dangers.

René Dubos, microbiologist and experimental pathologist, was lately Professor at the Rockefeller University of New York City. These extracts are taken from his book *Mirage of Health*, published by Harper Colophan, New York (1979).

1.2

Feed a cold, starve a fever

Cecil Helman

The National Health Service, set up thirty-three years ago, was designed to bring the best of scientific medicine to the whole population. Much of the ill-health that had previously been borne, as one writer put it, in 'the imposed silence of poverty,' was now accessible to free health care. But what has been the impact of three decades of health education, television programmes about health, and easy access to doctors and hospitals, on traditional beliefs about illness? Whatever happened to folk remedies and old wives' tales?

A study I conducted on medical folklore in a north London suburb suggests that these folk beliefs about illness and health *can* survive the impact of scientific medicine, and in some cases may even be reinforced by this contact. This is important because in Britain the majority of ill-health—especially minor complaints—is dealt with outside the formal health care system.

In one recent study, Ruth Levitt estimated that about threequarters of abnormal symptoms are dealt with by patients themselves, their friends, family, or even the local pharmacist—without ever consulting a doctor. Self-medication is common (in some studies twice as common as the taking of prescribed medication), for a whole variety of conditions. Even after a doctor's prescription is issued, patients frequently use—or don't use—their drugs in ways that 'make sense' to them, rather than in ways the doctor intended. This 'non-compliance' has been estimated at 30 per cent, or more.

So how patients perceive ill-health and its treatment, both before and after seeing a doctor, depends on lay beliefs about what causes illness. There is an increasing amount of research into this; my own study tackled folk beliefs about some common, minor ailments—'chills', 'colds' and 'fever'. As both an anthropologist and a GP I was trying to find out the concepts underlying the often-heard aphorism, 'Feed a cold, starve a fever.'

It arises from a folk model, or scheme of classification, of illness which is widely accepted by the patients; and it relates to those conditions of impaired well-being which the patients perceive as disequilibrium, and regard as 'illness', and which concern perceived changes in body temperature—either 'hotter' than normal, or 'colder'. In general, these feelings of abnormal temperature change are purely subjective; they bear little or no relation to biomedical definitions of 'normal' body temperature as 98.4°F or 37°C, as measured orally on a thermometer. The conditions where the patient 'feels hot' are classified as *Fevers*, those where he 'feels cold' in his body are classified either as *Chills* or *Colds*. Both Fevers and Colds/Chills are states of being—both classified as abnormal—which, in the folk model have different causes, different effects, and thus require different treatments.

There are two important principles underlying this folk classification of 'illness-misfortune': (1) the relation of man with *nature*, i.e. with the natural environment, in Colds and Chills, and (2) the relation of man to man, which exists within human *society*, in Fevers.

To a large extent the area covered by the folk model—which I have set out schematically in Figure 1—corresponds to that area of disorders which biomedicine classifies as Infectious Diseases: that is, acute or chronic inflammatory conditions where the causative agent is known to be either a virus or a bacterium. These disorders, which occur very commonly in general practice, include disorders known as: upper respiratory tract infections;

	HOT	COLD
	(1) *Ear, Nose, and Throat* FEVER+NASAL CONGESTION OR DISCHARGE	**(1) *Ear, Nose, and Throat*** COLD+NASAL CONGESTION OR DISCHARGE, WATERY EYES, 'SINUS' CONGESTION
	(2) *Chest* FEVER+PRODUCTIVE COUGH	**(2) *Chest*** COLD+NON-PRODUCTIVE COUGH
WET	**(3) *Abdomen*** FEVER+DIARRHOEA AND ABDOMINAL DISCOMFORT	**(3) *Abdomen*** COLD+LOOSE STOOLS AND SLIGHT ABDOMINAL DISCOMFORT
	(4) *Urinary System* FEVER+URINARY FREQUENCY AND BURNING	**(4) *Urinary System*** COLD+SLIGHT URINARY FREQUENCY BUT NO PAIN
	(5) *Skin* FEVER+RASH+NASAL DISCHARGE OR COUGH	
DRY	FEVER+DRY SKIN, FLUSHED FACE, DRY THROAT, NON- PRODUCTIVE COUGH	COLD+SHIVERING, RIGOUR, MALAISE, VAGUE MUSCULAR ACHES

Figure 1 The Folk Classification of common 'Hot' and 'Cold' Symptoms.

influenza; coryza; bronchitis; pneumonia; sinusitis; urinary tract infections; gastroenteritis; childhood fevers (e.g. rubella); and several others. This classification overlaps, to some extent, the area covered by the folk model but as will be described there are significant differences. Illnesses associated with temperature change are common in all sections of the population, as are the often associated symptoms of cough or rhinitis. Cough is apparently the commonest symptom complained of in general practice,[1] and it is common even among those who do not consult the doctor: in Dunnell and Cartwright's study[2] 32 per cent of adults reported 'cough, catarrh, or phlegm' in a sample two-week period, while 18 per cent had suffered from 'cold, influenza, or rhinitis'. To describe the folk model it is necessary to adopt a diachronic approach: what follows is mainly the folk classification reported by older patients; those born during or since World War Two, while sharing the basic underlying classification, have introduced new elements, particularly with regard to the germ theory.

Structural Analysis of the Folk System

In Figure 1 I have listed the common groups of symptoms which relate to, or are accompanied by, perceived changes in body temperature. There are four diagnostic categories in all (see Figure 2); the basic division is between 'Hot' and 'Cold' conditions, but in addition there is a further division into 'Wet' and 'Dry' conditions. 'Wet' conditions are those where the temperature change is accompanied by other symptoms, and with a seemingly abnormal amount of 'Fluid' being present—either still within the body, or else emerging from its orifices; this 'Fluid' includes sputum, phlegm, nasal and sinus discharge, vomitus, urine, and loose stools. The symptoms here include nasal congestion or discharge, sinus congestion, productive coughs, 'congested' chests, diarrhoea, and urinary frequency. 'Dry' conditions are those where the abnormal temperature change is the only, or the paramount symptom—such as a subjective feeling of being cold, shivering or rigours on one hand—and a feeling of being 'hot', perhaps with a dry throat, flushed skin, slight unproductive cough, and possibly delirium, on the other. Skin rashes usually occur on the 'Hot' side of the classification. Other subsidiary symptoms—including pain—may occur in one form or another on both sides of the temperature division.

	HOT	COLD
	HOT	COLD
WET	WET	WET
	HOT	COLD
DRY	DRY	DRY

Figure 2

	HOT	COLD
	FEVER	COLD
WET	+	+
	FLUID	FLUID
DRY	FEVER	COLD

Figure 3

Thus there are four basic compartments into which common symptoms relating to temperature change can be fitted (see Figure 3): 'Hot/Wet' (Fever plus Fluid), 'Hot/Dry' (Fever), 'Cold/Wet' (Cold plus Fluid), and 'Cold/Dry' (Cold). Obviously these compartments are not watertight; there is always some overlap between divisions. In addition, not all conditions associated with abnormal temperature changes have been included; only the commonest, as encountered in general practice.

'Colds' and 'fevers' relate to two bodily states both perceived as being abnormal. The first is where you feel 'colder', the other 'hotter', than usual. But, in fact, both are subjective feelings, unconnected to actual measurements on a thermometer. Both can occur in a 'dry' form (the abnormal temperature change alone), or in a 'wet' form (where temperature change is associated with excess fluid). 'Wet' symptoms would include nasal congestion, 'runny noses', 'congested chests', coughing up mucus, diarrhoea or urinary frequency.

In *chills* and *colds*, the abnormal temperature change is usually seen as a by-product of one's personal battle with the natural environment—particularly with areas of lowered temperature. In this view, damp or rain ('cold/wet' conditions), or cold winds or draughts ('cold/dry'), can penetrate the boundary of the skin, and cause similar conditions within the body.

A cold, rainy day causes one to feel 'cold', with a runny nose. Sitting in a cold wind ('a draught') causes a feeling of coldness, though often without the excess fluid.

Wind at body temperature is not dangerous, and is merely 'fresh air'. Night air, however, is often considered dangerous by older patients. And 'the children get sick if you leave the bedroom windows open at night.'

Some areas of skin are seen as more vulnerable than others to penetration by environmental cold—particularly the top of the head, the back of the neck, and the feet. I found that 'colds' occurred when these areas were inadvertently exposed to draughts or damp—for example: 'getting your feet wet', 'walking around with damp hair', 'going out into the rain, without a hat on', or 'stepping into a puddle'. Elderly men, in particular, reported an increased vulnerability to 'head colds' after a haircut—when the back and top of the head are unprotected by their normal covering of hair.

Temperature changes between hot and cold environments were considered dangerous, especially the intermediate zone between the two temperatures—for example, 'going into a cold room after a hot bath', 'walking on a cold floor when you have a fever'. Changes in season were also risky—autumn, for example, where the 'hot' summer is changing to 'cold' winter. It was explained to me that 'summer colds' are more common since cheap air flights returned people suddenly from 'hot' Spain or Italy to 'cold' Britain, with disastrous results.

Cold, once it has entered the body, can move around. From damp feet it can migrate to cause a 'stomach chill', or it can shift even further upwards to cause 'a head cold' or 'sinus cold'. In general, *chills* occur below the waist ('stomach chill', 'bladder chill', 'kidney chill'), and *colds* above it ('a head cold', 'a cold in the sinuses', 'a cold in the chest').

Unlike fevers, cold and chills are more one's own responsibility. They are the result of carelessness, or lack of foresight—if 'you don't dress properly', 'allow your head to get wet', 'wash your hair when you don't feel well'. Colds are caused, as one middle-aged patient explained seriously, 'by doing something abnormal'.

So folk remedies for colds emphasise the return to 'normal' temperature and equilibrium, by treating 'cold' with 'hot'. Hot drinks, hot food, rest in a warm bed, and generating your own bodily heat by 'tonics' or food ('feed a cold . . .') were frequently advised. Other remedies stress the return from the 'wet' state to the 'dry' one: drying up the excess fluid by a variety of traditional remedies (goose fat was commonly used at one time), or patent decongestants bought from a chemist.

By contrast, *fevers* are thought to be due to invisible entities known—interchangeably—as 'germs', 'bugs' or 'viruses'. Some of these terms may be borrowed from modern medicine, but they are used and conceptualised in an entirely different way.

For example, 'germs' are described as living, invisible and malevolent entities. They have no free existence in nature, it seems, but exist only in or among people. They are thought of as occurring in a cloud of tiny particles, or as a tiny invisible 'insect'. They travel through the air between people, entering the body of their victim by one of the orifices (usually the mouth, or the nose, but also the ears, urethra, and so on). They signal their presence by causing a 'fever'. The germs that cause stomach upsets are more 'insect-like' than others ('a tummy bug'), and apparently larger in size.

Germs have personalities. These reveal themselves, or are expressed in, the sorts of symptoms they cause. 'I've got that germ, doctor, you know—the one that gives you the dry cough and the watery eyes,' or 'the one that gives you diarrhoea, and makes you bring up.' The germs are amoral in their selection of victims, but they can only cause harm once they do attack. There are no 'good' germs: *all* germs are bad, and patients do not differentiate between 'germs', 'bugs' and 'viruses'.

Once a germ enters the body, and causes a fever, it can move or expand to attack several parts of the body simultaneously. 'It's gone to my lungs,' 'I can feel it in my stomach,' 'It's moved to my chest', or, as one patient with a peptic ulcer said, 'I got the flu, but then it flew to the ulcer and that blew up.'

Because germs, unlike colds (at least to older patients), originate in other *people*, rather than in the natural environment, germ infection implies some sort of social relationship of whatever duration. Infection is an inherent risk in all relationships, though neither party is to blame if one 'picks up a germ.'

Cough up the muck

In that case, the victim is less blameworthy than in the case of a cold, and more able to mobilise sympathetic friends or relatives around him. One of the obligations of close relationships is to risk infection, if necessary, in looking after another person.

'Fevers' particularly attack the weak, the old, and the poor. This vulnerability of the poor is often explained away by their association with the dirt and disorder of poverty. 'Dirt' is seen as concentrated, or condensed, germs.

Like colds and chills, fevers can occur in the 'dry' ('feeling feverish', with a flushed skin, dry mouth) or 'wet' form (accompanied by excess catarrh, phlegm, urine). Folk remedies for fevers aim to return the victim from the 'hot' state to normal temperature; but also to move him (with the aid of *fluids* which 'flush out' or 'wash out' the germ) from the 'dry' state to the 'wet' state.

Fluids of one sort or another are used to 'wash out' the germ from the chest, so that a 'dry' cough can 'loosen', bringing with it the offending germ. A variety of fluids, like tea, hot water, and now patent cough mixtures, are used for 'getting it off your chest', 'coughing up the muck', 'getting it out of your system'.

Patients complain that a dry cough 'hasn't broken', or 'hasn't loosened', so that they can 'cough it off my chest'. 'I gargled with salt water to get the catarrh out,' one man said, 'and I always swallow a bit of it to loosen the cough.'

Fluids are also used as folk treatments for other hot/wet conditions, like diarrhoea, vomiting, or urinary frequency accompanied by a fever, to flush out the offending germ. Other folk remedies induce sweating, allowing you to 'sweat it out' of your system—in this case through the skin itself. Antibiotics are seen as powerful chemicals that kill germs *in situ*, with the body being the battlefield of this great clash. Both 'germs' and 'viruses' are seen as vulnerable to the effects of antibiotics.

Most people who use the words 'germs' or 'viruses' have never *seen* either of these entities. They have no perceptual evidence for their existence. So that they can be thought of more as hypotheses, or theories of causality. There is some similarity between these western ideas of 'germs', and the invisible, malign 'spirits' said to cause illness by people in non-western and non-industrialised societies.

There is a marked difference in lay views of colds and fevers between older patients, and those born since the second world war—who constitute the world's first 'antibiotic generation'. Younger patients are more likely to ascribe both fevers *and* colds to 'germs' or 'viruses'.

The Germ Theory is one example of a medical concept that has gradually influenced patients' ways of thinking about illness. 'Germs', as a cause of illness, have gradually spread to include many of the 'cold' conditions as well. Instead of 'a chill on the bladder', you have 'a germ in the water'; instead of 'a cold in the head', you have 'picked up a virus'.

One result of this is that the amount of personal responsibility for illness (as in old-fashioned 'colds') seems to have gradually declined. If more and more conditions are due to 'germs', then the victims are increasingly blameless, and more able to mobilise a caring community around themselves.

Illness seems to have become more *social* in its origin, effects and even treatment. Where you have 'germs' as a believed cause for illness, then you have a greater need of doctors and their remedies. There is also the slight sense of increased danger in social relationships—the threat of infection. Young mothers—more often than their own mothers would have—now ask, 'My child's got a cold; can she mix with other children?'

The metaphor of 'germs' as invisible forces 'out there' which cause suffering to the innocent, seems to have become a pervasive social metaphor. Pollution, radiation, and social changes 'of epidemic proportions', are all expressions of this.

The main meeting place between lay health beliefs and the medical profession, is usually the GP's surgery. In Britain, according to Ruth Levitt, the health service GP is the first point of contact for about 90 per cent of those who *do* seek medical help. In the surgery, both doctor and patient have to agree on what is wrong with the patient, and what should be done about it.

This involves a process of 'negotiation', whereby each party tries to influence the other about the outcome of the consultation, and the treatment to be given. One aspect of this is that, in order to get their patients' cooperation, GPs have to couch their diagnoses and treatment in concepts that *make sense* in terms of the patients' view of ill-health. This, in turn, may reinforce those same ideas.

A patient who presents a list of symptoms is often given a diagnosis couched in the everyday idiom of the folk model: 'You've picked up a germ,' 'You've got a flu bug,' 'It's a viral infection,' 'It's just a tummy bug—there's one going around,' 'You've got a germ in the water,' 'I'm afraid it's gone to your chest,' or 'Oh yes, is that the one where you've got a runny nose, watery eyes, and you lose your voice? I've seen a dozen already this week.'

More precise medical diagnoses are less commonly given, especially to uneducated patients. In many cases, these conditions are trivial, and self-limiting. They won't get worse; they will soon go away of their own accord; and no one else will catch them. A precise 'technical' diagnosis may be unnecessary, and in fact impossible. Not every cough and cold can be subjected to complex and expensive laboratory tests to identify the precise virus or bacteria causing it. The four-to-seven minute GP consultation time also makes more precise diagnoses impractical.

Many doctors do not, or cannot, differentiate between bacteria and viruses. So neither do patients. Bacteria *are* treatable by antibiotics but viruses are not. The distinction, however, has become blurred. Doctors reinforce this when they over-prescribe antibiotics generally—and particularly when they prescribe them for viral illnesses. This blurring strengthens the lay view that all 'germs' are bad; all are similar in nature; and all of them therefore susceptible to antibiotics. It also increases dependence on the doctor for prescribed treatment, even for minor complaints.

Receptionist power

Doctors' receptionists, who do a great deal of health counselling over the surgery telephone, can also help the process of reinforcing folk beliefs. As one receptionist was heard to say to a patient with diarrhoea and vomiting: 'Yes, there is a tummy bug going around. Starve yourself and take only sips of water for 24 hours. Otherwise, the more you feed it [the bug], the more it'll enjoy itself and cause diarrhoea and sickness.'

Not everything which GPs do in order to meet their patients' need to 'make sense' of the treatment given can be 'scientifically' justified. For example, it's been estimated that *six million gallons* of cough mixtures are prescribed in Britain every year under the NHS. (This excludes the vast amount bought over the counter.) Yet most medical textbooks cast doubt on the scientific efficacy of these preparations. Part of this ocean of cough mixture must represent the subtle pressure of patients' expectations on GPs to prescribe—in a modern form—the *liquids* believed to 'wash out' or 'flush out' the infection from one's chest.

We need to know more about how people understand their sickness, how they deal with it, and how they interpret medical treatment they are given. Because self-treatment and 'non-compliance' are so common, we also need to know what happens to health and illness *outside* the NHS.

Free access to GPs, and health education on the media, does not seem to have altered some of the traditional folk beliefs about illness. Obviously, medical concepts like the Germ Theory of disease are widely known to the lay public. But they may be understood in entirely a different way, and often in terms of a much older folk view of illness.

References

1. Morrell, D. C. Symptom interpretation in general practice, *J. Roy. Coll. Gen. Prac.*, 22, 297–309 (1972).
2. Dunnell, K. and Cartwright, A. *Medicine takers, prescribers and hoarders*, Routledge and Kegan Paul, London, p. 11 (1972).

Cecil G. Helman is both a general practitioner and a social anthropologist, and works in the Department of Social Anthropology, University College, London. This article is made up from one published in *New Society*, 222–224 (5 November 1981) and an extract from an article of the same title published in *Culture, Medicine and Psychiatry* 2, 107–137 (1978).

1.3

'Doing the Month': Confinement and Convalescence of Chinese Women after Childbirth

Barbara L. K. Pillsbury

In China traditional custom stipulates that a woman should be confined to the home for one full month of convalescence after giving birth to a child. During this time she is said to be 'sitting out the month' and is expected to observe a broad set of extremely restrictive prescriptions and proscriptions collectively referred to as 'doing the month' (zuo yuezi). The purpose of the present essay is to describe and analyze this practice of 'doing the month'. It will do so from three points of view corresponding to the three medical systems coexisting in China—folk medicine of the 'little tradition', classical Chinese medicine of the 'great tradition', and Western medicine.

First, from the ethnomedical folk perspective, this essay describes the practices and rationale for doing the month. Second, it analyzes these practices according to the logic of traditional Chinese medicine with its theories of somatic balance of *yin* and *yang*, hot and cold, wind and fire. Finally, it suggests that doing the month can be appraised in light of Western medical and nutritional knowledge to determine how some of the constituent practices may be either beneficial or detrimental to restoration of normal health. The original data upon which the study is based were gathered in interviews in Mandarin Chinese with laypersons, herbalists, and physicians in Taiwan and with physicians and laypersons from the People's Republic of China.

The chief questions to be addressed concern the extent to which this indigenous folk medical system has provided Chinese women with an efficacious set of health behaviors. We will conclude that certain practices of doing the month are indeed instrumental in restoring and maintaining health after parturition. Certain other postpartum practices, however, appear dysfunctional in the contemporary health environment. Why then do millions of Chinese women—despite Westernization, industrialization, women's liberation movements, and socialism—still adhere to such practices?

Cultural elaboration of the biological differences between male and female and of the biological changes both undergo during the life cycle is universal to all societies. What is not universal is the manner in which those same changes and processes are differently elaborated in various cultures—i.e. the degree to which they are made explicit and ritualized. The postpartum restoration to a normal state of health is one such process, and China is one such culture where this process has become highly elaborated. There the highly specific set of prescriptions and proscriptions that has evolved are believed to be directly responsible for the successful restoration of health and, if not adhered to, of grave consequence for the negligent woman.

From unremembered antiquity, a woman from the birth of her child until the moon has gone through a full cycle is said to be 'in the month'—the character for 'moon' and 'month' being one and the same. The room where the woman is supposed to remain in confinement is called the 'month room'.

At the end of this period, the month—or moon—is said to be 'full', a time to commemorate by inviting friends and relatives to a banquet and by 'drinking the full month wine'. It is significant that no other month of the Chinese calendar or of a Chinese person's life is referred to as '*the* month'. It is also significant, by way of comparison, that while a term exists in English for the postpartum adjustment period—puerperium—it is hardly a household word today and certainly no longer connotes the specificity of behavior that continues to characterize 'doing the month'. It may be precisely because puerperial behavior and its consequences do not constitute a prominent feature on the cognitive map of Western researchers that the latter have overlooked the subject in their wide-ranging investigations on health and medicine in China and that so very little exists on the subject in English.

'The month' begins with the child's birth either in the home or at a hospital. Throughout the countryside in the PRC [People's Republic of China] delivery reportedly takes place at home attended by a midwife who calls upon the nearby commune hospital when necessary. Home delivery is also the norm in rural Taiwan. In the cities, childbirth usually takes place in a hospital attended by doctors [who] are women because of the traditional female reluctance to have reproductive problems dealt with by men.

'Rules' and Folk Rationale for Doing the Month

The 'rules' and rationale for doing the month follow as they were explained to me, their order indicative of the relative emphasis given them by informants.

1. *Do not wash yourself and do not wash your hair for the entire month.*

In addition, one must neither wash the dishes or wash the clothes. In all cases, even the slightest contact with *cold* water is to be strictly avoided. The reason is that water causes wind to enter the body—through any of its joints, orifices, or possibly the soles of the feet—and thus gives rise in future years to asthma, arthritis, and chronic aches and pains. These can be cured only by a subsequent pregnancy following which the month is then done 'well', i.e. completely and properly.

Variations on the proscription against washing oneself include sponge baths with water that has been brought to full boil and cooled just to tolerable.

2. *Do not go outside for the entire month.*

The reason is that by exposing herself to the sun she automatically causes the gods to look down and catch sight of her. This shows extreme disrespect since the gods will see nothing there but a great mass of blood, the dirty birth blood.

3. *Do not eat any raw or any cold food.*

A woman 'in the month' must be extremely careful about what she eats. The fundamental guiding principle is that she must avoid all foods that are either raw or 'cold'.

'Cold' refers [not to temperature but] to the intrinsic nature of a food and includes turnips, Chinese cabbage, bamboo shoots, leafy green vegetables, and most fruits. Most Chinese women are shocked and disapproving when they hear of Western women drinking ice water during the month—and even immediately after parturition.

4. *Eat chicken.*

   In contrast to the above *pro*scribed foods, this is the single most emphatically *pre*-scribed food. Indigenous Taiwanese say it must be sesame-oil chicken. This noteworthy dish is prepared by slow simmering in large amounts of sesame oil (the variety made from black seeds) and rice wine. (The proportions cited tend to be about one cup sesame oil and three cups rice wine per chicken.) Chicken is 'hot' [as are] sesame oil and rice wine. Hot foods are good because they 'create fire' and thereby 'supplement', or restore health.

   Chicken soup, livers, kidneys [and] eggs are also prescribed. In addition, a woman in the month should eat extra meals—ideally, about five or six a day. Finally, her rice bowl must always be rinsed out with scalding water or she will experience constant diarrhoea.

5. *Do not be blown on by the wind.*

   A woman in the month must absolutely avoid all exposure to any wind or breeze [and] under no circumstance may she come into contact with 'wind' from a fan or air-condition-ing. A woman's joints all open up and remain open after childbirth. If the wind blows at her body it will get in and inevitably in the future she will develop rheumatism—literally, 'wind-and-moisture disease'.

6. *Do not walk and move around.*

   It is essential to stay in bed as much as possible. In bed one should lie flat on one's back. This is necessary for straightening out the back-bone from the sway-back shape it curved into during pregnancy.

7. *Do not go to other person's homes.*

   [A woman] after childbirth should remember that others may want to avoid her because of this fact.

8. *Do not get sick during the month.*

9. *Do not read or cry.*

10. *Do not have sexual intercourse during the month.*

11. *Do not eat at the table with the rest of the family.*

12. *Do not burn incense.*

   That is, do not go to any temple or anywhere else burn incense to the gods; to do so with dirty blood would be most disrespectful and offensive to them and again cause them to cause misfortune.

   A final but crucial condition that makes all the above possible is that a woman must have someone to 'accompany her in doing the month'. Traditionally this is the woman's mother-in-law.

   It is apparent that the prescriptions and proscriptions a woman is supposed to follow during the month are regarded as a curative therapy. In another sense—one which some Chinese view as considerably more important—the practices are also preventive measures.

Chinese Medical Theory as regards Doing the Month

It has been stated above that three medical systems have coexisted in China: folk medicine of the little tradition, Chinese medicine of the great tradition, and Western medicine. To a large extent they are resorted to interchangeably. Doing the month is clearly part of China's folk medical tradition. It is something 'everybody' does to get well and remain well after parturition, and its specialists generally are simply mothers, mothers-in-law, and older women who are experienced in such matters.

Chinese medicine of the great tradition, on the other hand, is a far more esoteric body of knowledge. According to lay opinion, directions for doing the month are not something that can be found in the classical texts of Chinese medicine.

Yet, within the context of traditional Chinese medical theory, pregnancy and childbirth leave the woman in a state of imbalance much like that of illness. According to this theory, a state of health is one in which the vital forces within the human body are in balance with each other as well as with the forces of the natural environment. A state of illness is one in which the body's vital forces are out of balance. Childbirth is clearly an event which leaves the female body in precisely this state of imbalance.

The theoretical basis of Chinese medicine was, in essence, worked out some two thousand years ago within the broad context of classical Chinese cosmology. Just as equilibrium, or harmony, within a continual cycle of fluctuating changes is viewed as the basic principle of the natural universe, so too the human individual is healthy when his or her basic life forces are in harmony and unhealthy when the harmony is disturbed. This is expressed in terms of the polar combination of *yin* and *yang* and the flow through the body of the vital life force, *ch'i* (sometimes translated as 'pneuma') in accordance with the alteration of the 'five evolutive phases'—wood, fire, earth, metal, and water. Any disturbance leads to illness and, if not rectified, even death.

The *yin* and *yang* principle divides phenomena of the universe—the macrocosm of which the individual is the microcosm—into two mutually supportive forces which remain in balance for the harmonious functioning of the universe, the social system, and the individual. *Yin* corresponds to cold, darkness, wetness, softness, quiescence, femininity, earth, moon, north, below, squareness, and even numbers. *Yang* corresponds to heat, brightness, dryness, hardness, activity, masculinity, heaven, sun, south, above, roundness, and odd numbers.

Maintaining the balance between *yang-ch'i* and *yin-ch'i* is a basic principle of Chinese internal medicine. Much of illness that originates from within the body—as opposed to from obvious accidents or social factors—is attributed to excessive 'coldness' or 'hotness' in the body.

Women, being *yin* in nature, have more of the cold principle and thus are more susceptible to illnesses that result from its excess—especially at the dangerous time of childbirth. This is verbalized as 'not enough hotness/fire'. [A woman's body is very weak after childbirth because her 'hotness' has been depleted.] If one's body is out of balance due to too much hotness, one ingests [foods] that are cold. But if one has too much cold (as does a woman 'in the month'), one needs [foods] that are hot and must avoid all products that are cold.

Circulation of blood in the body is, in this way, directly influenced by the foods one eats. Entry of cold wind can also create tumors, weakness, and pains—precisely the danger a woman faces during the month because then all her joints are 'opened up'. This results in arthritis ('joint inflammation') and rheumatism ('wind-moisture-disease').

Chinese medical theory, generally regarded as notably holistic, nevertheless embodies a familiar dichotomy (perhaps better expressed as a *yin–yang* complementarity). On the one hand is the idea of direct attack on the pathogen, the external disease agent. On the other hand is the idea of strengthening of the body's vital resistance to disease and illness. In direct contrast to the relative emphases in Western medicine, Chinese medicine has tended to emphasize the latter: preventive rather than curative. It is thus congruent with Chinese great tradition medicine that the folk practices of doing the month are perceived by those who carry them out as being extremely efficacious as preventive measures. Western practitioners, however, have different perceptions.

Western Medical Theory and Practitioners Regarding Doing the Month

Opinions of physicians trained in Western medicine tend to fall into one of three categories regarding the value of doing the month. First are American physicians who, unfamiliar with anything Chinese (but duly impressed by acupuncture), find the custom 'very strange indeed'. They acknowledge that, in fact, 'there might be some underlying benefit to it all'— such as 'getting the patient to eat well and take it easy'.

Second are Chinese physicians who have been educated in 'modern science' and tend to look down on things that are traditional and Chinese. They [often say] that doing the month violates principles of good health with its prohibitions against bathing and washing one's hair, that it has no scientific or theoretically sound basis, and that it is of little value.

Third are Chinese who, although trained in and practicing Western medicine, insist that *certain* aspects of doing the month do indeed make sense empirically—such as getting rest, avoiding exposure to drafts, and increasing protein consumption (the latter being especially important in families that cannot ordinarily afford much costly protein).

One female obstetrician explained 'It is important to rest and recover after childbirth rather than return immediately to the tasks most women are faced with. "Doing the month" is like a scheme that Chinese culture invented to force women to rest. If they were just told "Rest!" that wouldn't do the trick. So, many taboos and supersititons [*sic*] had to be developed and made an intrinsic part of the month to make certain that a woman would get sufficient rest and regain enough energy to be able to resume and continue her work in good health.'

In this sense then, doing the month as a *holistic* entity—a set of linked practices that constitute a *single* health behavior—does indeed appear to be efficacious. If the constituent practices are examined individually, however, we see that some are efficacious, some neutral, and others perhaps dysfunctional. The latter practices may well have been functional in an earlier period with a considerably higher infectious disease level, but appear to have become dysfunctional in today's improved health environment.

The prohibitions against bathing, washing one's hair, being outdoors, visiting other persons' homes, and exposing oneself to wind or circulating air may indeed have been efficacious in former days when the risk of exposure to communicable diseases was greater. At present, however, rigid adherence to these prohibitions for the entire duration of the month may in fact be dysfunctional.

The fact that many Chinese homes are not insulated against bone-chilling damp winters and do not have hot running water can make bathing and a wet head risky for persons in a weakened state of health. In addition, the relatively high pathogen content of the available water increases the threat of vaginal infection for women who sit or squat in the water to wash. Showers, which Western-trained physicians usually recommend instead of baths during this period, are not [available] in the majority of Chinese homes.

Modifications cited by Chinese women do indeed indicate awareness of the importance of boiling water for destroying pathogens and of avoiding vaginal contact with water immediately after parturition when lacerations of the genitalia have not yet healed. Modifications of the prohibition against sexual intercourse also indicate recognition of the importance of the lacerations healing without infection.

The Chinese notion that crying and reading and that exposure to wind or water during the month will result in future ailments is not a causal relationship characteristically propounded by Western medicine. Nor do Western physicians believe that wind enters the body through its joints. Yet Western medicine definitely cautions against incurring illnesses during the postpartum period and against eyestrain at this or at any other time. The Chinese belief that a woman's joints are 'opened up' during the month is also corroborated by the Western medical knowledge that a woman's ligaments are indeed expanded following parturition. Given that avoidance of crying also implies avoidance of circumstances likely to induce crying, then the attempt to create a cheerful atmosphere for the new mother is also desirable from the perspective of Western medicine.

The prohibition against washing clothes and dishes appears efficacious in helping the new mother to avoid overtaxing her limited energies in the performance of household tasks. The prohibition against walking and moving around appears similarly efficacious immediately after parturition, although rigid adherence to this prohibition would seem dysfunctional later in the month when, from the perspective of Western medicine, moderate physical activity is desirable.

The prescription to consume large amounts of food—especially chicken, eggs, and organ meats—appears extremely efficacious given that a large percentage of households cannot afford the costly animal protein except on special occasions. The rule to do so, however, does in fact seem to raise their protein intake to a level acceptable by Western nutritional standards. The prescription to eat sweet foods is efficacious not, as many Chinese women believe, because the body supposedly needs sweets after parturition but because consumption of sweets tends to keep salt intake low. The proscription against raw and cold foods and liquids is efficacious in that it demands everything be cooked or boiled, thereby destroying pathogenic micro-organisms that might otherwise be consumed.

Persistence and Integration

Doing the month is clearly a tightly integrated holistic set of practices firmly imbedded in Chinese culture. We have identified three major reasons why Chinese women carry them out: curing the pregnancy-induced imbalance, preventing future illness, and preventing future misfortune to themselves and those with whom they interact. In traditional China, and in traditional households today, the extreme emphasis on perpetuating the patrilineal descent line and the concomitant marriage rule of patrilocality have resulted in the arrangement of marriages by parents in order to bring into their households daughters-in-law who would obligingly produce male descendants. Until successful in this, pressure upon them is great—and channeled primarily through the mother-in-law. Birth of a daughter-in-law's first child, especially if male, means relaxation of tension and pressure and confirms her status as a member of the family. Under such circumstances, doing the month is clearly a reward, and an important role reversal takes place. Having been obliged from the day of marriage to wait hand and foot on and be at the beck and call of her mother-in-law, the mother of the newborn infant is now given sanction to lie idle in bed for an entire month—waited upon and pampered by the mother-in-law herself. It is she, the mother-in-law, who informants say traditionally 'accompanies' a woman in the month.

My observations of interpersonal interaction in Chinese households during the month give the impression that far more attention is lavished upon the mother, relative to the newborn infant, than in the United States. This extra attention their families and social networks show them while doing the month seems, in fact, to preclude Chinese women from experiencing postpartum depression as understood and so taken for granted by Americans—despite the fact that the same biological factors are operative for women of both cultural backgrounds. Neither the Chinese translations of the term 'postpartum depression' nor the concept itself makes much sense to the majority of my informants. 'You would just feel disappointed', explained one of them, 'only if each time it is a girl, because then you know the family is not pleased.'

I found only two Chinese women who report having had children without doing the month. Both are fairly well-to-do professional women who say they were too smart for all that old-fashioned Chinese nonsense—too smart, both say, for their own good. One now attributes a recent long and costly bout with bronchial infection to not having done the month and chastizes herself for foolishly disregarding the wisdom of the Chinese ages. The other, holder of an American doctoral degree, says she subsequently developed arthritis and, seven years after the birth of her earlier child, again became pregnant in order to do the month properly, thus successfully restoring her health.

Comparative Perspective and Conclusion

Is China unique in its emphasis on postpartum maternal care and its cultural ritualization of behavior and diet at this time? Certainly not. The West too once had its practices of 'lying in' and confinement that prevailed prior to this century's advances in therapeutic medicine and the accelerated monopolization of health care and knowledge in the hands of legally-identified professionals. Indeed, a comparative perspective not only affords better understanding of natality and maternity in China but the latter also affords a better understanding of this major life-cycle event both universally and in our own cultures as well.

Evidence from other societies together with this from China permits the hypothesis that, prior to a population's coming under the influence of the professionalization and therapeutic techniques of Western medicine, the time during a woman's life cycle when the greatest concern is shown for her health is the period immediately postpartum. A contingent hypothesis is that, wherever this is true, specific rules for diet modification (prescriptions and proscriptions, especially as related to 'hot' and 'cold' distinctions) are a major and essential part of the culturally-indicated maternal postnatal care and are more important than during the prenatal period.

For example, the Subanun of Mindanao in the Philippines are reported to 'focus a remarkable amount of ritual and medical attention' on a mother during her *gigetaw* (postpartum period) in contrast to the relative lack of formal ritualization of other biological life-cycle events.[1] Mayan Indians, for instance, like rural Taiwanese, restrict diet during pregnancy but not nearly so rigidly as immediately after parturition.[2] Indicative of the importance attached to the postpartum period is the assignment to it of a special name and fixed duration. The Zapotec Indian and generally widespread Latin American *cuarentena* ('quarantine') is 40 days, the Subanun *gigetaw* is 7–9 days, and the Mayan postpartum confinement lasts 20 days (equivalent to one round of the ancient Mayan calendar). As in China, Mayan, Zapotec, Subanun and Tzintzuntan (Mexican) women are all reported to follow diets modified for reasons of hot and cold, lactation, propitiating the supernatural, and future health.

A related hypothesis suggested by data from several cultures is that, where the postpartum is the time of greatest concern for female health, then the measures taken are regarded by members of the given culture as primarily preventive although they do in fact have certain therapeutic value as well. In this context the beliefs and practices of Chinese-American women are instructive. Data collected by myself in interviews with twenty-three young mothers of Chinese origin now resident in California indicate that their having 'done the month'—some 'quite well' and others 'only a little bit'—was motivated largely by concerns for their own future health (including appearance). They, and their mothers and mothers-in-law, tend to consider it the responsibility of the Western medical establishment to deliver the infant but their own personal responsibility to lay the foundation for good health in the future since, in their words, American hospitals and doctors 'don't care about' this.[3] It is indicative of the persistence of the traditional Chinese postpartum practices that numerous Chinese-American women hospitalized for childbirth reject hospital food, pour out cold liquids, have special dishes snuck in by Chinese visitors, and only dampen a towel to pretend having showered.

In summary, 100 per cent of over 100 Chinese and Chinese-Americans interviewed consider 'doing the month' efficacious for reasons of physical health, social relations (and thus mental health), or both. Chinese lay informants and Chinese physicians alike attribute this in part to its function of restoring health and putting somatic and social relations into balance. They emphasize especially its value as a preventive therapy—one which makes for future physiological and mental well-being and harmony. In light of Western medical knowledge, some of its practices are efficacious while others, which may once have been so, now appear dysfunctional. For most Chinese women, however, even though they too regard some aspects of it as not particularly efficacious or pleasant, doing the month appears to remain an integrated (and integrative) health behavior whose components are not so easily disassociated—or discarded. Nor should they be disregarded by health professionals, Chinese or Western.

References

1. Frake, C. and Frake, C. 'Postnatal care among the eastern Subanun', *The Silliman Journal*, 4(3) p. 207 (1957).
2. Cosminsky, S. 'Birth rituals and symbolism: a Quiche Maya–Black Carib comparison'. In Young, P. and Howe, J. (eds) *Ritual and symbol in Native Central America*, University of Oregon, pp. 107–123 (1976).
3. Leung, J. 'Effect of acculturation on nutritional practices of pregnant and lactating Chinese mothers in San Francisco', paper presented at the West Coast Nutritional Anthropologists' First Scientific Meeting, San Francisco (1977).

Barbara Pillsbury is an anthropologist working in the Dept. of Social Anthropology at San Diego State University. This article is an edited version of an article published in *Social Science and Medicine*, 12, 11–22 (1978).

1.4

The Hysterical Woman: Sex Roles and Role Conflict in 19th-Century America[1]

Carroll Smith-Rosenberg

The ideal female in nineteenth-century America was expected to be gentle and refined, sensitive and loving. She was the guardian of religion and spokeswoman for morality. Hers was the task of guiding the more worldly and more frequently tempted male past the maelstrom of atheism and uncontrolled sexuality. Her sphere was the hearth and the nursery: within it she was to bestow care and love, peace and joy. The American girl was taught at home, at school, and in the literature of the period that aggression, independence, self-assertion and curiosity were male traits, inappropriate for the weaker sex and her limited sphere. Dependent throughout her life, she was to reward her male protectors with affection and submission. At no time was she expected to achieve in any area considered important by men and thus highly valued by society. She was, in essence, to remain a child-woman, never developing the strengths and skills of adult autonomy. The stereotype of the middle class woman as emotional, pious, passive and nurturant was to become increasingly rigid throughout the nineteenth century.[2]

There were significant discontinuities and inconsistencies between such ideals of female socialization and the real world in which the American woman had to live. The ideal woman was emotional, dependent and gentle—a born follower. The ideal mother, then and now, was expected to be strong, self-reliant, protective, an efficient caretaker in relation to children and home. She was to manage the family's day-to-day finances, prepare foods, make clothes, compound drugs, serve as family nurse—and, in rural areas, as physician as well.[3] Especially in the nineteenth century, with its still primitive obstetrical practices and its high child mortality rates, she was expected to face severe bodily pain, disease and death—and still serve as the emotional support and strength of her family. As S. Weir Mitchell, the eminent Philadelphia neurologist wrote in the 1880s, 'We may be sure that our daughters will be more likely to have to face at some time the grim question of pain than the lads who grow up beside them . . . To most women . . . there comes a time when pain is a grim presence in their lives.' Yet, as Mitchell pointed out, it was boys whom society taught from early childhood on to bear pain stoically, while girls were encouraged to respond to pain and stress with tears and the expectation of elaborate sympathy.[4]

Contemporaries noted routinely in the 1870s, 1880s and 1890s that middle-class American girls seemed ill-prepared to assume the responsibilities and trials of marriage, motherhood and maturation. Frequently women, especially married women with children, complained of isolation, loneliness, and depression. Physicians reported a high incidence of nervous disease and hysteria among women who felt overwhelmed by the burdens of frequent pregnancies, the demands of children, the daily exertions of housekeeping and family management. The realities of adult life no longer permitted them to elaborate and exploit the role of fragile, sensitive and dependent child.

Not only was the Victorian woman increasingly ill-prepared for the trials of childbirth and childrearing, but changes were also at work within the larger society which were to make her particular socialization increasingly inappropriate. Reduced birth and mortality rates, growing population concentration in towns, cities and even in rural areas, a new, highly mobile economy, as well as new patterns of middle class aspiration—all reached into the family, altering that institution, affecting domestic relations and increasing the normal quantity of intra-familial stress. Women lived longer; they married later and less often. They spent less and less time in the primary processing of food, cloth and clothing. Increasingly, both middle and lower class women took jobs outside the home until their marriages—or permanently if unable to secure a husband. By the post-Civil War years, family limitation had become a real option within the decision-making process of every family.

Despite such basic social, economic and demographic changes, however, the family and gender role socialization remained relatively inflexible. It is quite possible that many women experienced a significant level of anxiety when forced to confront or adapt in one way or another to these changes. Thus hysteria may have served as one option or tactic offering particular women otherwise unable to respond to these changes a chance to redefine or restructure their place within the family.

So far this discussion of role socialization and stress has emphasized primarily the malaise and dissatisfaction of the middle class woman. It is only a covert romanticism, however, which permits us to assume that the lower class or farm woman, because her economic functions within her family were more vital than those of her decorative and economically secure urban sisters, escaped their sense of frustration, conflict or confusion. Normative prescriptions of proper womanly behavior were certainly internalized by many poorer women. The desire to marry and the belief that a woman's social status came not from the exercise of her own talents and efforts but from her ability to attract a competent male protector were as universal among lower class and farm women as among middle and upper class urban women. For some of these women—as for their urban middle class sisters—the traditional female role proved functional, bringing material and psychic rewards. But for some it did not. The discontinuity between the child and adult female roles, along with the failure to develop substantial ego strengths, crossed class and geographic barriers—as did hysteria itself. Physicians connected with almshouses, and later in the century with urban hospitals and dispensaries, often reported hysteria among immigrant and tenement house women. Sex differentiation and class distinctions both play a role in American social history, yet hysteria seems to have followed a psychic fault line corresponding more to distinctions of gender than to those of class.

Against this background of possible role conflict and discontinuity, what were the presenting symptoms of the female hysteric in nineteenth-century America? While physicians agreed that hysteria could afflict persons of both sexes and of all ages and economic classes (the male hysteric was an accepted clinical entity by the late nineteenth century), they reported that hysteria was most frequent among women between the ages of 15 and 40 and of the urban middle and upper middle classes. Symptoms were highly varied. As early as the seventeenth century, indeed, Sydenham had remarked that 'the frequency of hysteria is no less remarkable than the multiformity of the shapes it puts on. Few maladies are not imitated by it; whatever part of the body it attacks, it will create the proper symptom of that part.'[5] The nineteenth-century physician could only concur. There were complaints of nervousness, depression, the tendency to tears and chronic fatigue, or of disabling pain. Not a few women thus afflicted showed a remarkable willingness to submit to long-term, painful therapy—to electric shock treatment, to blistering, to multiple operations, even to amputations.

The most characteristic and dramatic symptom, however, was the hysterical 'fit'. Mimicking an epileptic seizure, these fits often occurred with shocking suddenness. At other times they 'came on' gradually, announcing their approach with a general feeling of depression, nervousness, crying or lassitude. Such seizures, physicians generally agreed, were precipitated by a sudden or deeply felt emotion—fear, shock, a sudden death, marital disappointment—or by physical trauma. It began with pain and tension, most frequently in the 'uterine area'. The sufferer alternately sobbed and laughed violently, complained of palpitations of the heart, clawed her throat as if strangling and, at times, abruptly lost the power of hearing and speech. A death-like trance might follow, lasting hours, even days. At other times violent convulsions—sometimes accompanied by hallucinations—seized her body. 'Let the reader imagine,' New York physician E. H. Dixon wrote in the 1840s, 'the patient writhing like a serpent upon the floor, rending her garments to tatters, plucking out handsful of hair, and striking her person with violence—with contorted and swollen countenance and fixed eyes resisting every effort of bystanders to control her . . .' Finally the fit subsided; the patient, exhausted and sore, fell into a restful sleep.

During the first half of the nineteenth century physicians described hysteria principally though not exclusively in terms of such episodes. Symptoms such as paralysis and contracture were believed to be caused by seizures and categorized as infraseizure symptoms. Beginning in mid-century, however, physicians became increasingly flexible in their diagnosis of hysteria and gradually the fit declined in significance as a pathognomonic symptom. Dr Robert Carter, a widely-read British authority on hysteria, insisted in 1852 that at least one hysterical seizure must have occurred to justify a diagnosis of hysteria. But, he admitted, this seizure might be so minor as to have escaped the notice even of the patient herself; no subsequent seizures were necessary. This was clearly a transitional position. By the last third of the nineteenth century the seizure was no longer the central phenomenon defining hysteria: physicians had categorized hysterical symptoms which included virtually every known human ill. They ranged from loss of sensation in part, half or all of the body, loss of taste, smell, hearing, or vision, numbness of the skin, inability to swallow, nausea, headaches, pain in the breast, knees, hip, spine or neck, as well as contracture or paralysis of virtually any extremity.

Hysterical symptoms were not limited to the physical. An hysterical female character gradually began to emerge in the nineteenth-century medical literature, one based on interpretations of mood and personality rather than on discrete physical symptoms—one which grew closely to resemble twentieth-century definitions of the 'hysterical personality'. Doctors commonly described hysterical women as highly impressionistic, suggestible, and narcissistic. Highly labile, their moods changed suddenly, dramatically, and for seemingly inconsequential reasons. Doctors complained that the hysterical woman was egocentric in the extreme, her involvement with others superficial and tangential. While the hysterical woman might appear to physicians and relatives as quite sexually aroused or attractive, she was, doctors cautioned, essentially asexual and not uncommonly frigid.

Depression also appears as a common theme. Hysterical symptoms not infrequently followed a death in the family, a miscarriage, some financial setback which forced the patient to become self-supporting; or they were seen by the patient as related to some long-term, unsatisfying life situation— a tired school teacher, a mother unable to cope with the demands of a large family. Most of these women took to their beds because of pain, paralysis or general weakness. Some remained there for years.

The medical profession's response to the hysterical woman was at best ambivalent. Many doctors—and indeed, a significant proportion of society at large—tended to be caustic, if not punitive towards the hysterical woman. This resentment seems rooted in two factors: first, the baffling and elusive nature of hysteria itself, and second, the relation which existed in the physicians' minds between their categorizing of hysteria as a disease and the role women were expected to play in society. These patients did not function as women were expected to function, and, as we shall see, the physician who treated them felt threatened both as a professional and as a rejected male. He was the therapist thwarted, the child untended, the husband denied nurturance and sex.

During the second half of the nineteenth century, the newly established germ theory and discoveries by neurologists and anatomists for the first time made an insistence on disease specificity a *sine qua non* for scientific respectability. Neurology was just becoming accepted as a speciality, and in its search for acceptance it was particularly dependent on the establishment of firm, somatically based disease entities. If hysteria *was* a disease, and not the imposition of self-pitying women striving to avoid their traditional roles and responsibilities—as was frequently charged—it must be a disease with a specific etiology and a predictable course. In the period 1870 to 1900, especially, it was felt to be a disease rooted in some specific organic malfunction.

Hysteria, of course, lacked all such disease characteristics. Contracture or paralysis could occur without muscular atrophy or change in skin temperature. The hysteric might mimic tuberculosis, heart attacks, blindness or hip disease, while lungs, heart, eyes and hips remained in perfect health. The physician had only his patient's statement that she could not move or was wracked with pain. If concerned and sympathetic, he faced a puzzling dilemma. Equally frustrating and medically inexplicable were the sudden changes in the hysteric's symptoms. Paralysis or anaesthesia could shift from one side of the body to the other, from one limb to another. Headaches would replace contracture of a limb, loss of voice, the inability to taste. How could a physician prescribe for such ephemeral symptoms? 'Few practitioners desire the management of hysterics,' one eminent gynecologist, Samuel Ashwell, wrote in 1833. 'Its symptoms are so varied and obscure, so contradictory and changeable, and if by chance several of them, or even a single one be relieved, numerous others almost immediately spring into existence.'

Yet physicians, especially newly established neurologists with urban practices, were besieged by patients who appeared to be sincere, respectable women sorely afflicted with pain, paralysis or uncontrollable 'nervous fits'. 'Looking at the pain evoked by ideas and beliefs,' S. Weir Mitchell, America's leading expert on hysteria wrote in 1885, 'we are hardly wise to stamp these pains as non-existent.'[6] Despite the tendency of many physicians to contemptuously dismiss the hysterical patient when no organic lesions could be found, neurologists such as Mitchell, George M. Beard, or Charles L. Dana sympathized with these patients and sought to alleviate their symptoms.

Such pioneer specialists were therefore in the position of having defined hysteria as a legitimate disease entity, and the hysterical woman as sick, when they were painfully aware that no organic etiology had yet been found. Cautiously, they sought to formally define hysteria in terms appropriately mechanistic. Some late nineteenth-century physicians, for example, still placing a traditional emphasis on hysteria's uterine origins, argued that hysteria resulted from 'the reflex effects of utero-ovarian irritation'. Others, reflecting George M. Beard's work on neurasthenia, defined hysteria as a functional disease caused either by 'metabolic or nutritional changes in the cellular elements of the central nervous system'. All such explanations were but hypothetical gropings for an organic explanation—still a necessity if they were to legitimate hysteria as a disease.

The fear that hysteria might after all be only a functional or 'ideational' disease—to use a nineteenth-century term—and therefore not really a disease at all, underlies much of the writing on hysteria as well as the physicians' own attitudes toward their patients. These hysterical women might after all be only clever frauds and sensation-seekers—morally delinquent and, for the physician, professionally embarrassing.

Not surprisingly, a compensatory sense of superiority and hostility permeated many physicians' discussions of the nature and etiology of hysteria. Except when called upon to provide a hypothetical organic etiology, physicians saw hysteria as caused either by the indolent, vapid and unconstructive life of the fashionable middle and upper class woman, or by the ignorant, exhausting and sensual life of the lower or working class woman. Neither were flattering etiologies. Both denied the hysteric the sympathy granted to sufferers from unquestionably organic ailments.

Hysteria, S. Weir Mitchell warned, occurred in women who had never developed habitual restraint and 'rational endurance'—who had early lost their power of 'self rule'. 'The mind and body are deteriorated by the force of evil habit,' Charles Lockwood wrote in 1895, 'morbid thought and morbid impulse run through the poor, weak, unresisting brain, until all mental control is lost, and the poor sufferer is . . . at the mercy of . . . evil and unrestrained passions, appetites and morbid thoughts and impulses.'

In an age when will, control, and hard work were fundamental social values, this hypothetical etiology necessarily implied a negative evaluation of those who succumbed to hysteria. Such women were described as weak, capricious and, perhaps most important, morbidly suggestible. Their intellectual abilities were meager, their powers of concentration eroded by years of self-indulgence and narcissistic introspection. Hysterical women were, in effect, children, and ill-behaved, difficult children at that. 'They have in fact,' Robert Carter wrote, 'all the instability of childhood, joined to the vices and passions of adult age . . .'

Many nineteenth-century critics felt that this emotional regression and instability was rooted in woman's very nature. The female nervous system, doctors argued, was physiologically more sensitive and thus more difficult to subject to the will. Some physicians assumed as well that women's blood was 'thinner' than man's, causing nutritional inadequacies in the central nervous system and an inability to store nervous energy—a weakness, Mary Putnam Jacobi stressed, women shared with children. Most commonly, a woman's emotional states generally, and hysteria in particular, were believed to have the closest ties to her reproductive cycle. Hysteria commenced with puberty and ended with menopause, while ailments as varied as menstrual pain and irregularity, prolapsed or tipped uterus, uterine tumor, vaginal infections and discharges, sterility, could all—doctors were certain—cause hysteria. Indeed, the first question routinely asked hysterical women was 'are your courses regular?' Thus a woman's very physiology and anatomy predisposed her to hysteria; it was, as Thomas Laycock put it, 'the natural state' in a female, a 'morbid state' in the male.

Hysteria could also result from a secret and less forgivable form of sexuality. Throughout the nineteenth century, physicians believed that masturbation was widespread among America's females and a frequent cause of hysteria and insanity. As early as 1846, E. H. Dixon reported that masturbation caused hysteria 'among females even in society where physical and intellectual culture would seem to present the strongest barriers against its incursions. . . .' Masturbation was only one form of sexual indulgence. Hysteria, another physician reported, was found commonly among prostitutes, while virtually all physicians agreed that even within marriage sexual excess could easily lead to hysteria.

Expectedly, conscious anger and hostility marked the response of a good many doctors to their hysterical patients. Even the concerned and genteel S. Weir Mitchell, confident of his remarkable record in curing hysteria, described hysterical women as 'the pests of many households, who constitute the despair of physicians, and who furnish those annoying examples of despotic selfishness, which wreck the constitutions of nurses and devoted relatives, and in unconscious or half-conscious self-indulgence destroy the comfort of everyone about them.' He concluded by quoting Oliver Wendell Holmes' acid judgment that 'a hysterical girl is a vampire who sucks the blood of the healthy people about her.'

Hysteria as a chronic, dramatic and socially accepted sick role could thus provide some alleviation of conflict and tension, but the hysteric purchased her escape from the emotional—and frequently—from the sexual demands of her life only at the cost of pain, disability, and an intensification of woman's traditional passivity and dependence. Indeed a complex interplay existed between the character traits assigned women in Victorian society and the characteristic symptoms of the nineteenth-century hysteric: dependency, fragility, emotionality, narcissism. (Hysteria has, after all, been called in that century and this a stark caricature of femininity.) Not surprisingly the hysteric's peculiar passive aggression and her exploitive dependency often functioned to cue a corresponding hostility in the men who cared for her or lived with her. Whether father, husband, or physician, they reacted with ambivalence and in many cases with hostility to her aggressive and never-ending demands.

What inferences concerning woman's role and female–male relationships can be drawn from this description of nineteenth-century hysteria and of medical attitudes toward the female patient? What insights does it allow into patterns of stress and resolution within the traditional nuclear family?

Because traditional medical wisdom had defined hysteria as a disease, its victims could expect to be treated as sick and thus to elicit a particular set of responses—the right to be seen and treated by a physician, to stay in bed and thus be relieved of their normal day-to-day responsibilities, to enjoy the special prerogatives, indulgences, and sympathy the sick role entailed. Hysteria thus became one way in which conventional women could express—in most cases unconsciously—dissatisfaction with one or several aspects of their lives.

The effect of hysteria upon the family and traditional sex role differentiation was disruptive in the extreme. The hysterical woman virtually ceased to function within the family. No longer did she devote herself to the needs of others, acting as self-sacrificing wife, mother, or daughter. Through her hysteria she could and in fact did force others to assume those functions. Household activities were reoriented to answer the hysterical woman's importunate needs. Children were hushed, rooms darkened, entertaining suspended, a devoted nurse recruited. Fortunes might be spent on medical bills or for drugs and operations. Worry and concern bowed the husband's shoulders; his home had suddenly become a hospital and he a nurse. Through her illness, the bedridden woman came to dominate her family to an extent that would have been considered inappropriate—indeed shrewish—in a healthy woman. Taking to one's bed, especially when suffering from dramatic and ever-visible symptoms, might also have functioned as a mode of passive aggression, especially in a milieu in which weakness was rewarded and in which women had since childhood been taught not to express overt aggression. Consciously or unconsciously, she had thus opted out of her traditional role.

Women did not accomplish this redefinition of domestic roles without the aid of the men in their family. Doctors commented that the hysteric's husband and family often, and unfortunately, rewarded her symptoms with elaborate sympathy. 'The hysteric's credit is usually first established,' as one astute mid-century clinician pointed out, 'by those who have, at least, the wish to believe them.' Husbands and fathers were not alone in their cooperation; the physician often played a complex and in a sense emotionally compromising role in legitimizing the female hysteric's behavior. As an impartial and a professionally skilled observer, he was empowered to judge whether or not a particular woman had the right to withdraw from her socially allotted duties. At the same time, these physicians accepted as correct, indeed as biologically inevitable, the structure of the Victorian family and the division of sex roles within it. He excused the woman only in the belief that she was ill and that she would make every effort to get well and resume her accustomed role. It was the transitory and unavoidable nature of the sick role that made it acceptable to family and physician as an alternate mode of female behavior.[7]

The doctor's ambivalence toward the hysterical woman, already rooted as we have seen in professional and sexual uncertainties, may well have been reinforced by this complicitory role within the family. It was for this reason that the disease's erratic pattern, its chronic nature, its lack of a determinable organic etiology, and the patient's seeming failure of will, so angered him. Even if she were not a conscious malingerer, she might well be guilty of self-indulgence and moral delinquency. By diagnosing her as ill, he had in effect created or permitted the hysterical woman to create a bond between himself and her. Within the family configuration he had sided with her against her husband or other male family members—men with whom he would normally have identified.

The quintessential sexual nature of hysteria further complicated the doctor's professional stance. As we have already seen, the hysterical patient in her role as woman may well have mobilized whatever ambivalence towards sex a particular physician felt. In a number of cases, moreover, the physician also played the role of oedipal father figure to the patient's child-woman role, and in such instances his complicity was not only moral and intellectual but sexual as well. These doctors had become part of a domestic triangle—a husband's rival, the fatherly attendant of a daughter. This intra-family role may therefore go far to explain the particularly strident and suspicious tone which characterized much of the clinical discussion of hysteria. Physicians were concerned with—and condemned— the power which chronic illness such as hysteria gave a woman over her family. Many women, doctors noted with annoyance, enjoyed this power and showed no inclination to get well: it is hardly coincidental that most late-nineteenth-century authorities agreed that removal from her family was a necessary first step in attempting to cure the hysterical patient.[8]

Not only did the physician condemn the hysteric's power within her family, he was clearly sensitive to her as a threat to his own prestige and authority. It is evident from their writings that many doctors felt themselves to be locked in a power struggle with their hysterical patients. Such women, doctors claimed, used their symptoms as weapons in asserting autonomy in relation to their physician; in continued illness was their victory. Indeed, much of the medical literature on hysteria is devoted to providing doctors with the means of winning this war of wills. Physicians felt that they must dominate the hysteric's will; only in this way, they wrote, could they bring about her permanent cure. 'Do not flatter yourselves . . . that you gain an easy victory,' Dr L. C. Grey told a medical school class in 1888:

> On the contrary, you must expect to have your temper, your ingenuity, your nerves tested to a degree that cannot be surpassed even by the greatest surgical operations. I maintain that the man who has the nerve and the tact to conquer some of these grave cases of hysteria has the nerve and the tact that will make him equal to the great emergencies of life. Your patient must be taught day by day . . . by steady resolute, iron-willed determination and tact—that combination which the French . . . call "the iron

hand beneath the velvet glove."[9]

Much of the treatment prescribed by physicians for hysteria reflects, in its draconic severity, their need to exert control—and, when thwarted, their impulse to punish. Doctors frequently recommended suffocating hysterical women until their fits stopped, beating them across the face and body with wet towels, ridiculing and exposing them in front of family and friends, showering them with icy water. 'The mode adopted to arrest this curious malady,' a physician connected with a large mental hospital wrote,

> consists in making some strong and sudden impression on the mind through . . . the most potent of all impressions, fear . . .
>
>   Ridicule to a woman of sensitive mind, is a powerful weapon . . . but there is no emotion equal to fear and the threat of personal chastisement . . . They will listen to the voice of authority.[10]

When, on the other hand, the hysterical patient proved tractable, gave up her fits or paralyses and accepted the physician as saviour and moral guide, he no longer had to appear in the posture of chastising father. He could respond to his hysterical patient with fondness, sympathy, and praise. No longer was she thwarting him with 'temper, tears, tricks, and tantrums'—as one doctor chose to title a study of hysteria.

Thomas Addis Emmett, pioneer gynecological specialist, recalled with ingenuous candor his mode of treating hysterics:

> the patient . . . was a child in my hands. In some respects the power gained was not unlike that obtained over a wild beast except that in one case the domination would be due to fear, while with my patient as a rule, it would be the desire to please me and to merit my approval from the effort she would make to gain her self-control. I have at times been depressed with the responsibility attending the blind influence I have often been able to gain over the nervous women under my influence.[11]

Not surprisingly, S. Weir Mitchell ended one of his treatises on hysteria with the comment that doctors, who knew and understood all women's petty weaknesses, who could govern and forgive them, made the best husbands.

The hysterical female thus emerges from the essentially male medical literature of the nineteenth century as a 'child-woman', highly impressionable, labile, superficially sexual, exhibitionistic, given to dramatic body language and grand gestures, with strong dependency needs and decided ego weaknesses. She resembled in many ways the personality type referred to by Guze in 1967 as a 'hysterical personality', or by Kernberg in 1968 as an 'infantile personality'.[12] But in a very literal sense these characteristics of the hysteric were merely hypertrophied versions of traits and behavior commonly reinforced in female children and adolescents. At a time when American society accepted egalitarian democracy and free will as transcendent social values, women, as we have seen, were nevertheless routinely socialized to fill a weak, dependent and severely limited social role. They were sharply discouraged from expressing competition or mastery in such 'masculine' areas as physical skill, strength and courage, or in academic or commercial pursuits, while at the same time they were encouraged to be coquettish, entertaining, non-threatening and nurturant. Overt anger and violence were forbidden as unfeminine and vulgar. The effect of this socialization was to teach women to have a low evaluation of themselves, to significantly restrict their ego functions to low prestige areas, to depend on others and to altruistically wish not for their own worldly success, but for that of their male supporters.

Notes and References

1. Supported by grants from the National Institute of Health and the Grant Foundation, New York.

2. For a basic secondary source, see Barbara Welter, 'The Cult of True Womanhood' *The American Quarterly* **XVIII** pp. 151–171, (1966).
3. For an excellent secondary account of the southern woman's domestic life, see Anne Firor Scott, *The Southern Lady*, University of Chicago Press, Chicago, (1970).
4. S. Weir Mitchell, *Doctor and Patient*, J. B. Lippincott Company, Philadelphia, pp. 84, 92 (1887).
5. Thomas Sydenham, 'Epistolatory Dissertation', in *The Works of Thomas Sydenham, M.D. . . . with a Life of the Author*, Latham, R. G. (ed) 2 vols. New Sydenham Society, London, **II**, p. 85 (1850).
6. S. Weir Mitchell, *Lectures on the Diseases of The Nervous System, Especially in Women*, 2nd edn, Lea Brothers & Co., Philadelphia, (1885).
7. For an exposition of this argument, see Erving Goffman, 'Insanity of Place', *Psychiatry* **XXXII** 357–388 (1969). (An extract from this article is also in this Reader.)
8. The fact that the physician was at the same time employed and paid by the woman or her family—in a period when the profession was far more competitive than it is in mid-twentieth century America—implies a much higher level of stress and ambiguity.
9. Grey, L. C. 'Clinical lecture', (1888) 132.
10. Skey, F. C. *Hysteria*, A. Simpson, New York, 60.
11. Emmett, Thomas A. *Incidents of my Life*, G. P. Putnam's Sons, New York, 210 (1911).
12. Samuel Guze, 'The Diagnosis of Hysteria: What are We Trying to Do', *American Journal of Psychiatry*, **CXXIV**, 494–498 (1967); Otto Kernberg, 'Borderline Personality Organization', *Journal of the American Psychoanalytical Association*, **XV**, 641–685 (1967).

Carroll Smith-Rosenberg is Assistant Professor working in the Department of History and Psychiatry, University of Pennsylvania. These extracts are from an article originally published in *Social Research*, 39, 652–672 (1972).

1.5

The Causes of Disease: Women Talking

Mildred Blaxter

It is a common finding that one of the things which most concerns patients, when they are given a diagnosis, is to know not simply the name of their disease but also its cause.

The analysis presented here relates to the concepts of cause expressed by one group of the population during long tape-recorded discussions of health and illness. These are 46 women in middle-age, all in semi-skilled or unskilled manual social classes, living in a Scottish city. The questions being asked are: What diseases were mentioned by the women? Was there much speculation about cause? What categories of cause were most popular? Were the etiological models similar to those of medical science, either in principle or in detail? Do the answers to these questions offer any insight about the way in which this group typically reacts to illness, or any useful information to doctors attempting to diagnose their diseases or treat their ill-health? And always, of course, one must ask how far this group is expressing the special beliefs of a particular subculture, and how far it is possible to offer generalisations about the way in which people think about the causes of disease.

Method

The 46 women were interviewed in their own homes as the 'grandmothers' of a group of young families in which the health care of children was being studied.[1] For the other purposes of the research, they were selected as belonging to a close and distinct group of working-class families, neither geographically nor socially mobile; a group amongst whom an identifiable subculture might be expected.

The data do not consist of the answers to predetermined questions, but rather of 1–2 hour conversations during which, in the general context of health and illness, the women themselves chose which diseases they would talk about, or what stories they would tell. Upon this material, a verbal and content analysis is imposed in an attempt to derive models of the structure of their thinking. Every mention of a named disease was extracted from the transcripts. Every instance was then examined to see whether cause was explicitly or implicitly stated, and the causes for each disease were allotted to data-derived categories.

This form of analysis permits the examination not only of consistency within the group, but also of consistency within each woman's discussion. In fact, many explanations for the occurrence of a disease may be tried out, offered as alternatives, or changed according to context, even within the space of one conversation; acknowledgement of this more truly represents the nature of the women's 'knowledge'.

It must be made clear that this analysis is not of a more complicated concept, that of generalised 'illness'. The distinction between disease and illness has frequently been made[2-4] and the terms are being used in the manner defined, for instance, by Helman:[5] diseases are 'the named pathological entities that make up the medical model of ill-health'; illness 'refers to the subjective response of the patient to being unwell'.

The explanatory models which laymen use are commonly thought of as models of illness, in contrast to the models of disease with which medical science operates.[6-8] This is, however, an over-simplification: patients, too, have models of disease, which are a part (though not the whole) of their concept of illness. The analysis here relates to only one aspect of the patients' knowledge of disease, but it is one which may be an important component of their concept of illness, and may have crucial implications for their illness behaviour.

It must also be clear that the concern is not, primarily, with whether this knowledge is scientifically right or wrong: the intention is not simply to investigate the ways in which the women are misinformed. The main emphasis is upon the structure of the women's thinking, and its similarity or difference when compared with the models of medical science.

Diseases and Categories of Cause

All the diseases mentioned by the 46 women are listed in Table 1. The list demonstrates, perhaps, something of the environment and socio-medical history of the group: these are middle-aged women talking, and there is an emphasis on chest conditions, on the diseases of poverty and a cold, damp climate and on infectious diseases, as well as on the more serious common diseases (cancer, heart disease) which one might expect to be prominent.

A simple preliminary point which must be made is to note how frequent the discussion of cause was. There are 587 examples of named diseases in these 46 transcripts. It was judged that in 432 of these instances, some imputation of the cause of the disease was explicitly or implicitly expressed.

Table 2 shows which diseases were most commonly mentioned *without* discussion of cause. For some of these, the disease was probably considered too common or trivial for the cause to be worthy of discussion, or the cause too obvious. Other reasons may apply to, for instance, cancer or tuberculosis, which will be considered later.

These instances were much fewer than those in which there was some discussion of cause, however. The categories into which these causes appeared most easily to fall are shown in Table 3, and each will be discussed in turn.

The lists of diseases put into each category must make it clear that (childhood infections apart) there were few conditions where agreement about causes was high. Bronchitis, for instance, appears in almost every category.

Table 1 Diseases mentioned (46 women)

	No. of women
TB (consumption, shadow on the lung, etc.)	36
Measles, german measles	36
Bronchitis	34
Cancer (tumor, breast amputation, etc.)	28
Heart disease (attack, angina, etc.)	28
Cold, chill	24
Whooping cough	21
Asthma	18
Ulcer, chronic stomach trouble	17
Chickenpox	14
Laryngitis, tonsillitis	14
Arterial disease (coronary, thrombosis, etc.)	12
Migraine: chronic headache	12
Eczema, dermatitis, skin disease	12
Pneumonia	12
Cystitis, kidney disease	12
Mumps	11
Scarlet fever	11
Depression (nerves, breakdown, etc.)	11
Diphtheria	11
Rheumatism, rheumatics	11
Slipped disc (worn disc, vertebrae)	11
Gynaecological problems, fibroids	11
High blood pressure	10
Arthritis	10
Flu, influenza	10

Fewer than 10 instances in order of frequency: diabetes, convulsions, gastroenteritis, sinusitis, appendicitis, deafness, rheumatic fever, piles, congenital abnormalities, epilepsy, meningitis, anaemia, allergy, gallbladder disease, glandular fever, sciatica, fibrositis, hernia, leukaemia, thyroid disease, abscess in breast, ovarian cyst, peritonitis, mental retardation, bowel disease, varicose veins, pleurisy, jaundice, eye disease, hay fever, polio, croup, thrush, rickets, pancreatitis, Parkinson's Disease, St Vitus Dance, phlebitis, osteomyelitis, gangrene, presenile dementia, hiatus hernia, pyloric stenosis, Hodgkin's Disease, Pink's Disease, syphilis, 'brittle bones', 'lazy muscle', 'tennis elbow'.

Table 2 Diseases most frequently mentioned without discussion of cause (46 women)

	No. of women
Cancer	20
Tuberculosis	16
Cold	15
Heart disease	9
Tonsilitis	8
Stomach conditions	8
Pneumonia	7
Congenital abnormalities	6
Cystitis	6
Bronchitis	6
Appendicitis	6
Rheumatic fever	5

Childhood infectious diseases are omitted, since it can be presumed that there was general agreement that they came into the category of 'infection'.

Table 3 Categories of cause, and the diseases attributed to them (46 women). For the most frequently mentioned diseases in each category, the number of women using this category of cause for this disease is given in parentheses

1. *Infection* 126 instances
    Childhood infections, not always explicitly referred to as measles, mumps, whooping cough, chickenpox, german measles, scarlet fever, diphtheria; also: influenza (12), gastroenteritis (4), cold (4), cystitis (4) and tuberculosis, polio, jaundice, tonsilitis, glandular fever, pneumonia
2. *Heredity or familial tendencies* 55 instances
    Asthma (8), heart disease (5), tuberculosis (5), bronchitis (4), diabetes (4), eczema (4); also: high blood pressure, thrombosis, rheumatism, arthritis, sinusitis, stomach disease, cancer, tonsilitis, meningitis, presenile dementia, pyloric stenosis, 'lazy muscle'
3. *Agents in the environment: 'poisons', working condition, climate* 48 instances
    Bronchitis (8), cold (6), tuberculosis (6); also: flu, high blood pressure, rheumatism, sciatica, slipped disc, sinusitis, cancer, eczema, asthma, tonsilitis, pneumonia, diptheria, scarlet fever, measles, arthritis, pleurisy, breast abscess, Hodgkin's, Parkinson's, varicose veins, thrush
    Drugs or the contraceptive pill 13 instances
    Headache (3), gynaecological problems (3), birth abnormalities (3); also: stomach disease, 'nerves', heart disease
4. *Secondary to other diseases* 42 instances
    Bronchitis (9), heart disease (8), epilepsy and convulsions (5), pneumonia (4), deafness (4); also: headache, thrombosis, rheumatic fever, arthritis, cancer, tuberculosis, kidney disease, rheumatism, glandular fever
5. *Stress, strain and worry* 27 instances
    Migraine and headache (5), stomach disease (5), heart disease (4); also: depression and 'nerves', bronchitis, thrombosis, asthma, slipped disc, birth abnormalities, thyroid disease, St Vitus Dance
6. *Caused by childbearing, menopause* 27 instances
    Gynaecological problems (9), menopausal syndrome (5), piles (4); also: bronchitis, headache, anaemia, kidney disease, jaundice, bowel disease, uterine infection
7. *Secondary to trauma or to surgery* 25 instances
    Arthritis (4); also: rheumatism, rickets, slipped disc, osteomyelitis, meningitis, cancer, tuberculosis, appendicitis, hernia, asthma, stomach disease, thrombosis, presenile dementia, depression, ovarian cyst, eye disease, bronchitis
8. *Neglect, the constraints of poverty* 19 instances
    Tuberculosis (4), stomach disease (3); also: bronchitis, heart disease, high blood pressure, thrombosis, rheumatism, arthritis, asthma, cold, gastroenteritis, pleurisy, peritonitis
9. *Inherent susceptibility, individual and not hereditary* 18 instances
    Depression, 'nerves' (4), bronchitis (3), cold (3); also: influenza, sinusitis, asthma, stomach disease, tonsillitis, St Vitus Dance
10. *Behaviour, own responsibility* 18 instances
    Bronchitis (6), diabetes (3), high blood pressure (3); also: heart disease, cancer, slipped disc, arthritis, rheumatism
11. *Ageing, natural degeneration* 14 instances
    Rheumatism (6), slipped disc (5); also: arthritis, gynaecological problems

Infection and the Environment

Infection is the most important category of cause, if the very frequent mentions of childhood infectious diseases are included. Measles, mumps, whooping cough and chickenpox were commonly spoken of dismissively as inevitable in the past and, with the possible exception of whooping cough, not too troublesome now. Some other conditions recognised as infectious—diphtheria, scarlet fever, tuberculosis, gastroenteritis—had, however, been greatly feared and the importance of infectious disease to these families 40 or so years ago, when the women were children, is eloquently demonstrated by their descriptions of avoidance rituals. One, referring to a farmhouse with stone-flagged floors, said:

> My father wouldn't allow carpet in the house. But one mat was all that was allowed and that was at the fireside. And if there was anybody coming in it was lifted. Because my father said they took in the germs on their feet.

When they had children of their own, this fear of 'germs' continued, and even now one woman described how she boiled all her dishes now and then ('A'thing into the broth pot an' just let them boil awa!') or used strong domestic disinfectant in her bath: 'Oh, I'm an awfu' case for germs! I dinna believe in germs!'

Infections are associated, as a category, with the environment because there were certain environments or climatic conditions in which germs flourished, and it was sometimes not clear whether it was the environment *per se* that was being indicted or whether the women were referring to an infection. Certainly there were particular types of weather—damp, changeable, 'clammy' or hot—which were 'good for' germs and certain environmental circumstances—damp housing, changes of temperature—which made one more susceptible to infections.

There were many other conditions, however, when it was clearly agents and conditions in the environment which caused diseases not seen as infections. The popularity of 'external' causes—'something in the water', 'dampness in these houses'—appeared to represent a very natural desire on the women's part to allot 'blame'. To find a cause in the environment was more acceptable than to locate responsibility in one's own body, and an obvious way of rationalising the unknown. In any case, the women's lives truly presented many candidates for an environmental explanation of ill-health—an unkind climate, often poor housing and work in unpleasant conditions.

There were also some specific 'poisons' in the general environment that might be blamed for disease—petrol from cars, impurities in food or water. On the whole, however, this type of explanation had little prominence: the women were not concerned with the modern 'pure air' or 'unadulterated food' lobbies. The possibility that prescribed drugs, especially the contraceptive pill, might cause disease is another causal category of a similar kind.

Heredity and Familial Tendencies

It can be noted from Table 3 that the second most 'popular' category of cause, after infection, was heredity or family susceptibility. This was given much more weight than medical science might give it and was applied to a very wide variety of diseases. A distinction between 'hereditary' and 'familial' is not easy to make, though sometimes diseases were spoken of very clearly as inherited and at other times the women were definitely distinguishing between familial tendencies and hereditary diseases. They were faced with the fact that, since families in the past had been very large and certain diseases had been very prevalent, there was a high likelihood that patterns could be found. Rarely, they might recognise that random (or environmentally associated) similarities might occur: an example is a woman who said:

> Bronchial asthma's nae an inherited disease, it's something that starts in you yoursel'. I didnae take it from my father. It just so happens I followed in my father's footsteps.

More commonly, they might argue that similarities proved that a disease *must* be hereditary: as another woman said, 'They say ulcers is nae hereditary', but the fact that four children of a family had suffered from them, 'even thae two lassies in Australia', made her reluctant to accept this, for obviously it could not be diet or environment.

Family weakness or susceptibility often resided in particular parts of the body:

> His mother, my husband's, her mother before that and further down the line, all had awful legs. They've all been bothered wi' their legs.

Commonly, too, families had for generations been bothered with their chests or stomachs.

The liking for hereditary or familial 'weakness' as an explanation can easily be explained as a liking for continuity, a firm, long-term family identity. The women might not have much in the way of material prosperity to boast of, but they did belong to large, close families and, as one woman said, 'we're all built of an impression on our ancestors, aren't we?' Also, the emphasis on 'family failings' was, in part, a way of expressing the inevitability of disease. To explore familial patterns was a source of worry, but at the same time, it was to some extent comforting, for it meant that no responsibility for one's own diseases need be assumed.

Stress, Strain and Psychological Explanations

As Table 3 shows, stress and strain was one of the most popular categories of cause. The women were very conscious of a mind/body link, which led them not only to favour 'mind over matter' maxims for the management of illness, but also to favour psychological explanations for the cause of disease. Thus, of blood pressure, 'It's a nervous trouble, it's worry'; of stomach pain, 'It's because I'm all tensed up'; of ulcers, 'I should think worry is the cause'. Stress was especially blamed for headaches and migraine. Stress and overwork were also commonly mentioned as the cause of heart disease. A particular stress or shock (wartime bombs, bereavement) could also be the psychological, rather than the mechanical, cause of disease (St Vitus' Dance, coronary disease, thrombosis). One woman explained a stroke thus:

> I'd an awful lot of stress with my husband dying, and looking after my mum, and I went out to work . . . I wisnae home here until evening and by the time I did housework and bed—I was up early in the morning again. I think it just began that it got too much.

There were many other sophisticated analyses of how disease could be caused not only by strain but also by anger, resentment, frustration and despair.

It must be added that, although they themselves were happy to offer 'stress' or 'nerves' explanations, they sometimes resented it when doctors attempted to impose such explanations upon them. Such theories of cause were acceptable only when they were based on the detailed knowledge which they themselves had of the interrelations between life events and symptoms.

Disease which is Secondary to Trauma or Surgery

As Table 3 shows, causes of lesser importance, but nevertheless distinct categories, were the results of trauma or surgery. Both appeared to be thought of as assaults upon the body, unnatural openings, breakings, insults which might leave weaknesses or permanent gaps in defences against the environment. Since injury would more usually affect the bones and joints, the diseases that could follow might be arthritis, rheumatism, rickets, osteomyelitis; since surgery unnaturally stressed or exposed the organs of the body, a wide variety of conditions such as asthma, bronchitis, ulcers, thrombosis, might attack these organs. One woman expressed this very explicitly:

> I think that everyone that has an operation—when the body's opened up—they always have a cough after it . . . Once you're opened up the cold sets in.

In this way the women were of course attempting to provide what seemed to be rational explanations for the common experience of ill-health following traumatic events.

Behaviour: Neglect: The Constraints of Poverty

There is only a small number of instances, as Table 3 shows, where the women were willing to admit that disease was entirely self-inflicted. 'Rushing around' might be the cause of 'blood pressure'; several women described the cause of diabetes as overfondness for sugar, and a few said that not eating properly ('rushed meals, no vegetables') might result in stomach ulcers. Overweight was suggested by a few women as the cause of high blood pressure or heart attacks (but not many, for a high proportion were overweight themselves) and smoking was occasionally mentioned as a cause of bronchitis (but rarely, for almost all the women smoked).

One might also neglect one's health in a way that was irresponsible. In most of the examples where 'neglect' was being offered as a cause, however, self-responsibility was explicitly denied. Yes, it was this behaviour that caused the disease, but in the circumstances no one could behave differently. These 'neglect' explanations appear to belong rather to a category of the 'constraints of poverty', the life circumstances which made care of one's health and treatment for one's illnesses impossible.

On the other hand, there were many accounts of poverty in the past, especially in the women's own childhoods, which were not seen as particularly relevant to life-long health. Some women were adamant that poverty of itself, or poor living conditions, had nothing to do with the prevalence of disease. They preferred to think of disease as striking rich and poor alike:

> I dinna think their surroundings has onything to dee wi' it. I mean, you could have ony God's amount of money and the best of everything to give them, and you could hae the most unhealthiest child in the world. An' you could have nothing, an' hae to work an' bring them up yourself, an' you'll find you've got the healthiest kids.

Individual Susceptibility

A quite small but important category of cause has been given the same 'individual susceptibility'. This refers to diseases which were not thought of as hereditary or even familial, but which attacked an inborn or inherent 'weakness'. The sufferer was in a sense responsible for these illnesses, but they were inevitable: there was nothing one could do to avoid them, given one's personal makeup. This explanation was commonly applied to bronchitis, 'flu, colds and asthma, and the women said such things as 'I'm just the type', 'It's excitement, just her temperament', or 'There's nothing can stop that, if you're going to take it'. This was a common explanation for nervous conditions, 'breakdown', or depression. There was also a concept of readiness to take disease that appeared to be similar to an idea of immune status.

The Ageing Process: 'Natural' Degeneration: Stages of Life

A conspicuous feature of the women's general norms of 'health' was an acceptance of poor health as a natural feature of the ageing process and an accelerated time-scale for 'getting on now'. Though only in their late 40s and 50s, they frequently spoke of themselves as older than their years. As one woman typically said:

> I'm getting on in years, so I'm not really bothered now. See, I'm 47. I say, och, it's a waste of time. If they canna do nothing about it, they canna do nothing about it—I dinna like to fight with them.

However, it can be noted from Table 3 that there were very few *diseases* which they were willing to attribute to ageing or to natural degenerative processes: this was not a popular category of cause for specific ailments. Some conditions were, of course, attributed to natural events of a woman's life, childbearing or the menopause. Childbearing had left them with many gynaecological problems, they believed, and a few women were complaining of menopausal syndromes or talked of this as an illness they had gone through. On the whole, however, this was not as frequently mentioned as might have been expected.

Diseases Mentioned Without Cause: Cancer and Tuberculosis

It is not surprising that cancer and tuberculosis are two of the diseases most frequently mentioned in these transcripts, but it is interesting that they are also the most frequently mentioned without discussion of cause. They were also the two for which there was a wide variety of synonyms, as though the name itself were taboo.

When the cause of tuberculosis was discussed or imputed, a wide variety of etiologies was offered. Only three women explicitly indicated their recognition that the disease was infectious. A few causal agents in the environment were offered—materials in a factory, working in the pits, exposure to gas during the First World War—but only a few of the women associated tuberculosis clearly with poverty. If they did, however, they saw the cause as lying within the stresses and neglect of health brought about by the living conditions, rather than directly due to poor nutrition or the risk of infection.

There was much less detailed discussion of cancer. It was almost universally cited as the disease which was dreaded nowadays, but we can only record—without any good explanation—that few women talked about it at length. The women gave the impression of *preferring* to believe that cancer was quite randomly caused: 'it could happen to anyone'. It seems possible that the relative lack of discussion, given the salience of cancer as judged by the number of times the disease was mentioned, was due not only to the fact that they believed the cause to be unknown (a fact which did not deter discussion of many other diseases) but also to a specific reluctance to talk about it. Cancer was, as TB had been, a condition to which a superstitious dread adhered, as well as a rational and understandable fear—to talk about it was to invoke it, to speak briefly or in a lowered voice was to leave it sleeping.

Secondary Diseases: Chains of Cause: Consistence of Explanations

So far, causes have been discussed as though they were single. This is, of course, to some extent a misrepresentation, since neither in contemporary medical science, nor in the thinking of these women, is it suggested that the concept of single causes was paramount.

As Table 3 shows, diseases which were secondary to another condition, described as usually, or sometimes, or in the instance under discussion caused by another disease, were in fact the third most common category. Thus bronchitis was described as being caused by 'flu, cold, whooping cough, 'a scarred lung', or heart disease by measles, mumps, rheumatic fever, bronchitis ('the chronic bronchitis weakened the heart'). The most common disease which could lead to others was measles, which was thought to be the cause of such varied conditions as deafness, squints and arthritis as well as heart disease.

Usually, the women were individually consistent about ascription of cause, and there were only a few instances where they stated categorically that the cause was of one sort in one part of the interview, and another sort later in the interview. However, they did of course recognise that there might be several *alternative* causes for a particular disease, and Table 3 inevitably conceals the fact that one individual might offer a selection of causes. In these discussions the women were obviously thinking in terms of causal agents, which required initial susceptibility to take effect, and also required precipitating factors. As one woman said of cancer, 'Everyone's got it, but it needs something to set it off.' They were, in fact, using models very similar to those of advanced medical science.

In their often elaborate chains of cause the women were going further than medical science, however. There appeared to be a positive strain towards accounting for their present bodily state, or describing their accumulated experience, by connecting together the relevant health events. It did not seem reasonable to them to suppose that one part of their body had gone wrong at one stage, and another part at some other time, in a totally random fashion. Although they accepted the idea of disease striking randomly to some extent, in any case they preferred other models. Thus, they believed that their childhood experiences, their pregnancies and deliveries, their work and environment and the major illnesses they had suffered must all be connected. This was particularly true of chronic diseases. Some trivial illnesses could be seen as temporary and outside the self. But those diseases which were always present were part of identity. They had to accommodate pain or restriction of function into their middle-aged selves, just as they had to accommodate grey hair or thickened waistlines—these were permanent parts of personality, and ascribing chains of cause to illnesses was part of a process of accounting for their identities.

Conclusion

It can be concluded, in answer to the questions posed at the beginning of this article, that ideas about cause were a very important component of the models of disease held by this particular social group. Their 'preferred' categories of cause can be shown to be a product of their particular social situation. Their general models of causal processes, painstakingly derived from their experience as they saw it, were often scientifically wrong in detail, but were not in principle unscientific.

It is obvious that the 'folk' concepts of this group of women can be seen as in *opposition* to scientific medicine only on a very narrow and outmoded view of medical theory—only if it is supposed that medicine still prefers single causes, views psyche and soma dichotomously, has a narrow definition of heredity, or regards disease and behaviour as discrete. Though medical theory may be complex, however, medical practice, treating that which is before it, may seem to oversimplify. Concepts of disease become relevant to 'illness' and its management because the subjective chains of cause which the woman perceived may have been quite different from the clinical cause, though no less logically derived.

These women's beliefs about cause could be demonstrated to have a direct effect upon their help-seeking behaviour. Just as a respondent of Koos[9] said, many years ago, 'If I knew how I did it—say from lifting a bucket of coal—I might not go [to the doctor] as quick as if I didn't know where it came from', so these women might say 'If I got another pain I wid just take it was the menopause again.'

On the other hand, there are many examples of the women worrying over symptoms, consulting again and again, because (although they had been given a diagnosis) they had not been given a *cause* or at least one which they found acceptable. People have to inhabit their bodies, and their physical identity is part of themselves. Particularly as they grow older, they have a need to account for this identity, to draw together all that they have experienced. This body is their inheritance, it is the result of the events of their life, and it is their constraint.

In their discussions of medical consultation, the women sometimes conveyed a sense of despair at the impossibility of making known the whole. A consultation presents incompatible obligations: to be brief and helpful, not waste time which is manifestly in short supply, and yet somehow to tell the story of a life in all its long detail.

In the surgery, the doctor's view of the disease process must be reconciled with the patient's. The diagnosis must make sense in terms of the patient's models or it will not be accepted. Doctors do use concepts and a vocabulary borrowed from lay models, as Helman[10] has noted, and patients can learn from their doctors, as some examples here have shown. The use of what are perceived of as lay models can create problems, however, if the considerable sophistication in the concepts of even poorly educated patients is underrated.

Acknowledgement

The greater part of the interviewing for this study was the expert work of Elizabeth Paterson, Research Fellow of the Institute of Medical Sociology, Aberdeen.

References

1. Blaxter, M. and Paterson, E. *Mothers and Daughters: a Three-Generational Study of Health Attitudes and Behaviour*, Heinemann, London (1982).
2. Fabrega, H. 'The scope of ethnomedical science', *Cult. Med. Psychiat.*, 189, 969 (1975).
3. Cassell, E. J. *The Healers Art*, Penguin, Harmondsworth (1978).
4. Erde, E. L. 'Philosophical considerations regarding defining "health", "disease", etc. and their bearing on medical practice', *Ethics Sci. Med.*, 6, 31 (1979).
5. Helman, C. G. 'Disease versus illness in general practice', *Jl. R. Coll. Gen. Pract.*, 31, 548 (1981).
6. Eisenberg, L. 'Disease and illness: distinction between professional and popular ideas of sickness', *Cult. Med. Psychiat.*, 1, 355 (1977).
7. Helman, C. G. 'Lay and medical attitudes to illness', *MIMS Magazine*, p. 51, (15 April 1980).
8. Snow, L. F., Johnson S. M. and Mayhew, H. E. 'The behavioural implications of some old wives' tales', *Obstet. Gynaec.*, 51, 727 (1978).
9. Koos, E. L. *The Health of Regionsville: What the People Thought and Did About it*, Columbia University Press, New York (1954).
10. Helman, C. G. 'Feed a cold, starve a fever', *Cult. Med. Psychiat.*, 1, 107 (1978).

Mildred Blaxter is a Research Fellow and sociologist at the University of East Anglia, Norwich. She was previously at the MRC Medical Sociology Unit, Aberdeen. This article is an edited version of a paper published in *Social Science and Medicine*, 17 (2) 59–69 (1983).

1.6

The History of Pernicious Anaemia from 1822 to the Present Day

Irvine Loudon

First of all the history of pernicious anaemia is discussed as an interesting story in its own right, starting with the earliest clinical reports which led to the recognition of the disease, and ending with recent views on its nature.

The story is then presented as a characteristic example of the way that advances in the theory and practice of medicine occur and are influenced, sometimes adversely, by currently fashionable ideas on the causation of disease.

It has always been obvious that if you were severely wounded, or lost blood for any other reason, you could become weak or ill or even die, and blood is essential for life. But the idea that the blood could be deficient, not from excessive bleeding, but from a disease of the blood *sui generis*, was essentially a concept of the early nineteenth century when the term anaemia first came into general use. Once anaemia was recognised as common it was found that most cases responded well to an adequate diet and medicine. Iron, which had been used as a tonic or stimulant for a long time, was soon recognised as the treatment of choice for anaemia.

In 1849, Thomas Addison (1793–1860), a physician at Guy's Hospital in London, published a brief account of a form of anaemia which was unusual. He called it 'A remarkable form of anaemia which, although incidentally noticed by various writers [Dr Combe in Edinburgh had described a case in 1822] has not attracted . . . the attention it really deserves.' This form of anaemia occurred, he wrote, in males aged twenty to sixty'. . . commencing insidiously and proceeding very slowly'; and it was invariably fatal. No treatment, not even iron, was of the slightest benefit.

As interest in pernicious anaemia grew through the late nineteenth and early twentieth century, cases were commonly seen in the wards of the hospitals because they were selected as examples of a particularly interesting disease. Within the community, however, pernicious anaemia, because it was fairly uncommon and affected people mostly towards the end of their lives, was not in quantitative terms a serious health problem.

At first, Addison's brief report attracted little attention until a Swiss doctor, Biermer, described some cases in 1872 of the same kind of anaemia and named it 'progressive pernicious anaemia'. After that, it became known as Addisonian pernicious anaemia, or, more briefly, pernicious anaemia.

Anaemia is by definition a deficiency in the number of red blood cells in the circulation, or a deficiency in haemoglobin (the oxygen-carrying pigment in the red cells), or both. Blood is formed in the bone marrow, and the red cells, after evolving through several stages to full maturity, are released into the circulation. After an average period of 120 days the obsolete red cells are destroyed. In health, production and destruction continue at the same rate, ensuring that the number of red cells in the circulation remains constant.

In order to understand the history and nature of pernicious anaemia, a simple analogy is helpful. The analogy is that of a car factory in a country where it is the only one, and no cars are imported. The factory (the bone-marrow) manufactures the cars (the red cells) which appear on the roads (the blood vessels) until they become worn out and are scrapped. Now, suppose there is a sudden deficiency in a vital piece of equipment used in the final stage of manufacture. At first, finished cars held in stock can be used up, but when that stock is exhausted the number of cars on the road begins to fall. Meanwhile the factory continues to produce cars that are nearly, but not quite, fit to be sold. A few of these incomplete cars slip past the inspectors and appear on the road, but soon break down. In the factory itself unfinished cars accumulate until, because they are crammed to capacity, some of the unfinished cars are broken up and stored as scrap iron. Meanwhile, the number of cars on the road falls gradually but relentlessly.

Advances in medicine in the 1850s, particularly the ability to estimate the number of red cells in the blood and measure the amount of the pigment haemoglobin, led to discoveries about pernicious anaemia similar to those in the imaginary car factory. Thus, in 1875 and 1876, Pepper in the USA and Cohnheim in Germany demonstrated that in cases of pernicious anaemia the number of red cells in the circulation was greatly diminished but the bone marrow was hyperplastic (=over active), overloaded with iron and packed with immature, abnormal precursors of the red cells. Moreover, the blood contained some abnormal red cells, corresponding to the unfinished cars that slipped past the inspectors.

Clearly, the bone marrow was responding to the anaemia by trying to manufacture red cells, but it lacked the ability to produce the finished product. It is interesting that in the first description of pernicious anaemia by Combe in 1822, he suggested the fault might lie in the digestive processes. However, proof of this did not come until the end of the nineteenth century. Then it was shown, first of all, that the stomachs of patients dying of pernicious anaemia were often atrophic (=wasted or worn out). This was followed by the finding that hydrochloric acid, present in normal gastric juices in abundance, was absent in cases of pernicious anaemia. The obvious conclusion, that pernicious anaemia was due to lack of hydrochloric acid, was soon shown to be untrue. Feeding hydrochloric acid by mouth did not cure it. Then it was suggested that the function of the acid in the stomach was to provide an antiseptic barrier, and that patients with pernicious anaemia were suffering from 'toxins' produced by swallowed bacteria, which poisoned the bone marrow. This theory can be found in textbooks published between 1910 and 1925.

Bacteriology was, at this time, a relatively new exciting branch of medical science. The temptation to attribute all diseases whose nature was obscure to bacterial sepsis or bacterial toxins was very strong. Thus it was widely believed that people could harbour toxin-producing bacteria in their tonsils, sinuses or teeth, even though these were, to all appearances, perfectly healthy; and that they could swallow these 'toxins' and become ill as a consequence. This was the theory of *focal sepsis*, and pernicious anaemia was for a time thought to be just such a disease. The unfortunate result was that a number of patients had healthy tonsils and teeth removed in obedience to a false theory. There were critics of this view of pernicious anaemia, but in general, the probability that a bone-marrow poisoned by toxins would appear hypoplastic (=under-active) rather than hyperplastic (=over-active) was ignored.

The next and most important stage of the story contains an element of luck, or at least trial and error. Whipple and his associates in the USA in 1920 carried out experiments that consisted of feeding various diets to dogs already made anaemic by bleeding them. They found that liver was the most effective food for stimulating new blood formation. This encouraged two other Americans, Minot and Murphy, in 1926 to try various diets, including liver in large quantities, on patients suffering from various kinds of anaemia. They found that cases of pernicious anaemia responded to liver in large quantities and some other foods (although not so well) including meat. These foods, it seemed, contained an anti-pernicious factor, but how this factor worked remained unknown. Whipple, Minot and Murphy were awarded a Nobel Prize for their work, and by 1928 an extract of liver which could be safely injected had been made and was soon brought into general use. Pernicious anaemia was, at last, treatable.

Treatment rapidly became available to all sections of the community and the hospital patients slowly dying of pernicious anaemia disappeared from the wards. As so often happens, when a really effective method of curing or preventing a medical disorder (but obviously not a surgical one) is discovered, it is nearly always a simple method that can be, and is, administered by general practitioners. Today, cases of pernicious anaemia are rarely seen in hospital wards, but every general practitioner has a number of cases for whose maintenance treatment he and his nursing staff are responsible.

Returning to the 1920s, the most imaginative and important advance was made by Castle in 1929. He postulated that blood formation required some dietary factor, found in high concentration in liver, which he called the *extrinsic* factor. However, the absorption of that factor was dependent on the secretion by the stomach of another factor, the *intrinsic* factor. Pernicious anaemia, Castle suggested, was a disorder of the stomach, and patients with pernicious anaemia had lost the ability to secrete not only hydrochloric acid (which was irrelevant to blood formation) but also the essential intrinsic factor. This proved to be correct. The most hopeful line of research was seen to be to try and isolate the extrinsic factor. This was done by 1948, when it was shown to be a vitamin and was named vitamin B_{12}. The nature of intrinsic factor is less important practically as it cannot be isolated and used in treatment, but the function of intrinsic factor is this. It 'escorts' the extrinsic factor (vitamin B_{12}) across the barrier of the wall of the gut, ensuring that all the B_{12} ingested in the diet is absorbed into the blood stream. In the absence of intrinsic factor (i.e. in pernicious anaemia) only a small percentage of ingested B_{12} can be absorbed by a process of slow diffusion across the gut wall. Thus by eating a diet with huge quantities of B_{12}, the patient with pernicious anaemia may just be able to absorb enough to stop the anaemia from getting any worse, but he has to continue to do so, day after day. What is the function of this vitamin B_{12}? Vitamin B_{12} is not so much an essential constituent of red cells; it is more a component required for certain chemical processes involved in the manufacture of normal red cells. The equivalent in the analogy of the car factory would be that the cars remained unfinished because a certain machine-tool was lacking and that tool was essential for finishing the manufacture of the car. To continue the analogy, there were plenty of the machine-tools available outside the factory gates, but the process of getting them through the factory gates and to the work bench had broken down. In this analogy the factory gates represent the stomach. *Pernicious anaemia is essentially a disease of the stomach made manifest through its effects on the blood.*

What does this mean in terms of medical practice today? Pernicious anaemia is rare below the age of 35; most cases occur at age 60 or over. It is found in 1 in every 250 people aged 60 in the United Kingdom, but there are large regional variations. Thus, it is more than three times as common in Scotland as it is in the South-east of England. It is much less common in the population as a whole than the ordinary iron deficiency anaemia by a ratio of about 9 to 1. It can occur in both sexes, not, as Addison thought, in males only. The usual history is that a patient is seen who is tired, often breathless and very pale; usually the pallor is described as of a lemon-yellow tint, but Addison's original description of the 'colour of bad wax' is much better. Pernicious anaemia is suspected, and a sample of blood is taken for examination. The blood shows a marked reduction in the number of red cells and the presence of some abnormal red cells (the unfinished cars which escaped on to the roads). The amount of vitamin B_{12} in the blood can be estimated, and in pernicious anaemia this is abnormally low. There are now known to be a number of diseases similar to pernicious anaemia, which are called as a group the megaloblastic anaemias. To be absolutely certain the patient really is suffering from Addisonian pernicious anaemia, the gastric contents can be examined and the absence of hydrochloric acid confirmed, and a specimen of bone-marrow can be examined for the characteristic appearance found in pernicious anaemia. Because treatment has to be life-long, and the characteristic signs disappear once treatment has begun, the tests must be completed first. Once the diagnosis is certain, vitamin B_{12} is given by injection and, once the blood has returned to normal, continued permanently. The injections are given regularly every three months, or more often if blood tests show it to be necessary. The commencement of treatment is the equivalent of removing the obstruction to the admission of machine-tools at the factory gates. In the analogy, the obvious result would be the sudden appearance on the roads of a large number of new, finished cars. Brand new cars would, for a while, form a much larger percentage of the total than usual. So it is with pernicious anaemia. The administration of vitamin B_{12} leads to a sudden rise in the number of new red cells. These are slightly different from ordinary red cells and are called reticulocytes. There are always some reticulocytes in the blood, just as there are always some new cars on the roads, but the rise in the percentage of reticulocytes when vitamin B_{12} is injected (the 'reticulocyte response') is further confirmation of the diagnosis of pernicious anaemia. Not only the blood, but also the bone marrow, rapidly return to normal. Usually the illness has come on so slowly and for such a long time that the patient has almost forgotten what it feels like to be well. For this reason, the treatment of pernicious anaemia can be one of the most striking and dramatic of all medical treatments as the patient is rapidly transformed back to health.

The history of pernicious anaemia is an unusually rich example of the nature of bio-medical advances, and of the historical periods in which they have taken place. It began as a clinical observation in the first half of the nineteenth century by astute physicians who recognised there was a 'new' form of anaemia different from the majority of cases. All advances at this time came from bed-side observation and post-mortem studies. The next stage occurred in the era of laboratory investigations, in the second half of the nineteenth century, when blood counts became available. This allowed the various kinds of anaemia to be identified and classified with a new certainty. Progress to this stage had followed a logical path but had provided no treatment for a fatal disease.

The next stage depended on the use of biochemical tests in the investigation of disease and also illustrated the importance of chance observations. It was the analysis of gastric juices that led to the unexpected discovery of 'achlorhydria' (=absence of hydrochloric acid) as an invariable feature of pernicious anaemia. This in turn led to three developments of a kind so common in medical research:
1. First it indicated, correctly, that the cause of pernicious anaemia lay in the stomach.
2. Second, it suggested (incorrectly) that pernicious anaemia could be cured by administering hydrochloric acid; in other words, that the acid was the missing factor.
3. When that failed, it led to the unfortunate theory of bacterial toxins as the cause, and

the subjection of many patients to the unnecessary removal of tonsils and teeth. Persistence of this kind of error was due to the popularity of a general theory of focal sepsis, then in vogue.

The next stage depended in the beginning on animal experiments, for it was Whipple's work on experimental anaemia that led to the discovery that liver contained the anti-pernicious anaemia factor.

Often, medical research is seen as the slow but steady progression through a logical series of steps. More often, it is actually a series of sudden jumps, some false (such as the focal sepsis theory), but others of outstanding importance. Often the sudden jumps seem obvious in retrospect, but Castle's theory of an extrinsic *and* an intrinsic factor was an example of a brilliant imaginative leap, and he confirmed the hypothesis by showing that ground beef (also a rich source of vitamin B_{12}) partially digested in the stomach of a 'normal' man induced a remission when fed to a patient with pernicious anaemia. The experiment may not sound attractive, but it was conclusive. Something in the gastric juice of healthy people was essential for the complete absorption of anti-pernicious factor. After this, the story was essentially one of logical but painstaking biochemical research to isolate the extrinsic factor: vitamin B_{12}.

It is easy to present the history of pernicious anaemia as one of the 'triumphs of biomedical research'. But one of the fashionable criticisms of modern medicine is that all too often it treats only the symptoms of a disease and fails to discover the root cause. This could be said of pernicious anaemia. The cause of the atrophy of the stomach that results in the failure to secrete intrinsic factor and hydrochloric acid (and, incidentally, is associated with an increased incidence of cancer of the stomach) is unknown. It tends to run in families and is therefore said to be 'an inherited constitutional weakness'. But that is no explanation. Recent work suggests that pernicious anaemia is an example of the failure of 'self-recognition' by the immune systems of the body. This means that pernicious anaemia belongs to a group of diseases in which there is a great deal of current interest, the auto-immune diseases. It is a group that contains, for example, certain forms of arthritis. The body contains an immune system whose function is to protect the body against the invasion by any foreign substances, such as bacteria or toxins. To perform this function, the immune system has to be able to distinguish between normal body tissues, or 'self', and foreign material, or 'not self'. If the recognition process breaks down, then the immune system can attack certain parts of the body. It is a kind of civil war waged by the immune system, or a situation such as an army shelling soldiers belonging to its own side. Why a part of the stomach should fail to be recognised as self and thus be singled out for attack in pernicious anaemia, rather than some other organ, is unknown. Indeed, the stomach is, sometimes, not the only target. There is another feature of pernicious anaemia not mentioned so far and which only appears in a minority of cases, and then, usually, only in the later stages. Occasionally, this other condition can occur even without any anaemia, but, when it does, it is always associated with the same disorder of the stomach and with absence of hydrochloric acid. This disorder, which consists of patchy damage to parts of the spinal cord, is called sub-acute combined degeneration of the cord; it results in numbness and weakness, both progressive, in the limbs. Existing damage cannot be reversed, but all progress of this disorder is prevented by injections of vitamin B_{12}. Thus it can be said that the cause of pernicious anaemia and of the spinal cord disease associated with it is unknown. It can even be argued that treatment with vitamin B_{12}, when the inability of the patient to absorb that substance is by-passed by injections, is an example of symptomatic treatment. Therefore, it can be argued that pernicious anaemia is a treatable disease, but not a curable one, and that the 'root cause' remains a mystery. Arguments of this kind, for all their philosophical interest, pale into trivial insignificance when set against the practical experience of a patient who, suffering from the disease, is restored to health by a few injections a year. Nevertheless, research into the nature of pernicious anaemia will, and should, continue—better methods of treatment, or even prevention, may well be discovered.

References

Readers who wish to follow the history of pernicious anaemia from original sources will find the early description of a case by Combe in:

Combe, J. S. 'A history of a case of anaemia', *Transactions of the Medical-Chirurgical Society of Edinburgh,* **1**, 194 (1822).

and Addison's first report in:

Addison, T. 'Anaemia—disease of the supra-renal capsules', *The London Medical Gazette,* 3rd series, **8**, 517 (1849).

Minot and Murphy's work appeared in the *Journal of the American Medical Association,* **87**, 470 (1926).

Castle's discovery was published in the *American Journal of Medical Sciences* **178**, 748 (1929).

Very good summaries of the history of pernicious anaemia with full references can be found in:

Haden, R. L. 'Pernicious anaemia from Addison to folic acid', *Blood,* **3**, 22–31 (1948). The same issue of the journal, *Blood,* contains a reprint of Minot and Murphy's original paper.

Jacobs, A. 'Pernicious anaemia 1822–1929', *Archives of Internal Medicine,* **103**, 329–333 (1959).

Major, R. *Classic Descriptions of Disease,* 2nd edn. Charles C. Thomas, Springfield and Baltimore (1939). Contains under one cover the papers of Addison, Combe, and Minot and Murphy.

Irvine Loudon, a retired general practitioner, is currently a Research Fellow at the Wellcome Unit for the History of Medicine, University of Oxford. This article has not appeared in print before.

1.7

Magical Elements in Orthodox Medicine: Diabetes as a Medical Thought System

Tina Posner

This paper will look at the diagnosis and treatment of diabetes as a medical system within the wider medical system of orthodox Western medicine. I will attempt to examine the thinking behind the practice, and to show why the treatment can be viewed partly as a magical ritual. My starting-points are the presuppositional, analogical and circular nature of much scientific thought, and the rationality, within limits, of magical thought. Important theoretical considerations are Horton's argument that the crucial difference between traditional and scientific thinking is that the traditional thinker is unable even to imagine possible alternatives to his established theories; and the suggestions of writers such as Kuhn and Polanyi[1] that scientific thinkers, though they may admit alternatives, may none the less have a protective attitude towards established theory. Such protectiveness recalls Evans-Pritchard's discussion of the 'secondary elaboration' of the Azande in the face of the failure of their magic.[2]

I wish to take a definition of magic provided by Raymond Firth and use it as a framework within which to illustrate what I am calling the magical elements in the treatment of diabetes, as I have seen it and heard it spoken about. The illustrations will be drawn from my observations in a diabetic outpatient clinic and from interviews with doctors I have observed. These interviews were tape recorded. The observation was carried out in a large London teaching hospital. Notes were made of the doctor–patient interaction and parts of the conversation written down. Three doctors were observed. Since the time the paper was written, further observation has been carried out in another outpatient clinic and three other doctors subsequently interviewed. Firth[3] suggests that 'magic as commonly accepted' is 'a rite or verbal formula projecting man's desires into the external world on a theory of human control, to some practical end, but as far as we can see based on false premises'. I will talk about the theory of human control—the rationale of diabetic treatment—as it has been presented to me. I shall also discuss the treatment itself, viewed as a protective ritual.

The practical end of the treatment of diabetes is to eliminate the patient's symptoms; secondly, to normalise a biochemical parameter—the blood sugar level—defined as 'abnormal' in diabetics according to its distribution in the general population; and, finally, to prevent or retard the development of diabetic complications, which can include peripheral neuropathy—loss of feeling at the extremities, gangrene and possible amputation, death from coronary thrombosis or a stroke, vascular disease, renal failure, impotence and loss of sight resulting from cataract or retinopathy.

The basic premises of the theory of the medical control of diabetes are that it is right to reduce the raised blood sugar level to a level defined as 'normal', i.e. approximating the average in the general population, and to maintain it at such a level. Such a reduction, it is argued, serves to eliminate symptoms and prevent or retard complications. Control of diabetes—'control' is a key word in diabetic terminology—can be theoretically achieved and maintained by treatment with a diet eliminating sugar and restricting carbohydrate intake, or with a diet and tablets, or with a diet and insulin injections, depending on the severity of the diabetes.[4] Treatments will reduce a raised blood sugar level and relieve the patient of symptoms (such as excessive thirst and passing an increased volume of urine), associated with a high blood sugar level. The main rationale of treatment, however, is the prevention, or at least, retardation of complications, and treatment will be initiated even when the patient has no symptoms, or continued after the patient's symptoms have been relieved, in an attempt to keep the blood sugar level held to be normal and safe. In the usual way, treatment would be continued for the rest of the patient's life with the importance of 'good control' being constantly stressed.

The basic hypothesis that the diabetes can be controlled by attempting to normalise the blood sugar level with the treatment available is far from established, however. No direct correlation has been shown between the severity of the diabetes and the development of complications, or between the degree of 'control' and the development of complications. Patients with mild diabetes may develop severe complications. Patients who have apparently been 'well controlled' may also develop complications. It is generally admitted there is room for doubt. One doctor interviewed said: 'at the moment we haven't got any terribly good evidence that rigidly controlling diabetes will prevent complications'. Later in the interview he said 'the few studies that have been done on this problem *do* indicate that rigid control *does* prevent complications. The evidence is *not good*. But there is *some* evidence pointing that way. There is *no* evidence . . . that if you leave them out of control they get less complications.'[4] [Later he] said: 'Although we're not sure that we're doing good, until we've proved—until the answer has come out, most people think it's unethical not to control the diabetes rigidly.'

[Another] doctor whom I observed and subsequently interviewed was more open when I asked him about the side-effects of treatment. I had been asking him about the frequency of comas resulting from *low* blood sugar (hypoglycaemia, a complication of taking insulin), as compared with comas resulting from high blood sugar, i.e. untreated diabetes or diabetes completely out of 'control'. He said that *hypo*glycaemic attacks were 'much more common. It's the commonest of all the complications of diabetes.' 'In other words,' I said, 'it's treatment-induced. It's iatrogenic illness.' 'Treatment induced,' he replied, and quoted me a survey which had showed that in long-term diabetes the most common complication had proved to be hypoglycaemic attacks resulting from taking insulin.

A basic rationale of treatment, to reiterate, is that it will prevent or retard the development of the serious complications of diabetes, yet we have here an admission that the most common complication of diabetics on insulin is a result of treatment. It appears to be very difficult to get the blood sugar level just right by artificial means and often insulin treatment overdoes it, so that the patient has too low a blood sugar level rather than a level that is too high. A low blood sugar level affects mental capacity amongst other things.

Disadvantageous complications may also arise from the tablets prescribed in the treatment of diabetes, as one doctor put it to me, 'The bad effects are that we don't know really whether they [the tablets] stop you getting complications or whether they actually cause complications.' In reply to my questioning the justification of treating a patient with no symptoms with tablets, when there is some controversy about the possible ill effects of the tablets, doctors admitted that sticking strictly to a diet might well reduce the blood sugar level sufficiently in such cases. I asked one doctor what percentage of patients could be 'well controlled' on diet alone. He replied: 'A much greater proportion than, in fact, are at the moment. So, in fact, too many people are on tablets.' The reasons he gave for this situation were that the patients had not been given adequate dietary instruction; that it had not been emphasised to them how important diet is, and that the patients did not stick to the diet for one reason or another. Another doctor, in reply to my question about why there was comparatively little emphasis on diet in spite of its admitted importance and apparent efficacy and the possible ill effects of tablets, replied:

> I think for a number of reasons. Mainly doctors and patients feel that by giving tablets you're practising real medicine, or by giving insulin, and by putting someone on a diet you're not really practising real medicine . . . But there's lots of very good evidence that if you severely restrict the carbohydrate content of the diet you can control the diabetes in a large percentage of cases.[4]

There is widespread agreement that diet is an all-important aspect of treatment, but disagreement about the best dietary policy and considerable differences in dietary practice between diabetic clinics. It is only relatively recently that dieticians have been seen as other than 'glorified cooks' (as the dietician in the hospital where I was observing put it to me). They are one of the 'professions supplementary to medicine' and they are nearly always female. It could be said that the present status of dieticians in the eyes of doctors and patients is not in accordance with the importance that diet has in *theory* in the treatment of diabetes. Besides, the substance, so to speak, of the diet is out of the doctor's control. As one doctor put it: 'Diet is something that the layman can get to grips with and it's a form of medication that he can manipulate himself and he's always got some theories about it, most of which are non-scientifically based.' A prescription of tablets or injections can be controlled far more accurately by the doctor alone. And medicine is about tablets and injections of course, not menus!

I shall now consider efforts made to protect the hypothesis that controlling the diabetes by attempting to normalise the blood sugar level will prevent or retard complications. This claim is made in the face of the lack of good evidence to support it and the evidence of complications arising from the treatment itself.

Firstly, the medicine itself can be blamed. If the blood sugar is not at the desired level the most likely thing the doctor will do is to alter the prescribed tablets or insulin in some way—raising or lowering the dose or altering the type.

Secondly, the patient can be blamed. If he has not kept to the 'rules', how can he expect things to be all right? Even if the patient takes the tablets or insulin strictly according to prescription, it is highly unlikely that he will never, perhaps inadvertently, break his dietary taboos. Patients often blame themselves and supply dietary explanations for variations in their physiological state.

Then there are also the 'things we cannot control'. The mother of a boy being seen by the consultant asked: 'I wonder whether the ups and downs in the sugar are to do with his age?' The consultant replied: 'What you've got to understand is that there are three things we can control—the amount of insulin; the amount of food he eats; and the amount of exercise he gets. There are other things we can't control. We can never get it quite perfect.'

Blame can then be attributed to the inadequacy of the means of monitoring the patient's blood sugar level. One doctor pointed out:

If we're looking at diabetic control we ought to think of all the biochemical variables such as lipids, proteins, lipoproteins—hundreds of things really and one really ought to measure the whole spectrum to see (a) whether they're normal at a point value in time and (b) whether they're normal throughout the day, and obviously you just can't do this. So really ideally diabetic control is when the diabetic's biochemical variables are the same as yours or mine, and we never ever achieve it, and this may well be why diabetics still get complications when their sugars seem to be apparently in the normal range.

Writing about diabetics, Cochrane[5] makes the following points:

In general the treatment of mature diabetics would seem to be an example of the large-scale use of ineffective and possibly dangerous therapies in a particularly inefficient way. The cause of the sad situation seems to be the assumption that if some bio-chemical parameter is abnormally distributed in a defined group of people, 'normalizing' the distribution must do more good than harm. In mature diabetes it may well be the wrong parameter that is being altered.

In spite of awareness that other biochemical parameters are involved in this metabolic disorder which may be as, if not more, important, doctors feel they are 'very justified', indeed, that it would be 'unethical' not to attempt to normalise the blood sugar level which by definition is abnormal in diabetics. With the discovery of insulin, the blood sugar level could be lowered and to some extent, controlled. The whole specialism of diabetes grew up around this ability. Other relevant biochemical parameters are not at present under the doctor's control to anything like the same extent, although they can be measured. The blood sugar level and its regulation is, then, all important in the treatment of diabetes as it has evolved—treatment which can be viewed in part at least as a protective ritual to ward off the threat of complications arising.

I shall now examine parts of this ritual purporting to control the diabetes. The essential feature as far as the doctor is concerned is the monitoring and regulation of the blood sugar level. At the diabetic clinic under observation, this level was measured from a blood test at each visit. The patients often said 'How is my diabetes?', meaning 'What is my blood sugar?' [One] doctor's emphasis on the *symbolic* importance of the blood sugar level measurement is significant. In my observations and recordings in the outpatient clinic, I have noted many instances of the patient's diabetes being treated as if equivalent to his blood sugar level by both doctor and patient alike. [However] there is some recognition that the measurement of the blood sugar level at one point in time could well be unrepresentative, and that such a measurement could have drawbacks as a criterion of control of the diabetes.

Considerations of the medical construction of reality and claims to certainty[6] are very relevant here, and in the examination of the main diagnostic test for diabetes. One of the doctors I observed spoke to a patient of a 'special test which will *prove one way or the other* whether you have got diabetes'. The test he was referring to was the glucose tolerance test—a four-hour test during which the body's response to a large dose of glucose (administered orally or intravenously) is plotted by testing the blood sugar level. It was admitted to me that 'the definition of an abnormal glucose tolerance curve is variable depending on which centre you work at'. An experiment on prison inmates, where the experimenter could standardise the variable factors affecting the test to an extent impossible in normal circumstances, found that a large number of individuals were never diabetic, some were always diabetic, and some were sometimes diabetic and sometimes not, on routine criteria.

Arthur Mirsky[7] writing about the 'Certainties and Uncertainties in Diabetes Mellitus', suggested that:

Too frequently little or no consideration is given to the fact that the variation between successive tests in the same subject may be as great as the variation between subjects; that a test may be apparently abnormal one day and normal thereafter. Likewise, the influence of age, sex, prior diet, prior medication, posture, emotional state, physical activity, and many other factors is frequently disregarded in evaluating the clinical significance of a conventionally defined abnormal tolerance curve. Since the tolerance for glucose, as judged by standard criteria, decreases with age, all of us will become 'chemical' diabetics if we live long enough.

[To be] defined as diabetic according to the standard criteria [is to] be labelled and treated as 'diabetic'. This labelling may have an important bearing on the type of job which will be open to the patient thereafter, and, remember, it is assumed that once a diabetic always a diabetic—the label is permanent; and if his tests were only marginally abnormal they might have been normal had he come at another time; and who sets the criteria on which the tests are based? I heard one doctor say: 'Diabetes is what I say it is.' It is openly admitted that the NHS could not cope with the number of diabetics who would be found on a large-scale screening programme.

It is important to point out that it may be very misleading to think of all the patients classified as diabetic according to the standard tests, as having the same metabolic disorder. 'Diabetes is undoubtedly a group of diseases', I was told by one doctor. There is a definite distinction to be made between 'juvenile-onset' diabetics (in which the ability of the pancreas to produce insulin is very limited or absent); here, patients need insulin and would die without it sooner or later with *hyper-glycaemic* coma and ketoacidosis; and 'mature-onset' diabetes which normally occurs in a much milder form and sometimes may be a transient consequence of obesity and corrected by a suitable dietary, it seems.

Mirsky pointed out that vascular derangements occurred very frequently in diabetics and were regarded as complications of the metabolic disorder termed diabetes. As we have seen, a basic rationale of treatment of the diabetes is that 'good control' will have a preventative effect on the development of such complications. Often, however, vascular derangements occur among diabetics whose diabetes has been 'well controlled' and the manifestations of such pathological changes may be fully evident before the diabetes produces any symptoms.

How is it that the basic hypothesis we have been examining has not been seriously challenged and replaced? The definition of magic which we took at the beginning of this paper was 'rite or verbal formula projecting man's desires into the external world on a theory of human control, to some practical end, but as far as we can see based on false premises'. I have tried to show how the theory of the medical control of diabetes is based on unproven and, at the least, questionable premises. It has become evident that to some extent at least, acceptance of the basic hypothesis is a question of faith. Although evidence is not weighted heavily in favour of good control reducing complications, we all *secretly feel* that this is in fact the case, that if you can control the patient's diabetes as well as possible it *should* retard the development of complications. We all *secretly believe* this and *hope* about it, but there's no outstanding evidence that it is true. There have been a number of papers that support this, but a number of papers that don't support it.

I wish to suggest that the medical theory of the treatment of diabetes is a belief system which is sustained by certain medical assumptions and, like any other, by social, structural and cultural factors. The application of strictly scientific criteria to diagnosis and treatment would change the whole nature of the disease and the specialism which has grown up to treat it. Doctors involved in treating diabetes are faced with a situation of very great uncertainty. In many relevant areas they lack knowledge based on the firm foundations of statistically valid empirical research. Further uncertainty arises from the many factors beyond their control which effect the metabolic disorder defined as diabetes, and from the unpredictability of the onset of serious and life-threatening complications associated with the disorder. They have made it their job to treat a condition which they cannot cure and which may be degenerative. The need to feel that they can at least control it, and that there is something they can do which will help prevent complications is understandable. There is a predisposition to act rather than leave things alone and an assumption that the mistake of judging a sick person well is more to be avoided than judging a well person sick—a decision rule for handling situations of medical uncertainty described by Scheff,[9] who then suggested that the assumption on which this norm was based led to a situation where 'physicians and public typically over value medical treatment relative to non treatment as a course of action in the face of uncertainty and this overvaluation results in the creation as well as the prevention of impairment.'

'The function of magic', Malinowski[8] wrote, 'is to ritualize man's optimism.' Here we have doctors purporting to control diabetes, a metabolic disorder which they know involves a complex of biochemical parameters, through the manipulation of one such parameter over which they have incomplete control. Further, they insist that maintaining 'good control' of this parameter is essential to the prevention or at least retardation of complications associated with the disorder. If they are not convinced they are doing the right thing, then they 'feel', 'believe', and 'hope' they are. They have faith in the efficacy of their ritual.

I should like to end by quoting from a book by Francis Hsu[10] which discusses the measures taken to combat a cholera epidemic in a town in West China:

> . . . if we follow the thoughts and ways of a culture as expressed through the bearers of the culture, magic and real knowledge are not only intertwined, but may not even be distinguished, so that, for reaching one and the same end, the individual oscillates between one and the other, or resorts to both simultaneously, with the greatest facility and ease of mind . . . this lack of discrimination . . . is common to human behaviour in general . . . man fails to differentiate between magic and science not because he lacks any power of rationality, but because his behaviour in general is dictated by faith developed out of the pattern of his culture.

Notes and References

1. Kuhn, T. S. *The structure of scientific revolutions*, 2nd edn, University of Chicago Press (1970).
2. Evans-Pritchard, E. E. *Witchcraft, oracles and magic among the Azande*, Oxford University Press, London (1937). See also Horton, R. 'African traditional thought and Western science', in Wilson, B. R. (ed.) *Rationality*, Basil Blackwell, Oxford (1970).
3. Firth, R. *Human types*, revised edn, Merton Books, New York, p. 124 (1958).
4. Since the original publication of this article there have been further developments.

   As a result of epidemiological and dietary research, previous dietary recommendations have been overturned and the British Diabetic Association currently advocates an increase in the proportion of carbohydrate in a diabetic's diet, but this should be made up of complex rather than simple carbohydrate. See British Diabetic Association Nutrition Sub-Committee 'Dietary Recommendations for Diabetics for the 1980s'.

   The categorisation of diabetes has been altered so that a grey area between non-diabetic and diabetic is now recognised and called 'impaired glucose tolerance'. It is not yet clear whether this situation constitutes a significant threat to a person's future health. See World Health Organisation Expert Committee on Diabetes Mellitus, *Second Report* (1980).

   The empirical situation in regard to the level of control of the diabetes and the development of complications has become more complex. Since 1977 several key papers have been published showing that good control reduces the risk to the foetus in diabetic mothers and reduces, but does not eliminate, the risk of retinopathy and renal failure in insulin-dependent diabetes mellitus (25% diabetic population). How good control relates to the development of atherosclerosis (to which diabetics are prone) and to complications in non-insulin-dependent diabetes mellitus appears more complex and is still an unanswered problem.

5. Cochrane, A. L. *Effectiveness and Efficiency: random reflections on health services,* Nuffield Provincial Hospitals' Trust, pp. 56–7 (1972).

6. Maclean, U. *Patient Delay: some observations on medical claims to certainty,* Dept. of Community Medicine, University of Edinburgh (1974).

7. Mirsky, I. A. 'Certainties and uncertainties in Diabetes Mellitus'. In Ellenberg, M. and Ritkin, H. (eds) *Diabetes Mellitus: theory and practice,* McGraw-Hill, New York (1970).

8. Malinowski, B. *Magic, Science and Religion and other Essays,* Doubleday Anchor Books, New York, p. 90 (1925).

9. Scheff, T. J. 'Decision rules, types of error and their consequences in medical diagnosis', *Behavioural Science,* **8**, (1963).

10. Hsu, F. L. K. *Religion, Science and Human Crisis,* Routledge and Kegan Paul, London (1952).

Tina Posner is a social anthropologist working in the Department of Community Medicine and General Practice, University of Oxford. This article is an edited and amended article first published in Dingwall, R., Heath, C., Reid, M. and Stacey, M. (eds) *Health Care and Health Knowledge,* Croom Helm, London, pp. 142–158 (1977).

Part 2

Influences on health and disease

Introduction

What factors influence patterns of health and disease? The answers to this question reflect many things: a particular historical or political perspective; the frame of reference provided by an academic discipline; the relative importance attached to individual action or social process. Inevitably, just as the answers reflect these things, so too do the many ways in which the question is posed, and the nature of the evidence considered.

For Frederick Engels, revolutionary communist and close colleague of Karl Marx, the question followed on from his analysis of nineteenth-century English society. Unfettered capitalism was transforming cities like Manchester into the workshops of the world, producing explosive rates of urban growth and stark extremes of wealth and poverty. *The Conditions of the Working Classes in England* was first published in 1845, in German. Almost fifty years passed before an English edition appeared. In it, Engels set about the systematic documentation of the consequences of this upheaval for that part of the population—the majority—to whom the benefits of industrialisation must have seemed far from obvious. In the extract included here, which deals with health, Engels portrays the squalor of existence and the disparities between social classes in death and disease. What marks out his portrait as unique, however, is not the facts themselves (which were in large part culled from official reports) but his repeated stress on the nature of the society which could produce these conditions. The bourgeoisie, 'interested in maintaining and prolonging this disorder', has created these victims and stands accused by Engels of deliberate 'murder'. Although Engels' political conclusions are as disputed now as in the 1840s, his description is generally accepted as a valuable historical document.

In *Inside the Inner City* Paul Harrison provides a journalist's account of Hackney in the 1980s which seems to question whether the passage of time has changed very much. The symptoms he documents—bad housing, poor working conditions, bad health, poverty, powerlessness—seem to be different only in that their context is not expansion but decline. 'Society' is still the generator of inequality, and the inner city is its dark side, inhabited by helpless prisoners without options or choice.

Social inequalities are, of course, relative to time and place, but the similarity of the accounts given by Engels and Harrison might well lead one to forget that in the period separating them, life expectancy approximately doubled and infant mortality declined dramatically. Richard Titmuss, historian, social policy theorist, and a key intellectual influence on the formation of the post-war welfare state in the UK, never let go of his belief in the power of 'consciously directed social change'. In 'The position of women' he explores the implications of increasing life-expectancy and the remarkable decline in the birth-rate since the Victorian era. The falling birth-rate and declining family size documented by Titmuss are attributed by him to an increase in women's control of their own fertility, resulting in striking changes in family-building habits. And, as so often in Titmuss' work, the essay builds from the present a vision of the future and the new problems it is likely to pose. Written in 1952, Titmuss' essay might be seen as reflecting an optimism historically specific to the beginning of the long post-war boom, whereas Harrison's survey was carried out during the most prolonged post-war recession. Nevertheless, the primacy that both give to social factors in explaining patterns of health and disease only accentuates the contrast between Harrison's bleak pessimism and Titmuss' confidence in progress.

George Brown is a medical sociologist who has written widely on mental illness. In 'Depression: a sociological view', Brown presents an aetiology of a particular condition: depression. Again, emphasis is placed on the social context. He claims that the connection between the social environment and depression is mediated by a wide range of factors. These can be represented by a causal model consisting of three components: provoking agents, such as major life-events or difficulties; vulnerability factors, for example, the absence of intimate relationships with others; and symptom formation factors, such as the childhood loss of a parent; all of which may influence the type and severity of depression. But despite the convincing empirical evidence which Brown provides of the importance of social class, lifestage and provoking agents in influencing the prevalence and distribution of psychiatric disorders, such sociological ideas emphasising the current environment have made little impact on psychiatric teaching— as he himself acknowledges.

It is not always obvious why a particular view of the factors influencing health and disease patterns—for example, the sociological view of depression—fail to make headway in the world. Perhaps one reason is that the conclusions to which a particular view leads, no matter how well empirically supported, may go against one's intuitive beliefs. A good example of this is provided by the research of the economist Amartya Sen into the factors influencing the occurrence of famines. Based on close study of a number of famines, Sen's conclusion is that famines need not imply the existence of any food shortage, and that it is misleading to focus on food supply in trying to explain their occurrence. In the extract from his book *Poverty and Famines* reproduced here, Sen develops his concept of food 'entitlement' as the primary influence on the onset, duration and distribution of famine, that is, legal, economic, political and social factors determine who has command over food.

Sen's version of the influences on famine incidence is focused firmly on the external environment. In fact, the attempt to find an external cause of disease is a tradition deeply embedded in the history of Western medicine. The career of the Nobel prize-winning immunologist, Sir MacFarlane Burnett, has been devoted to the development of an alternative to this tradition. In a lecture given in 1980 which summarised his views, 'Biomedical research: changes and opportunities', Burnett states this alternative. He claims that some genetic element is probably involved in every disease state, and genetic factors are likely to be relevant in influencing susceptibility to stress, infection, or even alcoholism and other forms of drug-abuse. Moreover, the same demographic changes which Titmuss welcomes as liberating women's position are what Burnett sees as responsible for 'an intolerable degree of genetic deterioration' in the long term. And, he argues, genetic research must be involved in formulating policies to counteract this.

Burnett's stress on the primary influence of genetic elements on patterns of health and disease has little in common with the social/environmental perspectives already encountered, save that the role of individual behaviour plays little part: the victim of disease is also the victim of either social circumstances or genetic make-up. These are decidedly not the conclusions reached by the Medical Services Study Group of the Royal College of Physicians. Of the 250 deaths examined by them among in-patients aged 1 to 50, they conclude that almost 40 per cent can be held as largely to blame for their own death, by choosing to smoke, drink, overeat, ignore medical advice or not comply with treatment, or by taking a more direct path to 'self-destruction', i.e. suicide. The extent to which these patients are held responsible for their own death is indicated by the Study Group's implicit view that the demands placed by such patients on health services are unreasonable and wasteful.

The 'policy' which follows from the conclusions of the Medical Services Study Group is that much more attention should be paid to the advice of doctors, notwithstanding the 'psychopathic' attitude to doctors attributed to many of these patients. Doctors are thereby allotted a potentially central influence over health and disease patterns. But their influence can also derive from their role in defining and legitimating the existence of disease. Richard Asher, a British physician, describes an entirely different form of self-produced illness: malingering, or the deliberate faking, production or encouragement of illness. The motives for this form of 'illness' are listed as fear, desire or escape, and, as Asher observes, the ingenuity of, for example, prisoners-of-war in faking illness is well-documented. However, there is also a 'borderland of malingering', where the purpose is not evident and the motives obscure; Munchausen's Syndrome, which is perhaps the most spectacular example provided by Asher, calls into question the ease with which a dividing line can be drawn between 'real' and 'fake' illness.

The articles in this part represent a wide range of views on what influences the patterns of health and disease. Some are irreconcilable with others, but some are differentiated largely by the rather arbitrary demarcations of academic disciplines. Overcoming these demarcations would not remove all conflicts of view, but would make the substance of such conflicts much clearer.

2.1

Health: 1844

Frederick Engels

When one individual inflicts bodily injury upon another, such injury that death results, we call the deed manslaughter; when the assailant knew in advance that the injury would be fatal, we call his deed murder. But when society places hundreds of proletarians in such a position that they inevitably meet a too early and an unnatural death, one which is quite as much a death by violence as that by the sword or bullet; when it deprives thousands of the necessaries of life, places them under conditions in which they *cannot* live—forces them, through the strong arm of the law, to remain in such conditions until that death ensues which is the inevitable consequence—knows that these thousands of victims must perish, and yet permits these conditions to remain, its deed is murder just as surely as the deed of the single individual; disguised, malicious murder, murder against which none can defend himself, which does not seem what it is, because no man sees the murderer, because the death of the victim seems a natural one, since the offence is more one of omission than of commission. But murder it remains.

The manner in which the great multitude of the poor is treated by society today is revolting. They are drawn into large cities where they breathe a poorer atmosphere than in the country; they are relegated to districts which, by reason of the method of construction, are worse ventilated than any others; they are deprived of all means of cleanliness, of water itself, since pipes are laid only when paid for, and the rivers so polluted that they are useless for such purposes; they are obliged to throw all offal and garbage, all dirty water, often all disgusting drainage and excrement into the streets, being without other means of disposing of them; they are thus compelled to infect the region of their own dwellings. Nor is this enough. All conceivable evils are heaped upon the heads of the poor. If the population of great cities is too dense in general, it is they in particular who are packed into the least space. As though the vitiated atmosphere of the streets were not enough, they are penned in dozens into single rooms, so that the air in which they breathe at night is enough in itself to stifle them. They are given damp dwellings, cellar dens that are not waterproof from below, or garrets that leak from above. Their houses are so built that the clammy air cannot escape. They are supplied bad, tattered, or rotten clothing, adulterated and indigestible food. They are exposed to the most exciting changes of mental condition, the most violent vibrations between hope and fear; they are hunted like game, and not permitted to attain peace of mind and quiet enjoyment of life. They are deprived of all enjoyments except that of sexual indulgence and drunkenness, are worked every day to the point of complete exhaustion of their mental and physical energies, and are thus constantly spurred on to the maddest excess in the only two enjoyments at their disposal. And if they surmount all this, they fall victims to want of work in a crisis when all the little is taken from them that had hitherto been vouchsafed them.

How is it possible, under such conditions, for the lower class to be healthy and long lived? What else can be expected than an excessive mortality, an unbroken series of epidemics, a progressive deterioration in the physique of the working population? Let us see how the facts stand.

That the bad air of London, and especially of the working-people's districts, is in the highest degree favourable to the development of consumption, the hectic appearance of great numbers of persons sufficiently indicates. If one roams the streets a little in the early morning, when the multitudes are on their way to their work, one is amazed at the number of persons who look wholly or half-consumptive, pale, lank, narrow-chested, hollow-eyed ghosts, whom one passes at every step, these languid, flabby faces, incapable of the slightest energetic expression.

In competition with consumption stand typhus, to say nothing of scarlet fever, a disease which brings most frightful devastation into the ranks of the working-class. This fever has the same character almost everywhere, and develops in nearly every case into specific typhus. According to the annual report of Dr Southwood Smith on the London Fever Hospital, the number of patients in 1843 was 1,462, or 418 more than in any previous year. Many of the patients were working-people from the country, who had endured the severest privation while migrating, and, after their arrival, had slept hungry and half-naked in the streets, and so fallen victims to the fever. These people were brought into the hospital in such a state of weakness, that unusual quantities of wine, cognac, and preparations of ammonia and other stimulants were required for their treatment; 16½ per cent of all patients died.

In Edinburgh and Glasgow it broke out in 1817, after the famine, and in 1826 and 1837 with especial violence, after the commercial crisis, subsiding somewhat each time after having raged about three years. In Edinburgh about 6,000 persons were attacked by the fever during the epidemic of 1817, and about 10,000 in that of 1837, and not only the number of persons attacked but the violence of the disease increased with each repetition.

But the fury of the epidemic in all former periods seems to have been child's play in comparison with its ravages after the crisis of 1842. One-sixth of the whole indigent population of Scotland was seized by the fever, and the infection was carried by wandering beggars with fearful rapidity from one locality to another. It did not reach the middle and upper classes of the population, yet in two months there were more fever cases than in twelve years before. In Glasgow, 12 per cent of the population were seized in the year 1843; 32,000 persons, of whom 32 per cent perished, while this mortality in Manchester and Liverpool does not ordinarily exceed 8 per cent.

When one remembers under what conditions the working-people live, when one thinks how crowded their dwellings are, how every nook and corner swarms with human beings, how sick and well sleep in the same room, in the same bed, the only wonder is that a contagious disease like this fever does not spread yet farther. And when one reflects how little medical assistance the sick have at command, how many are without any medical advice whatsoever, and ignorant of the most ordinary precautionary measures, the mortality seems actually small.

Another category of diseases arises directly from the food rather than the dwellings of the workers. The food of the labourer, indigestible enough in itself, is utterly unfit for young children, and he has neither means nor time to get his children more suitable food. Moreover, the custom of giving children spirits, and even opium, is very general; and these two influences, with the rest of the conditions of life prejudicial to bodily development, give rise to the most diverse affections of the digestive organs, leaving lifelong traces behind them. Scrofula is almost universal among the working-class, and scrofulous parents have scrofulous children, especially when the original influences continue in full force to operate upon the inherited tendency of the children. A second consequence of this insufficient bodily nourishment, during the years of growth and development, is rachitis, which is extremely common among the children of the working-class. The hardening of the bones is delayed, the development of the skeleton in general is restricted, and deformities of the legs and spinal column are frequent, in addition to the usual rachitic affections. How greatly all these evils are increased by the changes to which the workers are subject in consequence of fluctuations in trade, want of work, and the scanty wages in time of crisis, it is not necessary to dwell upon. Temporary want of sufficient food, to which almost every working-man is exposed at least once in the course of his life, only contributes to intensify the effect of his usually sufficient but bad diet.

Besides these, there are other influences which enfeeble the health of a great number of workers, intemperance most of all. All possible temptations, all allurements combine to bring the workers to drunkenness. Liquor is almost their only source of pleasure, and all things conspire to make it accessible to them. The working-man comes from his work tired, exhausted, finds his home comfortless, damp, dirty, repulsive; he has urgent need of recreation, he *must* have something to make work worth his trouble, to make the prospect of the next day endurable. Drunkenness has here ceased to be a vice, for which the vicious can be held responsible; it becomes a phenomenon, the necessary, inevitable effect of certain conditions upon an object possessed of no volition in relation to those conditions. They who have degraded the working-man to a mere object have the responsibility to bear.

Another source of physical mischief to the working-class lies in the impossibility of employing skilled physicians in cases of illness. English doctors charge high fees, and working-men are not in a position to pay them. They can therefore do nothing or are compelled to call in cheap charlatans, and use quack remedies, which do more harm than good. An immense number of such quacks thrive in every English town, securing their *clientèle* among the poor by means of advertisements, posters, and other such devices. Besides these, vast quantities of patent medicines are sold, for all conceivable ailments: Morrison's Pills, Parr's Life Pills, Dr Mainwaring's Pills, and a thousand other pills, essences, and balsams, all of which have the property of curing all the ills that flesh is heir to. It is by no means unusual for the manufacturer of Parr's Life Pills to sell twenty to twenty-five thousand boxes of these salutary pills in a week, and they are taken for constipation by this one, for diarrhoea by that one, for fever, weakness, and all possible ailments. As our German peasants are cupped or bled at certain seasons, so do the English working-people now consume patent medicines to their own injury and the great profit of the manufacturer. One of the most injurious of these patent medicines is a drink prepared with opiates, chiefly laudanum, under the name Godfrey's Cordial. Women who work at home, and have their own and other people's children to take care of, give them this drink to keep them quiet, and, as many believe, to strengthen them. They often begin to give this medicine to newly-born children, and continue, without knowing the effects of this 'heart's-ease', until the children die. The less susceptible the child's system to the action of the opium, the greater the quantities administered. When the cordial ceases to act, laudanum alone is given, often to the extent of fifteen to twenty drops at a dose. The Coroner of Nottingham testified before a Parliamentary Commission that one apothecary had, according to his own statement, used thirteen hundred-weight of laudanum in one year in the preparation of Godfrey's Cordial. The effects upon the children so treated may be readily imagined. They are pale, feeble, wilted, and usually die before completing the second year. The use of this cordial is very extensive in all great towns and industrial districts in the kingdom.

The result of all these influences is a general enfeeblement of the frame in the working-class. They are almost all weakly, of angular but not powerful build, lean, pale, and of relaxed fibre, with the exception of the muscles especially exercised in their work. Nearly all suffer from indigestion, and consequently from a more or less hypochondriac, melancholy, irritable, nervous condition. Their enfeebled constitutions are unable to resist disease, and are therefore seized by it on every occasion. Hence they age prematurely, and die early. On this point the mortality statistics supply unquestionable testimony.

According to the Report of Register-General Graham, the annual death-rate of all England and Wales is something less than 2¼ per cent. That is to say, out of forty-five persons, one dies every year. This was the average for the year 1839–40. In 1840–41 the mortality diminished somewhat, and the death-rate was but one in forty-six. But in the great cities the proportion is wholly different. I have before me official tables of mortality *(Manchester Guardian,* 31 July 1844), according to which the death-rate of several large towns is as follows: In Manchester, including Chorlton and Salford, 1 in 32.72; and excluding Chorlton and Salford, 1 in 30.75. In Liverpool, including West Derby (suburb), 31.90, and excluding West Derby, 29.00; while the average of all the districts of Cheshire, Lancashire, and Yorkshire cited, including a number of wholly or partially rural districts and many small towns, with a total population of 2,172,506 for the whole, is 1 death in 39.80 persons. How unfavourably the workers are placed in the great cities, the mortality for Prescott in Lancashire shows; a district inhabited by miners, and showing a lower sanitary condition than of the agricultural districts, mining being by no means a healthful occupation. But these miners live in the country, and the death-rate among them is but 1 in 47.54, or nearly 2½ per cent, better than that for all England. All these statements are based upon the mortality tables for 1843. Still higher is the death-rate in the Scotch cities; in Edinburgh, in 1838–39, 1 in 29; in 1831, in the Old Town alone, 1 in 22. In Glasgow, according to Dr Cowen, the average has been, since 1830, 1 in 30; and in single years, 1 in 22 to 24. That this enormous shortening of life falls chiefly upon the working-class, that the general average is improved by the smaller mortality of the upper and middle-classes, is attested upon all sides. One of the most recent depositions is that of a physician, Dr P. H. Holland, in Manchester, who investigated Chorlton-on-Medlock, a suburb of Manchester, under official commission. He divided the houses and streets into three classes each, and ascertained the following variations in the death-rate:

First class of Streets. Houses	I. class. Mortality	1 in 51
„ „ „ II. „ „ „	41
„ „ „ III. „ „ „	36
Second „ „ I. „ „ „	55
„ „ „ II. „ „ „	38
„ „ „ III. „ „ „	35
Third „ „ I. „ Wanting —	—
„ „ „ II. „ Mortality „	35
„ „ „ III. „ „ „	25

It is clear from other tables given by Holland that the mortality in the *streets* of the second class is 18 per cent greater, and in the streets of the third class 68 per cent greater than in those of the first class; that the mortality in the *houses* of the second class is 31 per cent greater, and in the third class 78 per cent greater than in those of the first class; that the mortality in those bad streets which were improved, decreased 25 per cent. He closes with the remark, very frank for an English bourgeois:[1]

> When we find the rate of mortality four times as high in some streets as in others, and twice as high in whole classes of streets as in other classes, and further find it is all

but invariably high in those streets which are in bad condition, and almost invariably low in those whose condition is good, we cannot resist the conclusion that multitudes of our fellow-creatures, *hundreds of our immediate neighbours,* are annually destroyed for want of the most evident precautions.

The death-rate is kept so high chiefly by the heavy mortality among young children in the working-class. The tender frame of a child is least able to withstand the unfavourable influences of an inferior lot in life; the neglect to which they are often subjected, when both parents work or one is dead, avenges itself promptly, and no one need wonder that in Manchester more than 57 per cent of the children of the working-class perish before the fifth year, while but 20 per cent of the children of the higher classes, and not quite 32 per cent of the children of all classes in the country die under five years of age.

Apart from the diverse diseases which are the necessary consequence of the present neglect and oppression of the poorer classes, there are other influences which contribute to increase the mortality among small children. In many families the wife, like the husband, has to work away from home, and the consequence is the total neglect of the children, who are either locked up or given out to be taken care of. It is, therefore, not to be wondered at if hundreds of them perish through all manner of accidents. Nowhere are so many children run over, nowhere are so many killed by falling, drowning, or burning, as in the great cities and towns of England. Deaths from burns and scalds are especially frequent, such a case occurring nearly every week during the winter months in Manchester, and very frequently in London, though little mention is made of them in the papers. I have at hand a copy of the *Weekly Dispatch* of 15 December 1844, according to which, in the week from 1 December to 7 December inclusive, *six* such cases occurred. These unhappy children, perishing in this terrible way, are victims of our social disorder, and of the property-holding classes interested in maintaining and prolonging this disorder. Yet one is left in doubt whether even this terribly torturing death is not a blessing for the children in rescuing them from a long life of toil and wretchedness, rich in suffering and poor in enjoyment. So far has it gone in England; and the bourgeoisie reads these things every day in the newspapers and takes no further trouble in the matter. But it cannot complain if, after the official and non-official testimony here cited which must be known to it, I broadly accuse it of social murder.

Reference

1. Report of Commission of Inquiry into the State of Large Towns and Populous Districts, First Report, 1844. Appendix.

Frederick Engels, son of a German textile manufacturer, came to Manchester in 1842 to work in his father's factory. In 1845, aged 25, he published *The Condition of the Working Class in England* in Leipzig. The first British edition did not appear until 1892. The extract reproduced here is drawn from the translation of the full work by the Institute of Marxism–Leninism, Moscow, published by Panther Books, London, 1969.

2.2

Inside the Inner City

Paul Harrison

The inner city is now, and is likely to remain, Britain's most dramatic and intractable social problem. [. . .] Three closely related factors define most of the problems of these areas. The first is that they are areas of older industry: clothing and textiles, shipbuilding, docking, and more recently, steel, cars and refining. They are often areas of former prosperity, now upstaged by changes in the pattern of world trade, in technology or in transport. The gradual decline in competitiveness of these industries is paralleled by a gradual shedding of labour and a relative decline in wage rates—and hence rising unemployment and falling incomes among residents. Often firms in these places have been bought up by larger companies or multinationals, or absorbed into vast nationalized monopolies, so that the destinies of local people and communities are increasingly controlled from outside. What determines their prosperity or misery is an impersonal calculus of profit or rationalization pursued regardless of social costs.

Second, these are areas of particularly bad housing, a mixture of old Victorian terraces, often built specifically to house manual workers and now reaching the end of their useful life, and more modern council housing, frequently of the worst possible design; an environment short of parks and access to countryside, full of dereliction and dehumanized concrete.

Third, these are areas with higher-than-average concentrations of manual workers, low-skilled, unskilled, or de-skilled as the industries they worked in have declined; areas of high unemployment and low incomes, where people are effectively stranded by their poverty, unable to travel to work outside the area, unable to afford private housing or to qualify for council housing elsewhere. People, like the places they live in, who were exploited for as long as there was profit in doing so and then abandoned to survive as best they could. The cheap housing in these areas also draws in other disadvantaged groups with low income or little capital: immigrants, single parents, the mentally and physically handicapped. At the same time the gradual decline of the area pushes out those with freedom to move—with savings, skills or educational qualifications. [. . .]

It is important not to consider the inner cities as unusual or isolated phenomena. The bulk of poverty, of bad housing, of declining industry, is in fact found outside the inner cities. Every urban area has some district of some size—even if it is only a single housing estate—that shares the interacting problems of concentrated poverty, unemployment, bad housing and crime of the larger inner city areas. Thus the inner city is less a precise geographical location than a mode of existence— more diffuse in some places, more concentrated in others—of the poor and disadvantaged. That is what makes it so hard to change, for it is not a surface wound that can be treated locally with a plaster, but the symptom of nationwide processes that create, and segregate, poverty.

The first of these diseases is a chaotic, unplanned process of economic advance, characteristic of British capitalism, that allows companies, private and public, to close down old plants regardless of the consequences for the people and communities that depend on them, in a callous, uncaring way, with little or no thought to prevention or mitigation. Related to this is the persistence of sharp class divisions between manual and non-manual workers, the 'educated' and the 'uneducated', and of long-lasting inequalities in wealth and income, all of these mapped in space in the marked segregation of middle-class and working-class areas. Added to this is the marginalization in British society of other groups—women, immigrants, the handicapped, the mentally ill, the unskilled and the under-educated—who are placed at a disadvantage by law, by social stigma, by discrimination, or by the changing requirements of the labour market.

All these wider structures generate large categories of disadvantaged people, who share a common problem of low income and therefore lowered freedom of choice. They are scattered widely across the country, found in greater numbers in the Celtic and northern regions, and in concentration in the inner city.

The inner city is therefore of far more than local interest. It is a very good place to learn about the destructive forces inherent in society. For the sake of concreteness and coherence I have chosen a single such area—Hackney. But this is intended to reflect the realities and problems of life for the poor within inner city areas and throughout Britain. [. . .]

There are many people who live in Hackney who will deny this: middle-class owner-occupiers will tell you aggressively that it is not at all such a bad place to live. And probably it is not, for people with cars, telephones, bank accounts and self-contained dwellings. They do not have to walk along dangerous streets with all the money they possess in their pockets, or queue for hours at bus stops, or search for unvandalized phones when someone falls ill. They do not have to share toilets or baths. They do not have to wrestle shopping and pushchairs up stairs or into lifts that often do not work. They do not have to suffer damp and cold. They do not have to be humiliated in social-security offices or wait months for essential repairs. Above all they are there by choice, not by compulsion. They can leave at any time they want: they do not have the sense of imprisonment, of closed options, that plagues those without the incomes or the saleable skills that would enable them to get out. Whether a place is tolerable to live in, or intolerable, depends on your income; that is as true of Britain as a whole as it is of Hackney. For the poor, the inner city is something akin to the Slough of Despond, a place so terrible that the only recourse seems to turn tail and run. Yet most of them lack the means of escape—the money to buy a house elsewhere, the skills or certificates to get a job elsewhere. [. . .]

The new Hackney began as a middle- to lower-middle-class suburb, but the poor quality of the construction soon led to social decline. Some of the larger houses intended for families with servants had to be let by the room almost as soon as they were built. Many terraced houses were built right from the start with multi-occupation in mind. [. . .]

Hackney's predicament has been shaped as much by the character of its local economy as by the state of its housing. Since the latter half of the nineteenth century the mainstays have been clothing, and to a lesser extent shoemaking and furniture. All three were notorious for 'sweating' their workers—that is, squeezing out a prodigious amount of labour for a minimal reward.

The nature of the local labour force lent itself readily to exploitation. First there were the wives of builders, labourers, dockers, porters—men in irregular, low-paid jobs for whom the wife's earnings were indispensable for survival. The sewing-machine allowed many of them to combine earning with their duties as mothers and housewives—albeit often at the cost of their own wellbeing and that of their children. The second source of labour was immigrants: the Jews, especially after the pogroms of 1881–86 in Russia and Poland; then, from the 1950s on, West Indians, Asians and Cypriots. Immigrant and female workers are harder to organize into unions than indigenous males and will generally accept lower wages. The rag trade was based—and still is—on the exploitation of female and immigrant labour. [. . .]

By 1900 then, the lines of Hackney's fate were already drawn. Bad housing meant low rents and low house prices, attracting people on low incomes— less skilled workers and immigrants. The local population in turn helped to determine the kind of employment that would predominate. Thus a vicious circle was outlined in which Hackney is still trapped; sweating industries pay low wages, and that, in its turn, ensures that the housing stock will deteriorate further because funds are not available to pay for the scale of repairs needed.

Eighty-odd years of the twentieth century, two world wars, massive efforts in public housing, a decade and a half of government programmes to help the inner cities—all these have made essentially no difference to Hackney's plight. Indeed it has worsened. The 1981 population of 180,000 was less than half the 1901 level. The building of Greater London Council housing in Outer London and Essex, and the growth of the new towns, gave many people a chance to move. Those who moved were mainly the most mobile: people with skills or school qualifications to offer employers, or with enough cash to buy houses elsewhere, the able-bodied in the twenty-five to forty-five age-group. They left behind many of the old, the unskilled, the handicapped.

Newcomers were moving in, too: as always, the lower-paid, the disadvantaged in various ways, and immigrants. Small businesses continued to arise out of their savings and ambitions—and to go under, too—but no sizeable new industries moved in. The Victorian housing stock continued to decay. Many slums were cleared by blitz or bulldozers, but the public housing that replaced them was in some respects worse. Local government was poor in resources, with a narrow and declining base on which to levy rates. Officers were reluctant to serve in Hackney and quick to move on to greener pastures. Educational results were spectacularly poor, perpetuating the shortage of qualified labour. Redevelopment, emigration and immigration progressively ate away at the community, the extended family and even the nuclear family. Socialization and social control of the young began to fail. Crime and vandalism blossomed. Good neighbourliness gave way to apathy or open conflict. [. . .]

The inner city is a precarious, shaky wall and most of its inhabitants and families are fragile Humpty-Dumptys. It is the entire complex of pressures acting on them that leads to their downfall. Social services and other helping agencies can only pick up the pieces and try to fit them together again. But they can only succeed on a lasting basis if the factors that led to the initial collapse are changed; if incomes, employment and housing are improved. If a patch-up job is done and the victim is propped up on the same unstable wall, he will certainly fall and break time after time.

The inner city, with its squalid housing, its atmosphere of decay, its endless conflicts, its threat of crime, is the worst conceivable environment for the mentally unstable. And yet the inner city attracts them and creates them and becomes, to some extent, a vast informal mental hospital, about as humane and caring as Bedlam, which in its famous heyday was sited within a stone's throw of modern Hackney. A 1973 study by the Hackney-based Psychiatric Rehabilitation Association found that, out of nineteen constituencies in northeast London and Sheffield, Hackney North and Hackney Central had, respectively, the second and the third highest discharge rates for schizophrenia. The North Hackney rate was 19.5 per 10,000 in 1968, almost double the national average. The study found that the discharge rate was very closely related to aspects of poverty, especially the unemployment rate, the proportion of unskilled workers, and the percentage of overcrowded and one-parent households. Hackney North and Hackney Central scored respectively second and third highest on a composite index of these factors.

There are two main theories to account for the connection between mental illness and poverty. The drift theory holds that those with a tendency towards mental instability will have a poor work record, pushing them gradually towards unskilled, insecure jobs. The stress theory suggests that the conditions of life in poor families generate mental illness. Almost certainly both are partly valid and work together to produce a concentration of mental disorder in the inner city. For the low income of unskilled workers pushes them to move into low-rent areas, while the multiple stresses of life in the inner city produce more mental problems, both of the more florid varieties and of the less visible kinds, such as depression, anxiety, nervous tension (all fully realistic in the circumstances) and phobias, obsessions and persecution complexes, which again frequently have a very real basis in the inner city. Recession intensifies the risks of most of these. Thus the principal aims of mental-health care—prevention and sustained rehabilitation—are quite impossible to achieve for most people in the inner city and even more so in a slump. [. . .]

All the inequalities of society, inequalities of power, status, income, conditions of work and housing, take their toll on the body as well as the mind. The general mechanism of stress has a potent effect: in nature it is adaptive, leading to either fight or flight. In human society, convention inhibits these natural responses, diverting them into redirected aggression and even into self-destruction. The body turns against itself, just as a rat that is involuntarily confined to the territory of another rat can die from stress. All the environmental sources of illness are stronger in poorer areas, and even more so in the inner city: smoking is more prevalent especially among women; diets contain more sugar, starch and fats because foods high in protein, minerals and vitamins are more expensive; damp and cold give rise to chest complaints and rheumatism; nervous tensions, air pollution, moulds from damp, all contribute to allergies, asthma, eczema; low birth weights are common because of poor maternal diet and smoking during pregnancy; there are more accidents in the home and on the street, from the use of paraffin heaters, lack of safe toys, absence of safe play facilities; injuries from family or street violence, and from work, are more common; there are health risks arising from poor refuse-disposal systems, shared toilets, ducted air heating; exhaustion from overwork and the effort of coping with stress leads to reduced resistance to other diseases. The inner city incubates illness, and attracts to itself those whose earning capacity is limited by long-standing illness.

Recession intensifies all the factors precipitating illness, by reducing incomes, and increasing malnutrition, damp and stress.

Personal health is one of the most telling and tragic indicators of the degree of inequality in Britain, and of its consequences. Comparing our lowest social group with our highest, we find that unskilled manual workers have three times the rate of limiting long-standing illness as professional and managerial types; four times the rate of mental illness; six times the rate of accidents at work; double the incidence of deafness; three times the incidence of total tooth loss; infant mortality two and a half times as high and stillbirth rates twice as high. Thus is inequality incised into the very flesh of the poor. And where the need is greatest the provision generally is poorest.

Primary health care in Hackney is no exception to the rule. It is not an area that would attract most doctors. There is a shortage of suitable premises, and the prospects of supplementing earnings from private practice are negligible. General practitioners have lists smaller than average, but that is more than made up for by the number of health complaints per person. Hackney GPs are older than average – one in four is over sixty – and half of them work alone rather than in health centres. Their surgeries are often behind dingy shop-fronts or on one floor of a terraced house. Many surgeries are open only four-teen hours a week, at times that do not suit working people (manual workers who take time off to see doctors usually lose pay). Many do not work an appointments system, so patients begin queueing out on the street, long before opening time, even on cold winter mornings.

Two-thirds of Hackney's GPs live outside the area. Hence getting hold of a doctor out of hours is more than usually difficult. The first problem is the phone. The phone is an essential but usually ignored element of our health system, taken for granted by the middle classes. But for the less affluent, who do not possess one, it is a constant tribulation, very much worsened by vandalism, and a nightmare in an emergency. [. . .]

Nor are the problems over once the doctor is seen, for prescriptions have to be taken to chemists and medicines collected. Pharmacists are a second element of the health system that is largely left to chance. Hackney has fewer chemists than a better-off area would have, and hardly any open after 7 p.m. When they are all closed, people have to embark on distressing and expensive voyages around London to find others that are open. [. . .]

In most deprived areas, hospital services would not make up for the deficiencies in primary health care. Hackney, because it is close to the centre of London, is well provided and benefits from specialized and teaching hospitals like the Queen Elizabeth Hospital for Children and Bart's. But a disproportionate share of the City and Hackney health district budget—91 per cent in 1979–80—was taken up by hospital services. A mere 6 per cent went on community health care, to provide health visitors, district nurses, child-health clinics, family-planning services and health centres. The hospital service itself was becom-ing more and more centralized partly because of budget restrictions, partly because of a misguided drive to rationalization. Centralization makes life easier for doctors and nurses, but more and more difficult for poor people in an area so badly provided with public and private transport as Hackney. For transport is the third unseen element of the health system and is the source of enormous distress and cost in time and money for the poor, tak-ing its toll of patients, and making supportive family visits that much more difficult.

Paul Harrison is a freelance writer and journalist based in London. This section comprises edited extracts from his book *Inside the Inner City. Life under the Cutting Edge*, published by Penguin (1983).

2.3

The Position of Women: Some Vital Statistics

Richard M. Titmuss

In a period when the possibilities of social progress and the practicability of applied social science are being questioned, it is a source of satisfaction to recall some of the achievements of the Women's Suffrage Movement in Britain. The development of the personal, legal and political liberties of half the population of the country within the span of less than eighty years stands as one of the supreme examples of consciously directed social change.

The purpose of this essay is twofold. First, to draw together some of the vital statistics of birth, marriage and death for the light they shed on the changes that have taken place since the beginning of the century in the social position of women. Second, to suggest that the accumulated effect of these changes now presents the makers of social policy with some new and fundamental problems.

The fall in the birth rate in Western societies is one of the dominating biological facts of the twentieth century. Viewed within the context of the long period of industrial change since the seventeenth century, it is the rapidity of this fall which is as remarkable as the extent of the fall over the past fifty years. By-and-large, these trends have been shaped by changes in the family building habits of the working-classes during the present century. From a mid-Victorian family size of six or more the average size of completed working-class families of marriages contracted in 1925–29 had fallen to just under two-and-a-half. For all classes, the proportion of couples having seven or more children during the second half of the nineteenth century was 43 per cent; for marriages contracted in 1925 this proportion had fallen to 2 per cent. It would probably be true to say that at the end of the century about half of all working-class wives over the age of forty had borne between seven and fifteen children. This contrast, remarkable as it is in average family size, is even more so in terms of the number of pregnancies—that is, when allowance is made for the losses from stillbirths, miscarriages and deaths in infancy experienced at the beginning of the century.

When this is done it would seem that the typical working-class mother of the 1890s, married in her teens or early twenties and experiencing ten pregnancies, spent fifteen years in a state of pregnancy and in nursing a child for the first year of its life. She was tied, for this period of time, to the wheel of childbearing. Today, for the typical mother, the time so spent would be about four years. A reduction of such magnitude in only two generations in the time devoted to childbearing represents nothing less than a revolutionary enlargement of freedom for women brought about by the power to control their own fertility.

What do these changes signify in terms of 'the forward view'—the vision that mothers now have and have had about their functions in the family and in the wider society? At the beginning of this century, the expectation of life of a woman aged twenty was forty-six years. Approximately one-third of this life expectancy was to be devoted to the physiological and emotional experiences of childbearing and maternal care in infancy. Today, the expectation of life of a woman aged twenty is fifty-five years. Of this longer expectation only about 7 per cent of the years to be lived will be concerned with childbearing and maternal care in infancy.

That the children of the large working-class families of fifty years ago helped to bring each other up must have been true; no single-handed mother of seven could have hoped to give to each child the standard of care, the quantity of time, the diffusion and concentration of thought that most children receive today. In this context, it is difficult to understand what is meant by those who generalize about the 'lost' functions of parents in the rearing of children. Certainly the children themselves, and especially girls, have lost some of these functions. But despite the help that the mother had from older children she could not expect to finish with the affairs of child care until she was in the middle-fifties. Only then would the youngest child have left school. By that time too her practical help and advice would be increasingly in demand as she presided over, as the embodiment of maternal wisdom, a growing number of grandchildren. In other words, by the time the full cycle of child care had run its course the mother had only a few more years to live—an analogous situation to the biological sequence for many species in the animal world. The typical working-class mother in the industrial towns in 1900 could expect, if she survived to fifty-five, to live not much more than another twelve years by the time she reached the comparative ease, the reproductive grazing field, of the middle fifties.

The situation today is remarkably different. Even though we have extended the number of years that a child spends at school and added to the psychological and social responsibilities of motherhood by raising the cultural norms of child upbringing, most mothers have largely concluded their maternal role by the age of forty. At this age, a woman can now expect to live thirty-six years. What these changes mean is that by the time the typical mother of today has virtually completed the cycle of motherhood she still has practically half her total life expectancy to live. For the generality of women in most societies of which we have any reliable records this a new situation. It presents an industrialized society, based on an extensive division of labour, on the early acquisition of occupational skills, on the personal achievement of status through educational and other channels which steadily narrow after the first ten years of adult life, with a host of new social problems. [. . .] These questions are being formed by the conjunction and combination of many forces. Changes in family building habits is one; changes in rates of dying since the nineteenth century is another.

It is common knowledge that there have been great reductions in mortality over the past fifty years, particularly in infancy and childhood where rates of dying have fallen by approximately 75 per cent. What is less well known is that death rates among women have been declining faster than among men. A comparison of the standardized mortality rates (which allow for differences in the age structure of the male and female populations) shows that the rate among men today exceeds that for women by about 50 per cent. This excess has accumulated steadily throughout the century. If rates of mortality are any guide to the general level of health of a population then these trends suggest that, since 1900, the health of women has improved, and is still improving, at a considerably faster rate than that of men.

The relative gains, as measured by death rates, of women over men apply to all age groups, but the really striking changes have taken place over the age of forty-five. This is shown by the percentage male excess at 10-year age groups for two periods:

	25–34	*35–44*	*45–54*	*55–64*	*65–74*	*75–84*	*85+*
1896–1900	15	22	29	24	17	13	9
1951–1955	28	28	62	91	65	37	20

Easily the greatest gains have been registered by women aged 45 to 74.

So far as Britain is concerned, a reasonable hypothesis would be that these improvements are in large part attributable to the decline in the size of the family since 1900. This receives support from the remarkable change, after 1930–32, in the relationship between the mortality of single women and that of married women. In Scotland, for instance, while the rates of single women in youth and early middle age fell by something like 25 per cent between 1930–32 (when they were lower than those for married women) and 1950–52, the rates for married women in the same age range fell by about 60 per cent by 1950–52. This fall put the rates for single women about 60 per cent in excess up to the age of forty-two.

Among married women, not only have the hazards of childbirth and the frequency of confinements been greatly diminished, but the number and proportion of mothers worn out by excessive childbearing and dying prematurely from such diseases as tuberculosis, pneumonia and so forth are but a fraction of what they were fifty years ago. Above all, the decline in the size of the family has meant, in terms of family economics, a rise in the standard of living of women which has probably been of more importance, by itself, than any change since 1900 in real earnings by manual workers. Nor would it be hard to argue that this factor was far more influential up to the Second World War than any additional benefits derived from the expansion of the social services and improvements in medical care.

Yet when one turns to the history of the Women's Movement in Britain it is odd to find that little attention was given to the problem of continuous childbearing with all its attendant evils of chronic ill-health and premature ageing. The social freedom of working-class women to control their own fertility was not an issue of any importance. Nevertheless, the Victorian myth about the biological inferiority of women was still powerful. For example, the manifesto of 1889, signed by Beatrice Webb, Mrs Humphrey Ward and others, protesting against Women's Suffrage, observed: 'We believe that the emancipating process has now reached the limits fixed by the physical constitution of women.'[1] Such an argument could hardly be brought forward today by those who oppose the principle of equal pay for women.

A more socially equal relationship was foreseen by the leaders of the Women's Movement but what they could hardly have envisaged is the rise in popularity of marriage since about 1911. Here we turn from the debatable field of value judgements about the quality of married life to the statistics of marriage distinguishing, as we must, between the amount of marriage taking place in a given population and the age at marriage.

As to the first, it is clear that for about forty years before 1911 marriage rates among women were declining. But somewhere around this time a change occurred; the amount of marriage began to increase. It has been increasing ever since, and in a striking fashion since the mid-1930s. An increase of nearly one-third between 1911 and 1954 in the proportion of women aged twenty to forty married represents, as the Registrar-General has said, 'a truly remarkable rise'.[2] Never before, in the history of English vital statistics, has there been such a high proportion of married women in the female population under the age of forty and, even more so, under the age of thirty. Since 1911 the proportion at age fifteen to nineteen has risen nearly fourfold; at age twenty to twenty-four it has more than doubled. Such figures as these hardly support the conclusion of the Royal Commission on Marriage and Divorce that 'matrimony is not so secure as it was fifty years ago'.[3]

More marriage has been accompanied by a great increase in the years of married life experienced by married couples. Declining death rates have not only lengthened marriage (and with earlier childbearing very substantially lengthened the years of married life during which there are no children to be cared for), but they have brought about a striking fall in the proportion of marriages broken by widowhood and widowerhood under the age of 60. It is highly probable that the proportion of broken marriages under the age of 60, marriages broken by death, desertion and divorce, is, in total, smaller today than at any time this century. It is also relevant to point out that the greater the amount of marriage becomes, the greater will be the chances that men and women, with impaired health and handicaps, physical and psychological, and unstable personalities will be exposed to the hazards of married life and child rearing. In other words, a wider range of personality and character variation may now be drawn into the ambit of marriage and parenthood. Formerly, this segment of the population (some part of which could be distinguishable by the incidence of acquired and inherited physical handicaps) might not have entered matrimony.* No interpretation of recent divorce statistics or of the facts about 'broken homes' can be satisfactory unless account is taken of this factor. And of the strikingly high rates of remarriage of divorced men and women in recent years. By 1955 this was in the region of threequarters.

Married life has been lengthened not only by declining mortality but by earlier marriage. It is a fact of the greatest social importance that for the past forty years a trend towards more youthful marriage has been in progress. In 1911 24 per cent of all girls aged twenty to twenty-four were married; by 1954 this proportion had risen to 52 per cent.† As a result of this trend and rising marriage rates the proportion of women still single at the age of thirty-five has fallen to only about 13 per cent. There are now fewer unmarried women aged fifteen to thirty-five in the country than at any time since 1881 when the total population was only 60 per cent of its present size. Yet 'the last generation in this country to reproduce itself completely was born as long ago as 1876 or thereabouts'.[4]

What broadly emerges from this incursion into the statistics of marriage is, first, a remarkable increase in the amount of marriage in the community; second, more and more youthful marriage—especially among women; third, a concentration of family building habits in the earlier years of married life; and, fourth, a substantial extension in the years of exposure to the strains and stresses of married life. All these changes have taken place during a period of increasing emancipation for women. Paradoxically, therefore, fewer social and legal restraints and more equality and freedom for women have been accompanied by an increase in the popularity of the marriage institution.

---

* Support for this thesis comes from the trend of mortality rates for married and single women since the 1930s. 'It is supposed,' wrote the Government Actuary, 'that those persons who marry are likely, on average, to be in better health than the unmarried; it was, therefore, to be anticipated that, as the number of spinsters became progressively smaller, a higher proportion of them would be of inferior vitality and that their mortality, relative to that of married women, would become heavier.' This expectation is borne out in a striking manner by the comparative mortality rates discussed in these paragraphs (*Registrar-General's Decennial Supplement*, England and Wales, Life Tables, 1951, pp. 14–15).

† According to a survey of 'Britain's six or seven leading marriage bureaux', conducted by *The Economist* in 1955, those who remain single and approach these agencies 'always want to marry a professional man, as do the heroines of women's magazine stories'. But 'it is the civil servants who really go like hot cakes, because of the pension'. (*The Economist*, August 27, 1955, pp. 678–9.)

To survey the changed position of women in English society from the standpoint of the vital statistics of birth, marriage and death raises a great many questions. While it has not been the purpose of this essay to analyse the causes of these changes, or to examine the modern family in sociological terms, it is nevertheless possible to discern from the bare facts the outlines of new social problems which, as yet, we have hardly begun to contemplate while other problems, long recognized, have now to be seen in a different frame of reference. The problem, for instance, of the dual roles of women in modern society; of the apparent conflict between motherhood and wage-earning which now has to be viewed in relation to the earlier and much more compressed span of life during which the responsibilities of motherhood are most intense. With an expectation of another thirty-five to forty years of life at the age of forty, with the responsibilities of child upbringing nearly fulfilled, with so many more alternative ways of spending money, with new opportunities and outlets in the field of leisure, the question of the rights of women to an emotionally satisfying and independent life appears in a new guise.

Yet, at present, practically all forms of educational and vocational training, along with entry to many pensionable occupations, are shut to the woman who has reached the age of forty. Motherhood and date of birth disqualify her, while the unthinking and unknowing may condemn her in moralizing terms for seeking work outside the home. Few subjects are more surrounded with prejudice and moral platitude than this; an approach which perhaps deepens the conflict for the women themselves about their roles as mothers, wives and wage-earners.

Already, it seems, more and more middle-aged mothers are seeking to find some solution to the social, economic and psychological problems which face them or may do so in the future. Dimly they may be perceiving the outline of these problems in the years ahead when the days of child upbringing are over. In the field of employment opportunities, as in so many other fields, new issues for social policy are taking shape as a consequence of these changes in the position of women in society. The problems for state policy which the women's movement of fifty years ago brought to the fore were largely political; those raised by the women's movements of today are largely social.

References

1. Strachey, R. *The Cause*, ?, p. 285 (1928).
2. *Registrar-General's Statistical Review*, England and Wales, 1940–45, Civil Text, Vol. II.
3. Report 1951–55, Cmd 9678, p. 24.
4. *Registrar-General's Statistical Review*, England and Wales, 1946–50, Civil Text, p. 83.

Richard M. Titmuss was an historian and social policy analyst. He was commissioned to write a volume of the Official History of the Second World War, published as *Problems in Social Policy* in 1950. He held the Chair of Social Administration at the London School of Economics and Political Science. He died, at the age of 65, in April 1973. 'The Position of Women' was originally given as the Millicent Fawcett Lecture at Bedford College, London, in 1952. It was published as Chapter 5 of *Essays on the Welfare State*, edited by R. M. Titmuss, Allen and Unwin, London (1958).

2.4

Depression: a Sociological View

George W. Brown

I have been asked for a personal statement about depression. Of all psychiatric conditions depression is perhaps the most fitting for a sociologist to study. It is an affliction of a person's sense of values; and an exploration of the way people give meaning to their world can be expected to throw some light on a condition whose central feature is a feeling that there is no meaning in the world, that the future is hopeless, and the self worthless. Around this three-fold sense of futility cluster different psychological and somatic symptoms none of which on their own are either sufficient or necessary for the diagnosis. But I will leave this aside and start at the heart of the matter—with aetiology.

I believe that depression is essentially a social phenomenon. (If this were not a personal statement I would say that present evidence does not make it unreasonable to hold this view.) I would not make the same claim for schizophrenia, though its onset and course are also greatly influenced by social factors. Society and depression are more fundamentally linked. I can envisage societies where depression is absent and others where the majority suffer from depression. While this is social science fiction something not too unlike it has been documented. At least a quarter of working-class women with children living in London suffer from a depressive disorder which, if they were to present themselves at an out-patient clinic, psychiatrists would accept as clinical depression; while women with children living in crofting households in the Outer Hebrides are practically free of depression no matter what their social class. (They do experience more anxiety conditions, but I believe that this is another story.) Moreover, I know of no compelling reason to believe that the many bodily correlates of depression such as those revealed by work on bioamines are any more than the *result* of social and psychological factors. This is not to deny the possible aetiological implications of recent biochemical research, nor the possible aetiological role of genetic and constitutional factors. But taking account of the need to explain differences in the rate of depression in whole populations, I do not think that there is likely to be any more than a very modest primary aetiological influence from biochemical processes, that is, from such processes alone. The evidence for such a primary role for psychological and social factors is certainly far more convincing.

Like most doing research in the field of depression I am firmly convinced of a multifactorial view: that factors at many levels can play a role in aetiology. But this perspective should not disguise the need to establish the *relative* contribution of the various levels. Lip-service tends to be given to a multifactorial view but often in practice, in teaching, in research, and in clinical work only a single class of factor is seriously considered. Ritual obeisance to many variables allows pursuit of one. A psychiatrist in 1967 who asserted that a woman attending his clinic could not be clinically depressed as her condition was clearly related to her bad housing was perhaps expressing in a somewhat unsophisticated way the same views as many of his colleagues. Clinicians understandably desire research that will justify intervention in clinical settings. They also want theories that would be both intellectually challenging and serve as a basis for their claims to professional expertise within medicine. The failure of sociological ideas and methods to make much of an impact on psychiatric teaching has meant that most psychiatrists see little intellectual challenge in a sociological approach concentrating on the current environment. This also means that many have remained tied to a narrow view of science in which only experimentation is given full honours.

Of course, during the last two decades there have been important changes not least due to the lead of Sir Aubrey Lewis. But social psychiatry still needs to devote more of its time to the heady and dangerous job of causal analysis in natural settings; only in this way is it likely to get the necessary challenge and impetus to develop measures and methods that will have the authority to influence psychiatry as a whole.

During the last eight years my colleagues and I have done our best to follow such a path: our ideas about depression cannot be said to diverge all that much from ideas expressed *somewhere* in the psychiatric literature. (Has any other discipline speculated quite so much?) Any claim to originality probably mainly rests on the way factors have been brought together on a causal model; and any claims to attention on the consideration we have given to methodological problems. Indeed the model is sufficiently well based for some interest to be shown in the theory that we have linked to it. But in what follows, model and theory should be kept distinct; claims made for our causal model cannot be made for our more speculative theory.

The job of creating such a model involves developing measures and research design so that a claim can be made that the factors, following the temporal order set out in the model (Figure 1), are in *some way* involved in bringing about depression. Obvious biases must be ruled out and objections that would trivialize the model must be met. (For example, while life-events do play a causal role they merely bring about a depressive disorder that would have occurred before long in any case without any pre-event occurring.) We have made some progress; certain kinds of severe life-events and difficulties do appear to bring about the majority of depressive disorders—both among women treated by psychiatrists and among

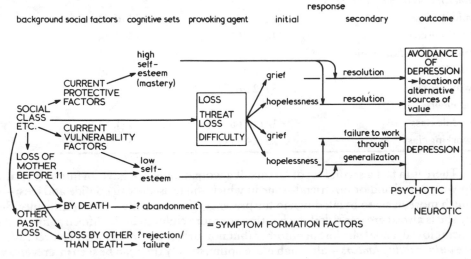

Figure 1 (key: CAPITALS=Causal model)

women found to be depressed after being selected at random from the general population (see Table 1). The kind of depression does not matter: these *provoking agents* are as

Table 1 Proportion with at least one severely threatening event or at least one major difficulty in the period before onset for patients and onset cases or interviews for 'normal' and 'borderline' women

	patients (N = 114) %	onset cases (N = 37) %	'normal' and 'borderline' women (N = 382) %
1 severe event alone	30 ⎫	41 ⎫	13 ⎫
2 severe event and major difficulty	31 ⎬ 75	24 ⎬ 89	6 ⎬ 30
3 major difficulty	14 ⎭	24 ⎭	11 ⎭
4 no severe event or major difficulty	25	11	70

strongly associated with the onset of psychotic as neurotic depressive conditions. Perhaps the most challenging claim of the model is that provoking agents (i.e., events and difficulties) are rarely sufficient to bring about depression—although they do determine *when* the disorders occur.

This is best illustrated by the way depression is linked to social class. Working-class women in London are not only far more likely to suffer from depression, they are also far more likely to develop a clear depressive disorder in the presence of a major life-event or difficulty (see Table 2). Something other than the provoking agent is at work.

Table 2 Percentage of women developing a psychiatric disorder (i.e. caseness) in year by life-stage, social class, and whether preceded by a severe event or major difficulty (chronic cases excluded)

	severe event/ major difficulty %	no severe event/ major difficulty %
women without child at home		
middle class	22 (7/32)	0 (0/62)
working class	10 (3/30)	2 (1/44)
women with child at home		
middle class	8 (3/36)	1 (1/80)
working class	31 (21/67)	1 (1/68)
all women		
middle class	15 (10/68)	1 (1/142)
working class	25 (24/97)	3 (2/112)

There is in fact a second set of factors. If a woman does not have an intimate relationship with a husband or boyfriend—one in which she feels she can confide and trust—she is much more likely to break down in the presence of a major life-event or difficulty. Similarly she is also at greater risk if she has three or more children under fifteen at home, if she is unemployed, and if she lost her mother (but not father) before the age of eleven. We call these *vulnerability factors*—although more optimistically they can be seen in a reverse way and called protective factors. None are capable of producing depression on their own, but they greatly increase chances of breakdown in the presence of a provoking agent (Table 3.) Some of the social class difference is explained by the fact that working class women in London experience more untoward life-events and difficulties—in this sense their lives are much tougher. But most of the class difference is due to their excess of vulnerability factors which put working-class women at risk for depression at the time of a major life-event or difficulty. The low rate of depression in the Outer Hebrides is probably due to the much greater degree of protection their culture and society gives these women—but this has still to be documented in detail.

Table 3 Proportion of women developing psychiatric disorder in the year among women who experienced a severe event or major difficulty by vulnerability factors (intimacy, employment status, early loss of mother and 3+ children under 15 at home)

		with event or difficulty			without event or difficulty		
'a'* intimacy relationship regardless	employed	(4/53)	9%	(9/88) 10%	(1/117)	1%	(2/193) 1%
	not employed	(5/45)	11%		(1/76)	1%	
non-'a'* intimacy relationship excluding early loss of mother or 3+ children under 15 living at home	employed	(6/39)	15%		(0/34)	0%	
	not employed	(7/23)	30%		(2/19)	11%	
non-'a'* intimacy relationship with early loss of mother or 3+ children under 15 living at home	employed	(5/8)	63%		(0/7)	0%	
	not employed	(6/6)	100%		(0/2)	0%	
		(33/164)	20%		(4/255) 2%		

*Essentially an 'a' intimacy relationship is one where the respondent reports a confiding relationship (where both partners can talk to each other about any personal matter) and this person is either a man or a member of the respondent's household.

Recently a third factor has been added to this model. While only loss of a mother before eleven increases the risk of a woman developing depression, other past losses of close relatives, largely in childhood and adolescence, influence the type and severity of depression. We call these *symptom formation* factors. Loss by *death* is strongly associated with psychotic-like depressive symptoms and their severity and *loss by other means* (e.g. parents separating) to neurotic-like depressive symptoms (and their severity). Only loss of mother before eleven plays two roles—as a vulnerability factor increasing risk of depression and as a symptom formation factor. Otherwise past loss merely determines the form and severity of a depressive disorder once it has occurred.

This is a rough outline of the model—stated without necessary caveats. But what does it all mean? What about theory? Consider employment and its protective role for women. Is it because it improves her economic circumstances, alleviates her boredom, keeps her occupied, brings her a greater variety of social contacts, or enhances her sense of personal worth? And just why should any of these aspects play a protective role? A causal model is not enough: theory is needed to explain what is happening. Theory unfortunately takes longer than a causal model to develop and to test. Any theory concerning the aetiology of depression has to deal with two crucial 'facts' provided by our model. First, that on the whole provoking life-events mainly involve major losses (if this term is allowed a certain licence to include events such as learning of a husband's infidelity); major difficulties and threats of loss can also at times bring about a depressive disorder. Something more than loss must be involved. Second, in the absence of a vulnerability factor such provoking agents rarely bring about depression. In other words, no matter how catastrophic a loss depression will not follow without the presence of at least one vulnerability factor.

We have speculated that low self-esteem is the common feature behind all four vulnerability factors and it is this that makes sense of the results. It is not loss itself that is important but the capacity of a woman to hope for better things once an event or difficulty has occurred. In response to a provoking agent relatively specific feelings of hopelessness are likely to occur: the person has usually lost an important source of value—something that may have been derived from a person, a role, or an idea. If this develops into a *general* feeling of hopelessness it may form the central feature of the depressive disorder itself; and Beck's triad of cognitions accompanies the well known affective and somatic symptoms of depression. Essential in any such generalization of hopelessness is a woman's ongoing self-esteem, her sense of her ability to control her world, and her confidence that alternative sources of value will be available. If the woman's self-esteem is low *before* the onset of any depression she will be less likely to be able to see herself as emerging from her privation. And, of course, once depression has occurred feelings of confidence and self-worth can sink even lower.

It must not be overlooked that an appraisal of general hopelessness may be entirely realistic: the future for many women *is* bleak. But given an event or difficulty, low self-esteem will increase the chances of such an interpretation of hopelessness. Here inner and outer worlds meet, and internal and external resources come together. And from there the sociologist must go on to build links with the wider cultural, economic, and political systems. Psychiatry cannot rest in the consulting room or even within the confines of a person's immediate social circle. Study of self-esteem cannot stop at the borders of a woman's personal world. For instance, may not feelings of low self-worth have something to do with the fact women are not paid for what many see as their central tasks? Do we take work seriously if it is not paid? The bitterness created by the recent attempts at wage control in all strata of male society suggest that more than economic considerations are involved in payment for work in our society.

While I have emphasized the role of the current environment our own results make it clear that this should not be taken too far—it is intended as a corrective. We carry with us our pasts. But I would again emphasize cognitive factors in explaining the effect of past loss. Loss of a mother before eleven, for instance, can be linked to the learning of uncontrollability, and through this low self-esteem. Martin Seligman's concept of learned helplessness has got a good deal in common with the way we have interpreted the role of vulnerability and protective factors. But unlike him I see no reason to restrict our model to so-called 'reactive' or 'neurotic' depressive conditions. The various vulnerability factors increase the risk of all types of depression; for example, among our patients those with neurotic-like depressive symptoms were no more likely to have more vulnerability factors or provoking agents than those with psychotic symptoms; we also have seen that past loss in childhood and adolescence can greatly influence the much later expression of psychotic or neurotic symptoms.

Here again I would emphasize a cognitive interpretation—in this instance, concerning long held perceptions of abandonment for psychotic as against rejection and failure for neurotic depressive symptoms.

But this is particularly speculative and I have at this point pursued our theoretical ideas enough. I will just finally add that we have also argued for a second, but less important, aetiological mechanism in which self-esteem is again implicated. Low self-esteem can inhibit a woman carrying out the necessary grief work after a major loss—and complications leading to depression are then likely to arise. This would also make it more difficult for her to take advantage of alternative sources of value that might be available.

It is probably unnecessary to make the obvious point that these processes will have biological correlates. It is possible that certain occurrences (e.g. early loss of mother, a depressive illness) may lead to more or less irreversible biochemical changes in the brain, thereby perhaps changing the mechanism of reward for the individual.

I am conscious of many gaps. I would have liked to explore the convergence of ideas about depression. There is, for instance, clearly a parallel between our sources of positive value and the psychologist's 'reinforcers', the psychoanalyst's 'narcissistic supplies', and the social scientist's concern with 'meaning'. I am also aware of my failure to deal with the perennial issue of diagnosis. Some psychiatrists may wish to dispute the label of depressive psychiatric disorder we have given to women in the community—very few of whom were receiving psychiatric help. I would point out that this is likely to place psychiatry in a perplexing intellectual and ethical dilemma. The women do not appear to differ in any essential way from many seen and treated in out-patient clinics. Is a psychiatric label to be restricted to those who manage to present themselves in such clinics? Fresh ideas and new research are required to clarify this issue. Another topic which needs much more exploration is the boundary between normal grief and depression.

But most of all I am conscious of my failure to convey in human terms what I believe to be involved in depression and in avoiding depression. I comfort myself that the reader of the *Bethlem and Maudsley Gazette* least requires such an account. But, if my talk of value resources, provoking agents, vulnerability factors, and protective factors has not lost you, Shakespeare may be able to illustrate our theory and to suggest the power of alternative sources of value to rescue a person from the onset of depression.

'When in disgrace with Fortune and men's eyes,
I all alone beweep my outcast state,
And trouble deaf heaven with my bootless cries,
And look upon my self and curse my fate,
Wishing me like to one more rich in hope,
Featured like him, like him with friends possessed,
Desiring this man's art, and that man's scope.
With what I most enjoy contented least,
Yet in these thoughts my self despising,
Haply I think on thee, and then my state,
(Like to the lark at break of day arising
From sullen earth) sings hymns at heaven's gate,
For thy sweet love remembered such wealth brings,

That then I scorn to change my state with kings.'
(Sonnet XXIX)

George Brown is a Medical Research Council External Staff Member and Honorary Professor of Sociology at Bedford College, London.

'Depression' was first published in the *Bethlem and Maudsley Gazette*, Summer 1977, pp 9–12. It was republished in *Basic Readings in Medical Sociology*, Tuckett, D. and Kaufert, J. M. (eds), Tavistock, London (1978).

2.5

Entitlements and Deprivation

Amartya K. Sen

Food and Entitlements

The view that famines are caused by food availability decline—the FAD view—[which is so widely used (explicitly or implicity)]—gives little clue to the causal mechanism of starvation, since it does not go into the *relationship* of people to food.

A food-centred view tells us rather little about starvation. It does not tell us how starvation can develop even without a decline in food availability. Nor does it tell us—even when starvation is accompanied by a fall in food supply—why some groups had to starve while others could feed themselves. The over-all food picture is too remote an economic variable to tell us much about starvation. On the other hand, if we look at the food going to *particular* groups, then of course we can say a good deal about starvation. But, then, one is not far from just describing the starvation itself, rather than explaining what happened. If some people had to starve, then clearly, they didn't have enough food, but the question is: *why* didn't they have food? What allows one group rather than another to get hold of the food that is there? These questions lead to the entitlement approach, going from economic phenomena into social, political, and legal issues.

A person's ability to command food—indeed, to command any commodity he wishes to acquire or retain—depends on the entitlement relations that govern possession and use in that society. It depends on what he owns, what exchange possibilities are offered to him, what is given to him free, and what is taken away from him. For example, a barber owns his labour power and some specialized skill, neither of which he can eat, and he has to sell his hairdressing service to earn income to buy food. His entitlement to food may collapse even without any change in food availability if for any reason the demand for hairdressing collapses and if he fails to find another job or any social security benefit. A general labourer has to earn his income by selling his labour power (or through social security benefit) before he can establish his command over food in a free-market economy; unemployment *without* public support will make him starve. A sharp change in the relative prices of haircuts, or labour power (i.e. wages) *vis-à-vis* food can make the food entitlements of the respective group fall below the starvation level. It is the totality of entitlement relations that governs whether a person will have the ability to acquire enough food to avoid starvation, and food supply is only one influence among many affecting his entitlement relations.

It is sometimes said that starvation may be caused not by food shortage but by the shortage of income and purchasing power. But the inadequacy of the income-centred view arises from the fact that it offers only a partial picture of the entitlement pattern, and starting the story with the shortage of income is to leave the tale half-told. People died because they didn't have the income to buy food, but how come they didn't have the income? What they can earn depends on what they can sell and at what price, and starting off with incomes leaves out that part of the entitlement picture. Furthermore, sometimes the income may be just 'notional', e.g. a peasant's possession of the foodgrains he has grown, and then the income-and-purchasing-power story is a bit oblique. To talk about his entitlement to the food he has grown is, of course, more direct. But the main advantage of the entitlement approach rests not in simplicity as such, but—as explained above—in providing a more comprehensive account of a person's ability to command commodities in general and food in particular.

The Poor: A Legitimate Category?

The entitlement approach requires the use of categories based on certain types of discrimination. A small peasant and a landless labourer may both be poor, but their fortunes are not tied together. In understanding the proneness to starvation of either we have to view them not as members of the huge army of 'the poor', but as members of particular classes, belonging to particular occupational groups, having different ownership endowments, and being governed by rather different entitlement relations. Classifying the population into the rich and the poor may serve some purpose in some context, but it is far too undiscriminating to be helpful in analysing starvation, famines, or even poverty.

The grossest category is, of course, the category of the entire population. It is on this that FAD concentrates, in checking food availability per head, and comes to grief. The entitlement approach not merely rejects such grossness; it demands much greater refinement of categories to be able to characterize entitlements of different groups, with each group putting together different people who have similar endowments and entitlements. As a category for causal analysis, 'the poor' isn't a very helpful one, since different groups sharing the same predicament of poverty get there in widely different ways. The contrast between the performances of different occupation groups in famine situations, even between groups that are all typically poor, indicates the need for avoiding gross categories such as the poor and the rich.

So much for causal analysis. But it might be thought that, while the category of the poor isn't very helpful in such causal analysis, it is useful in the *evaluation* of the extent of poverty in the nation. Indeed, the poor are usually huddled together for a head count in quantifying poverty. There is clearly some legitimacy in the category of the poor in this evaluative context in so far as there is a clear break in our concern about people at the 'poverty line'. On the other hand, even for evaluative purposes there is need for discrimination *among* the poor according to the severity of deprivation. In the head-count measure, the starving wreck counts no more than the barely poor, and it is easy to construct examples in which in an obvious sense there is an intensification of poverty while the head-count measure is unchanged or records a diminution. Thus, while the category of the poor has some legitimacy in the evaluative context, it is still far too gross a category and requires to be broken down.

World Food Availability and Starvation

The FAD approach applied to the food availability for the population of an entire country is a gross approach, lacking in relevant discrimination. What is a good deal more gross is the FAD approach applied to the population of the world as a whole. The balancing of world supply and world population has nevertheless received a lot of attention recently. While a fall in food availability per head for the world as a whole is neither a necessary nor a sufficient condition for intensification of hunger in the world, it has typically been assumed that the two *are* rather well correlated with each other. The evidence in favour of that assumption is not abundant, but it may be reasonable to suppose that, if the food availability per head were to go on persistently declining, starvation would be sooner or later accentuated. Different institutions and authors have provided estimates of 'short-falls' the 1980s and beyond, some more alarming than others.

I have little to add to this exacting exercise, except to point out the sensitivity of the results to the assumptions chosen and the remarkable lack of uniformity in the methodologies that have been thought to be appropriate. As far as the present is con-cerned—rather than the future—there is no real evidence of food supply falling behind population growth for the world as a whole, even though this has been observed for a number of countries. There is no outstripping of food growth by population expansion even when we look at the global picture leaving out the United States, which has been such a large supplier of food to other countries. The 'balance' in the future will depend on a var-iety of economic and political conditions, but there is as yet no indication that world popu-lation expansion has started gaining on the growth of world food supply.

But it is quite possible that severe famine conditions can develop for reasons that are not directly connected with food production at all. The entitlement approach places food production within a network of relationships, and shifts in some of these relations can pre-cipitate gigantic famines even without receiving any impulse from food production.

Some of the relations are simple (e.g. the peasant's entitlement to the food grown by him), while others are more complex (e.g. the nomad's entitlement to grain through exchange of animals, leading to a net gain in calories). Some involve the use of the market mechanism (e.g. selling craft products to buy food), while others depend on public policy (e.g. employment benefits, or relief in destitution camps). Some are affected by mac-roeconomic developments (e.g. demand-pull inflation), while others deal with local calamities (e.g. regional slump), or with microeconomic failures (e.g. denial of fishing rights to a particular community in a particular region). Some are much influenced by speculative activities, while others are not.

In considering food policy, what emerges is the importance of this angle of vision.

Market and Food Movements

Whether markets serve well the remedial function of curing famines by food movements has been the subject of a good deal of debating over centuries. Adam Smith took the view that it did, and that point of view was eloquently defended by Robert Malthus among others. These arguments in political economy were widely used by policy-makers, not least in the British Empire.

When a famine was developing in Gujerat in 1812, the Governor of Bombay turned down a proposal for moving food into an affected area by asserting the advisability of leav-ing such matters to the market mechanism, quoting 'the celebrated author of the *Wealth of Nations*', Warren Hastings, who had tackled a famine in Bengal in 1783–84 by using public channels for moving food into the region, was rapped on the knuckles by Colonel Baird-Smith for not having understood his Adam Smith, adding that Hastings could 'scarcely have been expected' to have absorbed Adam Smith so soon (1783) after the pub-lication (1776) of the *Wealth of Nations*. The basically non-interventionist famine policy in India lasted late into the nineteenth century, changing only around the last quarter of it.

Firm believers in the market mechanism were often disappointed by the failure of the market to deliver much. During the Orissa famine of 1865–66, Ravenshaw the Commissioner of Cuttack Division, expressed disappointment that private trade did not bring much food from outside which should have happened since 'under all ordinary rules of political economy the urgent demand for grain in the Cuttack division *ought to have created* a supply from other and more favoured parts'.

Adam Smith's proposition is, in fact, concerned with efficiency in meeting a market demand, but it says nothing on meeting a need that has not been translated into effective demand because of lack of market-based entitlement and shortage of purchasing power.

Indeed, in many famines complaints have been heard that, while famine was raging, food was being *exported* from the famine-stricken country or region. This was, in fact, the case in a relatively small scale in [the Ethiopian famine] Wollo in 1973, and also in [the] Bangladesh famine in 1974. It was a major political issue in the Irish famine of 1840s: 'In the long and troubled history of England and Ireland no issue provoked so much anger or so embittered relations between the two countries as the indisputable fact that huge quantities of food were exported from Ireland to England throughout the period when the people of Ireland were dying of starvation.' Such movements out of famine-stricken areas have been observed in Indian famines as well. In China, British refusal to ban rice exports from famine-affected Hunan was one of the causes of an uprising in 1906, and later a similar issue was involved in the famous Changsha rice riot of 1910.

Viewed from the entitlement angle, there is nothing extraordinary in the market mechanism taking food away from famine-stricken areas to elsewhere. Market demands are not reflections of biological needs or psychological desires, but choices based on exchange entitlement relations. If one doesn't have much to exchange, one can't demand very much, and may thus lose out in competition with others whose needs may be a good deal less acute, but whose entitlements are stronger. In fact, in a 'slump famine' such a tendency will be quite common, unless other regions have a more severe depression. Thus, food being *exported* from famine-stricken areas may be a 'natural' characteristic of the market which respects entitlement rather than needs.

Famines as Failures of Entitlement

The entitlement approach views famines as economic disasters, not as just crises. While famine victims share a common predicament, the economic forces leading to that predicament can be most diverse.

That famines can take place without a substantial food availability decline is of interest mainly because of the hold that the food availability approach has in the usual famine analysis. It has also led to disastrous policy failure in the past. The entitlement approach concentrates instead on the ability of different sections of the population to establish command over food, using the entitlement relations operating in that society depending on its legal, economic, political, and social characteristics.

I end with four general observations about the entitlement approach to famines. First, the entitlement approach provides a general framework for analysing famines rather than one particular hypothesis about their causation. There is, of course, a very *general* hypothesis underlying the approach, which is subject to empirical testing. It will be violated if starvation in famines is shown to arise not from entitlement failures but either from choice characteristics (e.g. people refusing to eat unfamiliar food which they are in a position to buy,[1] or people refusing to work[2]), or from non-entitlement transfers (e.g.

looting). But the main interest in the approach does not, I think, lie in checking *whether* most famines are related to entitlement failures, which I suspect would be found to be the case, but in characterizing the nature and *causes* of the entitlement failures where such failures occur. The contrast between different types of entitlement failures is important in understanding the precise causation of famines and in devising famine policies: anticipation, relief, and prevention.

Second, it is of interest that famines can arise in over-all *boom* conditions (as in Bengal in 1943) as well as in *slump* conditions (as in Ethiopia in 1974). Slump famines may appear to be less contrary to the 'common sense' about famines, even though it is, in fact, quite possible for such a slump to involve contraction of outputs *other than* those of food (e.g. of cash crops). Boom famines might seem particularly counter-intuitive; but, as discussed, famines can take place with increased output in general and of food in particular if the command system (e.g. market pull) shifts against some particular group. In this relative shift the process of the boom itself may play a major part if the boom takes the form of uneven expansion (for example favouring the urban population and leaving the rural labourers relatively behind). In the fight for market command over food, one group can suffer precisely from another group's prosperity, with the Devil taking the hindmost.

Third, it is important to distinguish between decline of food *availability* and that of *direct entitlement* to food. The former is concerned with how much food there is in the economy in question, while the latter deals with each food-grower's output of food which he is entitled to consume directly. In a peasant economy a crop failure would reduce both availability and the direct entitlement to food of the peasants. But in so far as the peasant typically lives on his own-grown food and has little ability to sell and buy additional food from the market anyway, the immediate reason for his starvation would be his direct entitlement failure rather than a decline in food availability in the market. Indeed, if his own crop fails while those of others do not, the total supply may be large while he starves. Similarly, if his crop is large while that of others goes down, he may still be able to do quite well despite the fall in total supply. The analytical contrast is important even though the two phenomena may happen simultaneously in a general crop failure. While such a crop failure may superficially look like just a crisis of food availability, something more than availability is involved. This is important to recognize also from the policy point of view, since just moving food into such an area will not help the affected population when what is required is the generation of food entitlement.

Finally, the focus on entitlement has the effect of emphasizing legal rights. Other relevant factors, for example market forces, can be seen as operating *through* a system of legal relations (ownership rights, contractual obligations, legal exchanges, etc.). The law stands between food availability and food entitlement. Starvation deaths can reflect legality with a vengeance.

Notes

1. However, anecdotal accounts of dietary inflexibilities can be less flexible than the dietary habits themselves, as judged by the following interesting statement by Dom Moraes, the distinguished poet: '. . . in India in the 1940s there was a famine in Bengal and millions of people died. During the famine, the British brought in a large amount of wheat. Now, the people of Bengal are traditionally rice eaters and they would not change their eating habits; they literally starved to death in front of shops and mobile units where wheat was available. Education must reach such people'. Education must, of course, reach all, but there is, in fact, little evidence of the hungry refusing any edible commodities during the Bengal famine. The explanation of people dying in front of shops has to be sought elsewhere, in particular in the shortage of

purchasing power and the minuteness of free distribution compared with the size of the hungry population queuing up for any food whatsoever.

2. Haile Selassie, the Emperor of Ethiopia, apparently provided the following remarkable analysis of the famine in his country in June 1973: 'Rich and poor have always existed and always will. Why? Because there are those that work . . . and those that prefer to do nothing . . . We have said that wealth has to be gained through hard work. We have said those who don't work starve.' They have indeed 'said' that for many centuries, in different lands.

Amartya K. Sen is Drummond Professor of Political Economy, All Souls College, Oxford. His work on famines formed part of the International Labour Office's World Employment Programme.

The above extract is taken from Chapter 10 of his *Poverty and Famines: An Essay on Entitlement and Deprivation*, Oxford University Press (1981).

2.6

Biomedical Research: Changes and Opportunities

Sir MacFarlane Burnet

The Lethal Diseases of Today's Affluent World

Today the great majority of human deaths are credited to three major groups: (1) cardiovascular degeneration and the associated accidents, strokes, acute heart attacks, etc.; (2) respiratory disease, largely as a terminal event of some chronic condition and often associated with cigarette smoking; and (3) cancer, including leukemia. This leaves a large list of 'other causes' in which chronic disease of the nervous system, peptic ulcers, and suicide are conspicuous. Keeping to the broadest possible approach, all of them appear to be diseases of multiple causation. The relevant factors can be broadly grouped under four headings:

1. Hippocrates taught that every disease has its own nature and arises from external causes; to a very considerable extent this attitude has continued throughout the history of Western medicine. Yet ever since Darwin looked at evolution and particularly after Mendelian genetics developed in the early twentieth century, physicians have become more and more interested in genetic aspects of disease. I have pushed that interest further than most and rightly or wrongly would hold that, within any fairly homogeneous community, much of the individuality in the medical history of people over 40 can be ascribed to the genetic diversity of human beings. Human life span, in so far as it can be dissociated from 'accidental' causes of death, has almost certainly a large genetic component which is most directly manifest in increased vulnerability, especially to death from casual infection. Genetically based susceptibilities also need to be considered in relation to a patient's response to infection, toxic agents, or drugs, and early recognition may be very helpful to both patient and physician. It is probably true that every disease state includes some genetic element in its causation, and in some groups, such as diabetes and the various conditions associated with high blood pressure, the association is clearly demonstrable.

2. The second important factor includes the conditions that are associated with somatic-genetic error. I have written extensively in recent years on this topic, especially in so far as it is concerned with the process of aging and with the origin of autoimmune disease and neoplastic conditions. Damage to DNA in somatic cells must occasionally occur at least from the time of birth onward. Sometimes the damage is irreversible and the cell dies. More often repair will be successful, giving a fully normal cell or, less happily, one which

has undergone mutation as a result of error in nucleotide sequence during the DNA repair process. Mutant cells and their descendants are to some degree abnormal and in general function less efficiently than normal. Elaboration of this theme can help to provide a useful approach to the basic nature of aging and the age-associated diseases, including cancer.

3. As I have already indicated, environmental factors are always to some degree concerned in the etiology of disease due mainly to genetic and somatic-genetic factors. Xeroderma pigmentosum is a striking example where in the absence of ultraviolet radiation none of the skin lesions would occur. In a quite different area, there is good reason to believe that paralytic polio and overt pulmonary tuberculosis depend more on the presence of individual genetic susceptibility to an initiated infection than to the virulence or dose of the infecting strain.

4. The effect of physical, mental, and emotional stress is almost universally held responsible for a considerable proportion of the 'diseases of civilization'. Deaths from the results of atherosclerosis and high blood pressure are commonly ascribed to stress. Genetic factors must be relevant here. In some individuals stress can be closely related to a fatal episode, but it is quite obvious that there are many persons who can remain healthy under stresses as great or greater than those that are seriously disabling for others.

Research on Disease of Intrinsic and Multiple Etiology

When we turn to disease and disability not referable mainly or primarily to the impact of the environment, the current needs for research can best be considered in terms of the main components of their multifactorial origin. Anatomical and functional abnormalities of genetic origin have been recognised as of medical importance for many years. Research at the biochemical level has been active over the last twenty years and is now complemented by more sophisticated epidemiological studies on the distribution of genetic disease or genetically based abnormalities. These make use of family studies on the incidence of disease in which two techniques are of special value: first, the comparison of identical twins with nonidentical twins and normal siblings, and second, investigations of adopted individuals involving comparison with their adoptive and biological parents. In the course of such essentially epidemiological work great use will normally be made of laboratory study, both of metabolites that may be relevant and of biochemical or immunological genetic markers, such as blood groups or HLA tissue groups.

I am deeply impressed with the need to clarify the implications of 'human' genetic diversity not only in the clinical field but also in relation to a host of socially important areas—crime, political terrorism, intelligence, leadership, the potentiality for special skills, etc. There are of course many difficulties in extending studies of this kind into highly sensitive areas such as those dealing with intelligence and aggression. Public opposition, however, will be less evident in medically oriented studies, and I should argue strongly for a steady increase in the volume of work on human genetic disease and of biochemical and immunological 'markers' that bear on medicine. The significance of the Rh blood groups and the HLA tissue antigens is well known; no doubt there are many other such genetic markers still to be discovered. At this point, I should like to interpolate a few examples from the genetics field which seem to call for further research at the present time.

Most experimental and clinical studies of genetic disease, inherited according to the standard Mendelian rules and therefore related to a single gene difference, have for rather obvious reasons concentrated on conditions in which a faulty structural gene can be recognized by the demonstrable absence or abnormality of a specific enzyme or by error in the amino acid sequence of the functional protein involved. Examples are galactosemia, phenylketonuria, and sickle cell haemogoblin disease.

But not more than 30 per cent of the DNA in the mammalian genome is identifiable as being present in structural genes. The remainder can be referred to as regulatory or control DNA, on the reasonable hypothesis that it is mainly concerned with the temporal sequence in which given structural genes are activated or repressed according to requirements during embryonic development or in various phases of mature functioning. In other words, regulatory DNA is a very complex 'administrative' system by which gene action, both structural and regulatory, is coordinated to the requirements of embryological development, the various types of mature functional activity, and potentially dangerous emergencies—notably trauma and microbial infection.

Regulatory DNA is not easy to study, but its importance is inescapable. Everything suggests that all types of DNA are subject to the same sorts of damage, are repaired in similar fashion, and are subject to similar types of informational error. It is equally certain that the genome in all somatic cells holds all or most of the regulatory information of the fertilized ovum.

I believe we could add at this point the probability or certainty that, in the neurological infrastructure on which human behavior develops, there are equivalent regulatory gene diversities which must have important influences on the individuality of intelligence, temperament, and social conformity among people.

I have a rather old-fashioned Galtonian dread of the genetic outcome of zero population growth with increasingly effective preventive medicine. As such, I believe that a major need is to study any examples where some particular allele has developed or been significantly increased in human gene pools over the historical period. We can briefly look at two candidates: the first is the high prevalence of the disease cystic fibrosis equivalent to the presence of the recessive gene involved in about 4 per cent of Caucasian people; the second is the linkage dysequilibrium of the haplotype HLA A1:B8.

Without offering any discussion of the basis for the conclusions, both can be looked at in the light of the classical example of sickle cell trait and sickle cell disease. They seem to represent the development and maintenance of an abnormal genetic pattern that favoured survival in a set of circumstances covering only a few hundred or a few thousand years—which of course is biologically a trivial period.

Marked change in those circumstances in our own time, that is to say, a very striking fall in the infant mortality from infection of all types and a great reduction by use of antibiotics in mortality from influenza, should in both instances eventually return the two sets of abnormal equilibria to the normal level.

On evolutionary grounds it seems inevitable that the great reduction in infantile mortality over the last 150 years must be associated with an increasing proportion of more susceptible children in the population as a whole, as a necessary result of the survival of those genetically more susceptible children, most of whom would have died in the nineteenth century. If civilization continues thus, an increasing proportion of children intrinsically more susceptible to lethal infections will be masked by modern preventive and therapeutic procedures. In the short-term view these may seem to be rather trivial topics, but in the very long term they may turn out to be prototypes of what I have spoken about as the inevitable result of the two-child family in which both offspring survive to reproductive age. Unless the whole accepted picture of the evolutionary process is wildly wrong, such a situation must lead us eventually to an intolerable degree of genetic degeneration. Sooner or later humanly directed measures to remedy the situation will be needed.

Fortunately the changes will be slow, and there is no call for precipitate action. I feel strongly that for the next 100 years at least we should be occupied in collecting and collating observational, experimental, and theoretical knowledge of human genetics. This knowledge will eventually make it possible to devise strategies to steer human evolution along lines which will have the same advantages for health and biological vigour as the historical evolutionary process but will do it without the 'slaughter of the innocents'. Even if eugenic measures are unthinkable today, they will probably be badly needed within the next two centuries. It is not too soon to begin a more active programme of research in human genetics oriented toward the problems of how, when public opinion will allow it, a vigorous attempt to counter clinically evident types of genetic deterioration can be initiated. One might speculate indefinitely about possible approaches that could be socially acceptable and, it is hoped, effective in the long term, but the time for that is still distant.

Self-inflicted disease

May I repeat here that the most urgently needed health measure in modern Western societies is one way or another to eliminate cigarette smoking. Every advanced country has taken what measures are possible in an egalitarian and permissive society, but to the best of my knowledge the mortality curve for lung cancer, though beginning to flatten out for males, has nowhere yet turned downward. In Australia we can say that mature males have almost stopped smoking, but the young are smoking more than ever, and in women of all ages the habit is increasing. The mortality curve for lung cancer in women is rising nearly parallel to what the male curve was doing a quarter of a century before.

As regards alcohol the position is complicated by the accepted finding that overall mortality is lower in well-controlled social drinkers than in total abstainers—though that does not necessarily prove that small amounts of alcohol are positively beneficial to health. The medical and social damage done by excessive drinking is proverbial; in Australia we are very much aware of the disastrous effect on aboriginal communities of the removal of all inhibitions on the supply of alcohol that coincided with their acceptance into full Australian citizenship.

Tobacco, alcohol, and cannabis are the traditional drugs of addiction to which heroin and other opiates, the psychedelic drugs and so on, have been added in this century. Research will have to be many-sided, and it may not produce the practical answers we desire. I am impressed with the evidence of genetic predisposition to alcoholism and with the studies that have shown wide genetically based differences between individuals in their capacity to handle most of the pharmaceutical agents that have been tested. Further research in these fields could perhaps lead to means of recognizing at an early stage individuals liable to develop addiction. Research into psychological and social factors related to initiation into drug use and subsequent addiction has been active in recent years, but little practical benefit can yet be perceived. Perhaps I am prejudiced in thinking that genetic and pharmaceutical studies will be more rewarding.

Rather similar approaches will be needed to the problems of overeating and obesity. On the one hand, combined genetic and metabolic studies can research the process by which fat is laid down and removed, but the compulsion to eat may have very much the character of an addiction, which calls for psychological and social approach.

I find the result of this brief summary of the needs and opportunities for effective mission-oriented research in the clinical-experimental field of medicine a little depressing. In every area there is a possibility of improving both the understanding of pathogenesis and the effectiveness of treatment, but it seems highly unlikely that anything approaching the dramatic effectiveness of medical research between 1920 and 1970 will ever result from any future fifty-year span.

The innate (genetic and somatic-genetic) disease conditions are becoming fairly well understood, but in a free democracy, with increasingly prevalent egalitarian and permissive attitudes, there is little room for optimism about even tentative preventive action. The significance of cigarette smoking as responsible for more than 90 per cent of primary bronchial carcinomas, by far the most lethal of common human cancers is known to every literate adult in the Western world. Self-motivated withdrawal from smoking is still too restricted to have made any real impact on the incidence of lung cancer death. In Australia, young people of both sexes seem to be smoking more than ever before despite a considerable propaganda effort in the schools. Some areas of advertising have been closed, but other equally effective avenues have flourished, notably the more publicized sponsorship of sporting events by cigarette companies.

Self-discipline has never been a widely prevalent human characteristic, and if this is needed (as it is) to counter the major disease-producing agents of the modern world, tobacco smoking, alcoholism and overeating, there is little likelihood of improving the current situation.

Direct preventive action against genetic disease is not yet a practical possibility apart from a modest amount of genetic counseling. Whether anything attempted in the future using some modernized eugenic approach will have any success is more than doubtful. Communities that cannot rid themselves of cigarette smoking are not going to take kindly to calls for unselfish cooperation in any programme to hinder human genetic deterioration.

The Pursuit of Knowledge for Its Own Sake

There is an equivocal attitude nowadays to what is variously called pure, basic, fundamental, or academic research, in which the investigator is primarily concerned with an understanding of some set of observable phenomena in scientific terms.

I believe that pure research aimed simply at the elucidation of things as they are, without any necessary bearing on the utility of the results for human comfort, profit, or power, is the most significant and desirable of human activities. I will not even add the usual qualification, 'unless its results are liable to be used for evil purposes.' No one can ever be certain that the use to be made of a new scientific discovery or a new paradigm will on balance be for good or evil. Most of us have come to realise that good and evil differ from one community to another and within the same community over a century or a decade. Any scholarly achievement which adds to the symmetry and completeness of our scientific picture of the universe is to be appreciated and cherished until it can be replaced or modified in the light of new discoveries or insights.

If man as the currently dominant form of life on earth is taken as the contemporary summit of evolution, it is easy to see that the central theme of evolution is progressive improvement in the capacity to handle information. In sequence we have the genetic control first of protein structure and subsequently of embryonic development and morphogenesis. Next comes a new level of information and control arising genetically, but to a large degree autonomous by way of local and systemic chemical (hormonal) communication within the organism. At yet higher levels we have the neuromuscular mechanisms that control and coordinate behavior. With the appearance of man we can continue the theme by mentioning, in sequence, (a) the development of consciousness and language; (b) the preservation of information in writing and more modern forms of communication; (c) calculating machines, machine tools, etc.; and (d) data-processing machines.

In the later stages of that sequence science has played a major part and however long the earth retains a biosphere science must remain a dominating factor in shaping the future course of human and posthuman evolution. If this viewpoint is adopted, the whole process of evolution—what I like to call the second sequence of creation—is meaningless unless it continues indefinitely or as long as our species and its descendants persist. This offers some justification for making the point that, given the virtual certainty that human lineage will retain its dominance of the biosphere and develop indefinitely increasing control of its environment, any human evolutionary change in the future will consciously or unconsciously be determined by man himself. It may be that for centuries the relevant activities will be for quite different purposes with no thought of modifying human characteristics. Eventually, however, some degree of intelligent control of the human gene pool must be superimposed on whatever spontaneous changes are taking place, though it may always need to have the quality of no more than gentle nudges away from visibly dangerous directions of change while still leaving scope for nature's own doings.

If progress in science and scholarship is the best criterion for social and demographic action, there seem to be four requirements that are highly relevant to the medical and biological aspects of human change over the long-term future. Let us remember that the useful time unit for evolutionary emergence of new mammalian species is a million years. Those long-term requirements seem to be:

1. To diminish and, if possible, reverse the degeneration of the gene pool that is inevitable in an uncontrolled zero-population-growth situation.

2. To provide environmental and social conditions conducive to good health in the individual and to stability and security in the community.

3. To recognize the great genetic diversity of human beings and to act appropriately.

4. To foster a global interest in human genetics and ecology, with full interchange of knowledge as it develops and cooperation in significant projects.

If such an approach is basically acceptable, one cannot help feeling that biomedical research of the future will continue to be very much as we know it. All that might change is the way in which the research is valued and supported.

Biological research must be aimed always toward the understanding of the human individual at all levels, genetic, developmental, cellular and morphological, psychological and biochemical, behavioural, social and linguistic—regarding both normal functioning and the malfunctioning that is associated with disease. There is a programme there that can look forward to a never-ending sequence of fresh focuses of special interest, that will change with changing human needs and, more importantly, with circumstances that make accessible study areas previously either unknown or misinterpreted. The understanding of man and his universe can never be complete. Error is in its own way basic to the whole evolutionary process. The role of the scholar and the healer will last for as long as our species survives.

Sir MacFarlane Burnet is retired and lives in Australia. He was formerly Director of the Walter and Eliza Hall Institute, and Professor Emeritus of Experimental Medicine, University of Melbourne. This extract is taken from the 1980 William S. Paley lecture on Science and Society, given at the Cornell Medical Center, New York. The full lecture was published in Perspectives in Biology and Medicine, 24 (4) 511–524 (Summer 1981).

2.7

Deaths under 50

Medical Services Study Group of the
Royal College of Physicians of London

Summary and conclusions

The Medical Services Study Group has started a collaborative study in the Mersey, West Midlands, and Grampian regions to examine the causes of death among medical inpatients aged 1 to 50. The cause of death was determined from the case notes and the consultant's opinion. The rate of ascertainment of cases was initially low, though it is increasing; despite this limitation an analysis of the first 250 cases showed one important finding. No fewer than 98 patients contributed to their own deaths through overeating, drinking, smoking, or not complying with treatment.

Introduction

The consultants in hospitals in the Merseyside and West Midlands regions were visited and told about the study. The project put forward was a broad one—namely, to look in detail at the causes and circumstances of all deaths of patients aged 1 to 50 years in medical wards. For this the information contained in the case notes and the consultant's opinion on the patient were needed.

After it had started the physicians in the Grampian Region asked to participate.

Ascertainment

The total population of the three regions under investigation is around 8 million—that is, about a sixth of the population of England and Wales. We would expect about 1,000 sets of case notes on medical patients dying in hospital each year.

From October 1977 to September 1978 over 400 were submitted. At present the rate of ascertainment is therefore about 50 per cent though there has been great variation between hospitals that promised support, some sending us all their deaths and some very few or none.

Results of analysis

The table shows the causes of death in the first 250 patients. Through studying the case notes in detail we have been able to assess the background to each case; in no fewer than 98 cases the patients contributed in large measure to their own deaths.

Summary of cause of death in the 250 patients surveyed

Causes of death	No. of cases	
Malignancies:		47
Carcinomas (primary site):		
Ampulla of Vater	1	
Breast	5	
Bronchitis	14	
Colon	2	
Stomach	3	
Undetermined	2	
Sarcomas	2	
Gliomas	4	
Myelomatosis	3	
Leukaemias	7	
Lymphomas	4	
Haematological conditions		7
Cardiovascular conditions		96
Myocardial infarction	31	
Cerebrovascular accidents	51	
Thromboembolic disease	7	
Miscellaneous	7	
Respiratory conditions		14
Asthma	6	
Respiratory failure	8	
Alimentary conditions		7
Crohn's disease	2	
Small intestine gangrene	4	
Oesophageal perforation	1	
Neurological conditions:		4
Multiple sclerosis	3	
Muscular dystrophy	1	
Infections:		25
Pneumonia	6	
Acute laryngoepiglottitis	3	
Encephalitis	6	
Meningitis	5	
Bacterial endocarditis	2	
Gastroenteritis	3	
Hepatic failure:		12
Cirrhosis	10	
Acute hepatic necrosis	2	
Renal failure		11
Chronic	8	
Acute	3	
Diabetes		2
Congenital abnormalities, brain damage at birth, etc.		10
Self-poisoning (1 accidental)		9
Others		6
Total		250

The 98 Cases of 'Self-Destruction'

Eight patients died from deliberate self-poisoning. In one there was no evidence of any previous psychiatric illness, but of the other seven, one had schizophrenia, one had a psychopathic personality, one was hopelessly dependent on alcohol, and the other four were depressives. Fashions in suicidal agents change and three used paraquat to kill themselves. One who died from barbiturate poisoning had had every conceivable treatment for schizophrenic depression: had been admitted for self-poisoning on three previous occasions; had slashed her wrists in an attempt to kill herself; and in her final illness had spent ten days in an intensive care unit. During her time in the intensive care unit she underwent 94 laboratory tests and 8 radiographic examinations—a sad example of the frequent inescapable commitment of skills and resources to patients beyond hope of being saved or restored to any worthwhile life.

Six of the 98 died from alcoholic cirrhosis of the liver, and another, whose liver disease was not primarily alcoholic in origin, accelerated his death by a high intake of alcohol. Though this group is small they exemplify the difficulty of helping alcoholics and the enormous demand they make on the health and social services. One 24-year-old man, who suffered cardiac arrest and irretrievable brain damage during acute alcoholic intoxication, occupied a bed in a teaching hospital for four months before he died, though it was clear from the outset that no recovery was possible.

Thirteen patients who died from carcinoma of the bronchus were strongly addicted to cigarettes, some smoking as many as 60 a day. Three other heavy cigarette smokers died from chronic airway obstruction and one from bronchopneumonia.

Among those whose death was attributable to myocardial infarction there were 25 with one or more causal factors within their own control. Twelve were grossly overweight; 22 smoked large numbers of cigarettes; two diabetics and two hypertensives did not comply with their treatment; and three others had had symptoms for a long time before they consulted a doctor.

Nine of the 98 patients delayed in seeking medical advice and in four this probably cost them their lives, for two died from gastroenteritis, one from meningococcal infection, and one from myxoedema. The patient with myxoedema had been ill for many years but had refused to see a doctor. Two of the other five might have survived and the remaining three lived longer had they sought help earlier.

Thirty-seven of the 98 patients refused admission to hospital, were unwilling to submit to investigation, discharged themselves from hospital, defaulted from diabetic clinics, or did not co-operate in taking medication. These attitudes were often encouraged by their spouses. It is impossible to quantify this factor, but certainly in many cases it was to some extent responsible for the fatal issue, while in others it hastened death. An anxious and nervous temperament was responsible in many instances but in others lack of co-operation seemed to stem from fecklessness or a psychopathic attitude to life and to doctors in particular. There was little to indicate that lack of intelligence played any significant part.

Discussion

Our initial finding will come as no surprise to the profession. Doctors have been saying for years that the causes of many of the killing diseases of middle life are not mysteries, but are contributed to by overeating, excess alcohol, and tobacco. Doctors' pronouncements tend not to be popular—some are contradictory and some are frankly disbelieved, and the disbelief is reinforced by the fact that the 'patient' often feels quite well. Health education is often derided ('It won't happen to me'), but there is an astonishing statistic which can stand much repetition. In 1930–32 the standard mortality ratio for ischaemic heart disease in social class I was 237 (normal 100). Over the next four decades it gradually fell to 88, but from 1951 to 1971 the crude mortality rate from ischaemic heart disease in all males almost doubled. Much the most likely explanation for this is that people in social class I do heed such advice whereas other groups do not.

The 'deaths under 50' project may be criticised on statistical grounds, but any bias in ascertaining the cases of 'self-destruction' is probably in the direction of under-reporting. The study's great merit lies in the fact that the information on causes of death is obtained from case notes and the clinicians' expert opinions, whereas in many surveys where the rate of ascertainment is better this information comes from death certificates.

'Deaths under 50' forms part of a report prepared by the Medical Services Study Group of the Royal College of Physicians of London. The report was compiled by Sir Cyril Clarke, director of the study group, and Dr George Whitfield, assistant director. A number of clinicians participated in the study. The full article was published in the *British Medical Journal*, 2, 1061–1062 (1978).

2.8

Malingering

Richard Asher

I define malingering as the imitation, production or encouragement of illness for a deliberate end. The patient is quite conscious of what he is doing and quite cognisant of why he is doing it. With that definition, pure malingering—the planned fraudulent faking of illness—is, in my experience, a very rare condition. Either that, or else I am a very gullible physician. I know I have been mistaken before now and it is possible that many malingerers have deceived me without being suspected.

True malingering is best classified by motives rather than by techniques—the principal prime movers being Fear, Desire and Escape.

Fear: fear of call-up, fear of overseas duty, fear of warfare.

Desire: desire for compensation, desire for a comfortable pension, desire for revenge against a surgeon for some (usually imagined) wrong. Desire for the comforts of hospital life. Desire to stay in the ward longer because one has fallen in love with the staff nurse.

Escape: escape from a prisoner-of-war camp by incurable disability, escape from prison by transfer to hospital, escape from an impending court case, escape from battle.

Malingering by prisoners of war has evolved a variety of ingenious techniques, even to the extent of passing borrowed albuminuric urine, secreted in a false bladder and passed in the presence of a suspicious German doctor, through a hand-carved and hand-painted penis of life-like verisimilitude.

It is well known that opposing forces try to weaken the enemy's army by dropping pamphlets persuading them to malinger. A particular pamphlet dropped in large numbers early in 1945 on English troops in Italy is worthy of your attention. Neatly produced in book-match form (to make it easy to hide), it opens with Three Golden Rules for Malingering which I do not think could be beaten:

1. You must make the impression you hate to be ill.
2. Make up your mind for one disease and stick to it.
3. Don't tell the doctor too much.

There is only time to give details about one of those. Here is how to have tuberculosis—according to the instruction book:

'First you must smoke excessively to acquire a cough. Then tell the doctor that you have lost weight, you do not feel well and that you cough a great deal. Say that sometimes you cough up streaks of blood. Sometimes you wake drenched with sweat. Stick to those symptoms, do not invent any new ones.'

Mental as well as physical disease can be simulated. Those with little experience of mental disease may learn with surprise that it is very hard to pretend to be mad. For instance, the peculiar distorted thinking of the schizophrenic is something a sane person cannot manage. An experiment was done in which twenty normal people were asked to feign insanity; they, and twenty genuinely psychotic patients, were interviewed by psychiatrists (who had no other means of telling which was which). The psychiatrists were able to pick out the malingerers in nearly 90 per cent of the cases.

I now pass to those cases of illness which, though self produced or prolonged, do not constitute malingering. They do not have so definite a purpose. I have grouped them together as The Borderland of Malingering.

The Borderland of Malingering

A. *Illness as a comfort.*
    (a) Hysteria.
    (b) The Proud Lonely Person (Lucy's disease).

B. *Illness as a hobby*
    (a) The Grand Tour Type (rich hypochondriac).
    (b) The Chronic Out-Patient (poor hypochondriac)
    (c) The Eccentric Hypochondriac (faddist).
    (d) The Chronic Convalescent (daren't recover).

C. *Illness as a profession*
    (a) Anorexia Nervosa.
    (b) The Chronic Artefactualists.
    (c) Munchausen's Syndrome.

Hysterics differ from malingerers because, although they may produce illness and enjoy it, they are unaware of what they are doing. They possess a capacity for self deception; they can wall off part of their mind so that it is impervious to self scrutiny. This process, dignified by psychiatrists with the term 'dissociation', is colloquially called 'kidding yourself'. Some cases of hysteria are very close to malingering. Others start as malingerers, and as they become better at kidding others, they finally succeed in kidding themselves, and become hysterics.

I have seen very little proven hysteria and I diagnose the condition only with diffidence. A fair proportion of 'hysterics' turn out to have organic disease, as many of us know to our cost.

Notice that among illness as a comfort I have put the proud, lonely person. Allow me to explain this. This pathetic type of case usually occurs in later life when praise and companionship are hard to come by. To lonely people a medical consultation may represent an event of great importance. It supplies that need to be noticed that exists in all human beings. A visit from the doctor allows them the illusion of seeking medical advice rather than companionship. A patient may be too proud to complain of loneliness, but there is no loss of pride in complaining of symptoms. Lonely people miss, not only companionship, but also the advice and criticism that go with it.

Turning to the hypochondriacs, first we have the rich hypochondriac. I call this one The Grand Tour Type, because she spends much of her time touring the larger cities in Europe visiting consultants. She always carries a large dossier, opinions from consultants, X-rays and laboratory reports; and usually a list of her own symptoms which she has carefully written out. During her tour she may have persuaded surgeons to remove some of her less essential organs. She has usually had her gall bladder and a quota of her pelvic organs removed by the time she reaches one's consulting room. To the consultant in private practice they are a familiar, tedious and lucrative burden.

The poor hypochondriac (or perpetual out-patient). Every hospital has a number of out-patients who have attended for many years. Whenever they are discharged from one department they turn up in another, thus acquiring a very large collection of documents, rivalling that of the rich hypochondriac although written on less luxurious writing paper and penned by less illustrious names. Though some have genuine chronic illness, many of them attend because they like the companionship of hospital; instead of going to the local public house for a glass of beer and a chat with the landlord, they go to the local hospital for a bottle of medicine and a chat with the other patients. One enlightened doctor tried the experiment of arranging out-patient sessions where the patients did not see the doctor at all unless they asked for him. It was a great success.

The eccentric hypochondriacs. These people like peculiar or unorthodox treatments. They believe with apostolic fervour in nature cures, osteopaths, astrologers and herbalists. Their preoccupation is more with treatment than with illness and they are harmless and often entertaining.

The chronic convalescent. When a patient has had longstanding organic disease for many years it becomes so familiar to him that it is almost a friend. If the illness is suddenly cured, he may feel deserted and friendless. He misses the familiar pain, the sympathetic enquiries of his friends and the security of his medical routine. He does not really want to get well; he has become a hypochondriac.

Now the last group: Illness as a profession. First, I consider anorexia nervosa. The reason why these people go to such lengths to avoid eating is rarely clear. They will resort to a variety of artifices to avoid food. They will hide food in their bed lockers, pour milk into their hot-water bottles and insist on starving in the midst of plenty.

The next group is that of the chronic artefactualists, who may spend years in self mutilation or the production of spurious fevers. Skin diseases are most favoured by the sufferers from chronic autogenous disease, but various other forms of self-damage are reported.

Lastly, Munchausen's syndrome. This is the strangest and rarest form of chronic autogenous disease. The patient with this syndrome is nearly always brought into hospital by police or bystanders, having collapsed in the street or on a bus with an apparently acute illness, supported by a plausible and yet dramatic history. Though his history seems most convincing at first, later his story is found to be largely false, and his symptoms and signs mostly spurious. He is discovered to have attended and deceived an astounding number of other hospitals. At several of them he may have been operated upon, and a large number of abdominal scars is often found. So skilfully do these people imitate acute illness that the diagnosis may be quite unsuspected until a passing doctor, ward sister or hospital porter says 'I know that man—we had him in St Quinidines last September. He says he's an ex-fighter pilot shot in the chest, in the last War, and he coughs up blood; or sometimes he's been shot through the head in the last war and has fits.'

Common varieties are:

(a) The abdominal type: laparotomophilia migrans.
(b) The bleeding type: haemorrhagica histrionica, colloquially called haematemesis merchants, haemoptysis merchants, and so on.
(c) The type specialising in faints, fits, convulsions and paralysis (neurologica diabolica).

These people differ from other chronic artefactualists in their constant progression from one hospital to another, often under a variety of false names, but nearly always telling the same false story, faking the same fictitious symptoms and submitting to innumerable operations and investigations. It seems that nothing can be done to prevent their continuing clinical depredations. Most doctors are so pleased if they succeed with detection and ejection they never think about protection. Though serious psychiatric studies of these people have been made, nobody can yet answer the two fundamental questions:

(a) Why do they do it?
(b) How can we stop them doing it?

All that can be said about them, and indeed about the whole subject of malingering, are these words of Robert Burns:

> But human bodies are such fools
> For all their colleges and schools
> That when no real ills do perplex them
> They make enough themselves to vex them.

The best explanation for all this self-manufactured disease is simply this: That human beings are such fools.

Richard Asher was a leading British physician who worked both in public health and hospital medicine from 1934 to 1963. This article is an extract from the book *Richard Asher Talking Sense*, a collection of his papers edited by Sir Francis Avery Jones, published by Pitman Medical (1972).

Part 3

The role of medicine

Introduction

During the first half of the nineteenth century there was systematic and vehement criticism of the effectiveness and humanity of medicine from both within and without the medical profession. This was the first era of 'therapeutic nihilism'. After that period, with the growth of a more scientific medicine, the prestige of the profession rose to new heights. But over the past twenty years, the role of medicine has once again been questioned. The critics have included economists and epidemiologists, feminists and sociologists, doctors and moral philosophers, social historians and theologians. They have focused on two particular issues—the effectiveness of medicine and the wider role of doctors in society. Clearly these subjects are inter-related, and several of the articles included in this part are concerned with both. It may be helpful, however, to consider them separately and see how the various perspectives either complement or contradict one another.

The effectiveness of medical practice

Assessment of the effectiveness of medicine has taken two main forms—historical analysis and evaluation of contemporary practice. The leading exponent of the former has been Thomas McKeown, a British doctor and demographer, who has argued that medicine played only a minor role in the dramatic decline in infectious diseases and in the growth of population in the UK since the seventeenth century. For McKeown, these changes resulted instead largely from improvements in nutrition and other social conditions.

Scepticism about the value of *contemporary* medical practice gained widespread attention, at least in the UK, with the publication in 1972 of a book entitled *Effectiveness and Efficiency*, written by the epidemiologist and doctor Archie Cochrane. His work was strongly influenced by his experiences in the Second World War, when he was captured and put in charge of medical care for his fellow prisoners. He had almost no medicines and yet, to his surprise, most of his patients made a full recovery. In his later work he went on to explore the dangers of simply assuming that medicine was necessarily effective in combating illness.

What has been the outcome of these criticisms of both the historical and the contemporary contribution of medicine? Most members of the medical establishment have not felt it necessary to respond. They consider the benefits resulting from their work to be obvious. However, a few doctors have attempted to systematically chronicle the achievements of biomedicine. Until his recent retirement, Paul Beeson was one of the leading physicians in the USA. While acknowledging the contribution of social improvements to the historical decline in mortality rates and accepting that medicine made mistakes in the past (such as the belief in the theory of focal infection), he is confident that 'biomedicine has achieved many important practical results' and that 'substantial advances have been made along the whole frontier of medical treatment'.

This confidence has received support from a seemingly unlikely ally—a Marxist doctor working in general practice in a small Welsh community, Julian Tudor Hart. Hart's concern has centred on the effect that criticism of medicine may have on the health care that communities, such as the one in which he works, receive. He fears such criticisms may unwittingly 'discourage support for public medical services' because, he claims, the critics are simply offering 'a passive scepticism'. He sees the lack of effectiveness of biomedicine as lying not in the subject itself but in its misapplication to curative rather than preventive goals.

Obviously this view is not shared by the so-called radical critics of contemporary medicine, as it does nothing to establish whether or not medical practice is effective. They argue that this can be achieved only by scrupulous scientific investigation and in particular the use of randomised controlled trials (RCT), such as that carried out in London in the late 1960s by David Piachaud and Jean Weddell. Apart from illustrating the method, this example demonstrates three other aspects: the need for economic, as well as medical appraisal; the practicality of introducing concepts of economics into the realms of clinical practice; and the danger of drawing policy conclusions before long-term follow-up has been carried out. Unlike the results after three years (reported in the article), there *were* significant differences in the relative effectiveness of the two procedures after five years, as the postscript reveals. This is not an argument against performing RCTs, simply a cautionary note about the difficulties involved.

Another area of potential difficulty concerns the ethics of RCTs. This is illustrated by the collage of articles, editorials and letters about a proposed trial to investigate the effect of vitamin supplements in preventing the occurrence of neural tube defects (such as spina bifida). The strength of feeling and the passions that such an issue provides can be seen in the material included in 'Ethical dilemmas in evaluation'.

The role of doctors in society

Recent years have witnessed a dramatic change in society's attitude to the role of doctors. Criticisms of doctors have arisen from a variety of standpoints—Marxist, feminist, Third World. They argue that, far from alleviating suffering and hardship, doctors act as agents of social control in maintaining the *status quo* (and, as such, the factors that cause ill-health). Doctors are able to do this, it is argued, because of the power relationship between themselves and the laity. It is this position of power which has enabled them to perpetuate the relative disadvantage suffered by members of the working class, women, ethnic minorities and other traditionally powerless groups. At their most extreme, these critiques have argued that doctors not only perpetuate existing structures but actually cause harm (iatrogenesis, or doctor-made disease). Probably the best known example of such a critique is the work of Ivan Illich. Illich, an Austrian theologian who has lived in Mexico since 1960, has argued that the ills of society result from individuals' loss of self-reliance, which in turn is a consequence of industrialisation. Thus, just as education becomes the province of teachers, so, equally undesirably, health has become the responsibility of doctors who now tyrannise the laity, causing more harm than good.

While Illich sees the basic struggle as one in which individuals must 'regain' their self-reliance and liberty from the oppressive nature of industrialisation, Vicente Navarro views it as a struggle against a particular mode of industrial society—capitalism. Navarro, an American doctor who comes from Spain originally, is one of the leading Marxist critics of modern medical care. He argues that doctors aid the capitalist process by promoting the view that illness results from decisions made by individuals. This, he argues, is far from the reality of most people's lives, who enjoy few, if any, opportunities to exercise free choice. In this situation, doctors are seen as an integral support for capitalism and therefore for the health-damaging nature of such an economic and social system. In the extract from his book *Medicine under Capitalism*, Navarro argues that increasing State intervention in health care is made necessary by the damage done to people's health by a capitalist system that produces great social inequalities.

Feminism provides a third critique of the role of doctors. Here a predominantly male medical profession is seen as oppressing women. As with the critiques of Illich and Navarro, this view is not confined to health and doctors, but is seen as a widespread feature of society. The article by the British sociologist, Ann Oakley, is taken from her book, *Women Confined*, a feminist study of women's experience of pregnancy and childbirth. In it she questions the benefits allegedly resulting from male doctors taking control of childbirth. For her, the main effect of such developments has been to reinforce women's social inferiority by manipulating their biology. In common with Navarro, doctors are seen as agents of an oppressive dominant ideology, which either wittingly or unwittingly they are helping to perpetuate.

The fourth view of the role of doctors considers their contribution in Third World countries. David Werner, an American biologist and teacher who spent many years living and working in Mexico, has argued that, although doctors are unwilling to work in rural areas of the Third World, they are also reluctant to relinquish medical control. In his book *Where There Is No Doctor* he has demonstrated that there is little or no need for doctors in such areas, and that the people would be more appropriately served by less highly qualified practitioners, whom he calls village health workers. Such workers, he feels, should be as involved in political activity to help bring about an end to oppressive inequities, as in traditional medical activity. This view is in sharp contrast to that held by Julian Tudor Hart who argues that doctors must occupy rather than desert those territories they have claimed for themselves but have been unable or unwilling to occupy. In other words, doctors should adopt a higher, rather than lower, profile and extend their influence over features of society which they presently ignore.

Hart's call to action is in marked contrast to the solutions proposed by the other authors. Ivan Illich seeks salvation through the limitation of the professional monopoly of doctors and the de-industrialisation of society. The industrial state would be transformed into a society free of the burden of iatrogenic disease and based on self-reliance and self-care. Vicente Navarro argues that for people to be truly free and self-governing, the state (and medicine) must be converted (in the words of Marx) 'from an organ superimposed upon society into one completely subordinated to it'. He views the self-help solution of Illich as reliant on a life-style theory of ill-health—a view rejected by a Marxist analysis. The feminist critique looks to changes in the patriarchal structure of society, in conjunction with other initiatives such as a central role for women doctors within the medical profession. And, as has already been mentioned, some critics of medicine in the Third World are seeking the development of alternatives to doctors—not as second-best substitutes but as being far more appropriate to needs. Village health workers are seen as being concerned not only for individuals, but for the whole community which 'they will serve, rather than bleed'.

Finally, how do the defenders of biomedicine view these criticisms of the role of doctors? They are largely silent on the topic—a silence that may reflect their lack of awareness of the growing clamour for change, or confidence in the knowledge that their position is safe and secure from the ravages of criticism.

3.1

The Medical Contribution

Thomas McKeown

Until recently it was accepted, almost without question, that the increase of population in the eighteenth century, and by inference later, was due to a decline of mortality brought about by medical advances. This conclusion was suggested by Talbot Griffith, who was impressed by developments in medicine in the eighteenth century. They included expansion of hospital, dispensary and midwifery services; notable changes in medical education; advances in understanding of physiology and anatomy; and introduction of a specific protective measure, innoculation against smallpox. Taken together these developments seemed impressive, and it is scarcely surprising that Griffith, like most others who considered the matter, should have concluded that they contributed substantially to health. This conclusion, however, results from failure to distinguish clearly between the interests of the doctor and the interests of the patient, a common error in the interpretation of medical history. From the point of view of a student or practitioner of medicine, increased knowledge of anatomy, physiology and morbid anatomy are naturally regarded as important professional advances. But from the point of view of the patient, none of these changes has any practical significance until such time as it contributes to preservation of health or recovery from illness. It is because there is often a considerable interval between acquisition of new knowledge and any demonstrable benefit to the patient, that we cannot accept changes in medical education and institutions as evidence of the immediate effectiveness of medical measures. To arrive at a reliable opinion we must look critically at the work of doctors, and enquire whether in the light of present-day knowledge it is likely to have contributed significantly to the health of their patients.

The obvious way to do this is to assess the contribution which immunization and therapy have made to the control of the infectious diseases associated with the decline of mortality. Since this can be done reliably only from the time when cause of death was certified, I shall examine the influence of medical measures in the post-registration period.

Airborne diseases

Tuberculosis Figure 1 shows the trend of mortality from respiratory tuberculosis in England and Wales since 1838. This is the disease which, if any, was critical for the fall of the death rate. It was much the largest single cause of death in the mid-nineteenth century, and it was associated with nearly a fifth of the total reduction of mortality since then.

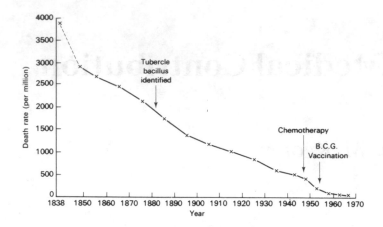

Figure 1 Respiratory tuberculosis: death rates, England and Wales

The time when effective medical measures became available is not in doubt. The tubercle bacillus was identified by Koch in 1882, but none of the treatments in use in the nineteenth or early twentieth century had a significant influence on the course of the disease. The many chemotherapeutic agents that were tried are now known to have been ineffective, as was also the collapse therapy practised from about 1920. Effective treatment began with the introduction of streptomycin in 1947, and immunization (BCG vaccination) was used in England and Wales on a substantial scale from 1954. By these dates mortality from tuberculosis had fallen to a small fraction of its level in 1848–54; indeed most of the decline (57 per cent) had taken place before the beginning of the present century. Nevertheless, there is no doubt about the contribution of chemotherapy, which was largely responsible for the rapid fall of mortality from the disease since 1950. Without this intervention the death rate would have continued to fall, but at a much slower rate.

Whooping cough   The trend of mortality from whooping cough is shown in Figure 2,

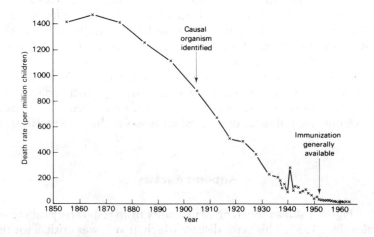

Figure 2 Whooping cough: death rates of children under 15, England and Wales

based on mean annual death rates of children under 15 in England and Wales. Mortality began to decline from the seventh decade of the nineteenth century, and the disease contributed 2.6 per cent to the reduction of the death rate from all causes.

Treatment by sulphonamides and, later, antibiotics was not available before 1938 and even now their effect on the course of the disease is questionable. Immunization was used widely after 1952; the protective effect is variable, and has been estimated to be between less than 20 and over 80 per cent. Clearly almost the whole of the decline of mortality from whooping cough occurred before the introduction of an effective medical measure.

Measles   Again Figure 3 is based on deaths of children under 15 in England and

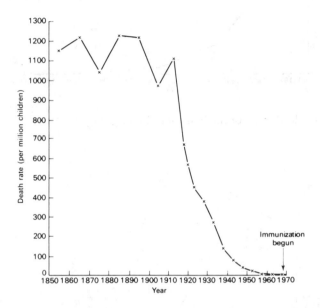

Figure 3 Measles: death rates of children under 15, England and Wales

Wales. The picture is among the most remarkable for any infectious disease. Mortality fell rapidly and continuously from about 1915. Effective specific measures have only recently become available in the form of immunization, and they can have had no significant effect on the death rate. However, mortality from measles is due largely to invasion by secondary organisms, which have been treated by chemotherapy since 1935. Eighty-two per cent of the decrease of deaths from the disease occurred before this time.

Scarlet fever   Because scarlet fever was grouped with diphtheria in the early years after registration of cause of death, the trend of mortality from the disease in children under 15 is shown from the seventh decade in Figure 4. There was no effective treatment before the use of prontosil in 1935. But even by the beginning of the century mortality from scarlet fever had fallen to a relatively low level, and between 1901 and 1971 it was associated with only 1.2 per cent of the total reduction of the death rate from all causes. Approximately 90 per cent of this improvement occurred before the use of the sulphonamides.

Diphtheria   Figure 5 is based on the mean annual death rate of children under 15, from the eighth decade of the nineteenth century. It is perhaps the infectious disease in which it is most difficult to assess precisely the time and influence of therapeutic measures.

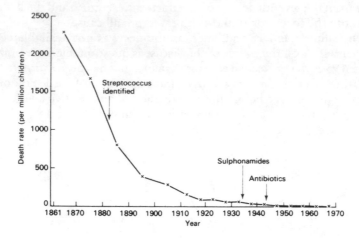

Figure 4 Scarlet fever: death rates of children under 15, England and Wales

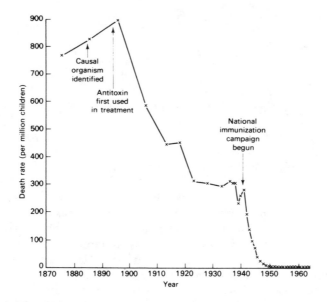

Figure 5 Diphtheria: death rates of children under 15, England and Wales

Antitoxin was used first in the late nineteenth century and has been the accepted form of treatment since then. It is believed to have reduced the case fatality rate, which fell from 8.2 per 100 notifications in 1916–25 to 5.4 in 1933–42, while notifications remained at an average level of about 50,000 per year. The mortality rate increased at the beginning of the last war but fell rapidly at about the time when national immunization began.

It is tempting to attribute much of the decline of diphtheria mortality between 1900 and 1931 to treatment by antitoxin and the rapid fall since 1941 to immunization. Nothing in

British experience is seriously inconsistent with this interpretation. However, experience in some other countries is not so impressive; for example there are American States where the reduction of mortality in the 1940s did not coincide with the immunization programme. Moreover, several other infections, particularly those that are airborne, declined in the same period in the absence of effective prophylaxis or treatment. While therefore it is usual, and probably reasonable, to attribute the fall of mortality from diphtheria in this century largely to medical measures, we cannot exclude the possibility that other influences also contributed, perhaps substantially.

Smallpox   The death rate from smallpox in the mid-nineteenth century was a good deal smaller than that of the infections already discussed, and the somewhat erratic trend of mortality since then is shown in Figure 6. Vaccination of infants was made compulsory in 1854 but the law was not enforced until 1871. From that time until 1898, when the conscientious objector's clause was introduced, almost all children were vaccinated. Most epidemiologists are agreed that we owe the decline of mortality from smallpox mainly to vaccination. Since the mid-nineteenth century the decrease has been associated with only 1.6 per cent of the reduction of the death rate from all causes.

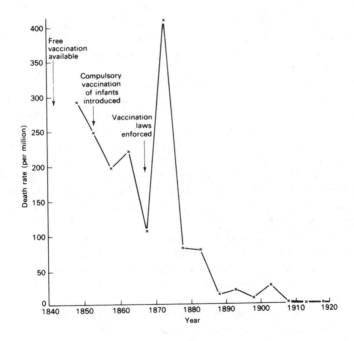

Figure 6 Smallpox: death rates, England and Wales

Infections of ear, pharynx and larynx   Together these diseases also were associated with only a small part (0.8 per cent) of the decrease of deaths. The main therapeutic influences have been chemotherapy and, in some ear infections, surgery. It is difficult to give a time from which surgical intervention can be said to have been beneficial, but in view of the small contribution made by these diseases it is perhaps not very important to assess it more precisely than by saying that one third of the decline (0.3 per cent of mortality from all causes in this century) occurred before the use of sulphonamides in 1935.

In summary, the airborne diseases accounted for two-fifths of the reduction of mortality from all causes from the mid-nineteenth century to 1971. Vaccination against smallpox was the only medical measure which contributed to the fall of deaths before 1900, and this disease was associated with only a small part (1.6 per cent) of the decrease of the death rate from all causes. In this century antitoxin probably lowered mortality from diphtheria, and surgery may have reduced deaths from ear infections, but together these influences had little effect on total deaths. With these exceptions, effective medical intervention began with the chemotherapeutic agents which became available after 1935, particularly the sulphonamides and antibiotics. By this time mortality from airborne infections had fallen to a small fraction of its level in the mid-nineteenth century; and even after the introduction of chemotherapy, with the important exception of tuberculosis, it is probably safe to conclude that immunization and therapy were not the main influences on the further decline of the death rate.

Water- and food-borne diseases

Cholera, diarrhoea and dysentry   In the mid-nineteenth century cholera was grouped with other diarrhoeal diseases in the Registrar General's classification; however, the last epidemic in Britain was in 1865, so from that time the contribution of cholera was negligible. Mortality from the diarrhoeal diseases fell in the late nineteenth century; it increased between 1901 and 1911 but then decreased rapidly.

It is unlikely that treatment had any appreciable effect on the outcome of the diseases before the use of intravenous therapy in the nineteen thirties, by which time 95 per cent of the improvement had occurred. For the main explanation of the decline of mortality we must turn to the hygienic measures which reduced exposure.

Non-respiratory tuberculosis   Non-respiratory tuberculosis was an important cause of death in the nineteenth century. Although mortality fell quite rapidly after 1901, there was still a considerable number of deaths in England and Wales (197) in 1971.

Interpretation of this trend is complicated by the fact that non-respiratory tuberculosis is due to both human and bovine infections; the abdominal cases are predominantly of bovine origin, whereas those involving other organs such as bones are often caused by the human organism. The human types can be interpreted in the same terms as the pulmonary disease, but a different explanation must be sought for the bovine infection. It is unlikely that treatment contributed significantly to the fall of mortality, since the level was already low when streptomycin—the first effective measure—was introduced in 1947.

Typhoid and typhus   Mortality from typhus fell rapidly in the late nineteenth century and there have been few deaths in the twentieth. It can be said without hesitation that specific medical measures had no influence on this decline.

The decline of the enteric fevers was also rapid, and began before the turn of the century, somewhat earlier than the fall of deaths from diarrhoea and dysentry. Effective treatment by chloramphenicol was not available until 1950, but by that time mortality from enteric fever was almost eliminated from England and Wales. Although immunization was used widely in the armed services during the war, its effectiveness is doubtful and it can have had little influence on the number of deaths.

In summary, the rapid decline of mortality from the diseases spread by water and food since the late nineteenth century owed little to medical measures. Immunization is relatively ineffective even today, and therapy of some value was not employed until about 1950, by which time the number of deaths had fallen to a very low level.

Other diseases due to micro-organisms

Convulsions and teething Most of the deaths included under these unsatisfactory terms were due to infectious diseases of childhood, for example to whooping cough, measles, otitis media, meningitis and gastro-enteritis. These infections are mainly airborne, and the general conclusions concerning the time and influence of immunization and therapy on airborne diseases may be accepted for them. That is to say, it is unlikely that medical measures had any significant effect on the frequency of death before the introduction of sulphonamides and antibiotics, and even after that time they were probably less important than other influences.

Syphilis Although syphilis was associated with only 0.3 per cent of the reduction of mortality from the mid-nineteenth century to 1971, it remained an important cause of sickness and death until about 1916, when salvarsan was made available free of charge to medical practitioners. From this time the number of deaths fell, and it was quite low in 1945 when penicillin largely replaced the arsenical preparations.

The decline of syphilis since its introduction to Europe in the fifteenth century was not due mainly to therapy, for after several centuries of exposure of the population the disease had changed to a milder form. Nevertheless it seems reasonable to attribute the reduction of mortality since 1901 essentially to treatment. It should of course be recognized that effective treatment, as in the case of tuberculosis, not only benefits those affected by the disease, but also reduces the number of persons who spread the infection. It seems right to regard this secondary effect as a further contribution of medical measures.

Appendicitis, peritonitis Mortality from these causes increased slightly during the nineteenth and early twentieth centuries—probably because of more accurate certification of cause of death—but declined after 1921. This improvement, which accounted for 0.4 per cent of the fall of death rate from all causes, can be attributed to treatment.

Puerperal fever The death rate from puerperal fever declined from the beginning of this century, but more rapidly after the introduction of the sulphonamides (1935) and, later, penicillin. It seems probable that the initial fall was due mainly to reduced exposure to infection, as the teaching of Semmelweis in the previous century began to improve the practice of the developing midwifery services; but from 1935 these services were greatly reinforced by chemotherapy. Both influences can be credited to medical interventions.

Other infections The 'other conditions' are a miscellaneous group, including some well recognized infectious diseases which caused few deaths, either because they were uncommon in this period (as in the case of malaria, tetanus, poliomyelitis and encephalitis) or because although common they were not often lethal (as in the case of mumps, chicken pox and rubella). They also include some relatively uncommon certified causes of death which are ill defined, such as abscess, phlegmon and pyaemia. In addition, there is a very small number of deaths due to worm parasites which, strictly, do not belong among conditions due to micro-organisms.

These infections were associated with 3.5 per cent of the fall of mortality between the mid-nineteenth century and 1971. In view of their varied aetiology it is not possible to assess accurately the major influences, but it is unlikely that therapy made much contribution before 1935. More than half of the reduction of deaths occurred before this time.

To summarize: except in the case of vaccination against smallpox (which was associated with 1.6 per cent of the decline of the death rate from 1848–54 to 1971), it is unlikely that immunization or therapy had a significant effect on mortality from infectious diseases before the twentieth century. Between 1900 and 1935 these measures contributed in some diseases: antitoxin in treatment of diphtheria; surgery in treatment of appendicitis, peritonitis and ear infections; salvarsan in treatment of syphilis; intravenous therapy in treatment of diarrhoeal diseases; passsive immunization against tetanus; and improved obstetric care resulting in prevention of puerperal fever. But even if these measures were responsible for the whole decline of mortality from these conditions after 1900—which clearly they were not—they would account for only a very small part of the decrease of deaths which occurred before 1935. From that time the first powerful chemotherapeutic agents—sulphonamides and, later, antibiotics—came into use, and they were supplemented by improved vaccines. However, they were certainly not the only influences which led to the continued fall of mortality. I conclude that immunization and treatment contributed little to the reduction of deaths from infectious diseases before 1935, and over the whole period since cause of death was first registered (in 1838) they were much less important than other influences.

Thomas McKeown was Professor of Social Medicine at the University of Birmingham from 1945 to 1977. This article is taken from Chapter 5 of his book *The Modern Rise of Population*, published by Edward Arnold, London (1976).

3.2

Effectiveness and Efficiency

A. L. Cochrane

The critical step forward which brought an experimental approach into clinical medicine can be variously dated. At any rate there is no doubt that the credit belongs to Sir Austin Bradford Hill. His ideas have only penetrated a small way into medicine, and they still have to revolutionize sociology, education, and penology. Each generation will, I hope, respect him more.

The basic idea, like most good things, is very simple. The randomized controlled trial (RCT) approaches the problem of the comparability of two groups the other way round. The idea is not to worry about the characteristics of the patients, but to be sure that the division of the patients into two groups is done by some method independent of human choice, i.e. by allocating according to some simple numerical device such as the order in which the patients come under treatment, or, more safely, by the use of random numbers. In this way the characteristics of the patients are randomized between the two groups, and it is possible to test the hypothesis that one treatment is better than another and express the results in the form of the probability of the differences found being due to chance or not.

The RCT is a very beautiful technique, of wide applicability, but as with everything else there are snags. When humans have to make observations there is always a possibility of bias. To reduce this possibility a modification has been introduced: the 'double-blind' randomized trial. In this neither the doctor nor the patients know which of the two treatments is being given. This eliminates the possibility of a great deal of bias, but one still has to be on one's guard.

There are other snags: first a purely statistical one. Many research units carry out hundreds of these so-called tests of significance in a year and it is often difficult to remember that, according to the level of significance chosen, 1 in 20 or 1 in 100 will be misleading. Another snag has been introduced by the current tendency to put too much emphasis on tests of significance. The results of such tests are very dependent on the number in the groups. With small numbers it is very easy to give the impression that a treatment is no more effective than a placebo, whereas in reality it is very difficult indeed to exclude the possibility of a small effect. Alternatively, with large numbers it is often possible to achieve a result that is statistically significant but may be clinically unimportant. All results must be examined very critically to avoid all the snags.

Another snag is that the technique is not always applicable for ethical reasons. There is, of course, no absolute medical ethic but the examples I quote here represent the majority of medical opinion at present, though I do not necessarily agree with them myself. They are: surgery for carcinoma of the lung, cytological tests for the prevention of cervical carcinoma, and dietetic therapy for phenylketonuria. No RCTs have ever been carried out to test the value of these standard therapies and tests. In the first two cases the RCT technique was not available when the surgical and medical innovations were made for carcinoma of the lung and cervix. By the time such RCTs were considered by medical scientists the one-time 'innovations' were embedded in clinical practice. Such trials would necessarily involve denying the routine procedure to half a group of patients and at this stage are nearly always termed unethical. It can be argued that it is ethically questionable to use on patients a procedure whose value is unknown, but the answer is that it is unethical not to do so if the patient will otherwise die or suffer severe disability and there is no alternative therapy. Such trials, it must be accepted, cannot be done in areas where the consensus of medical opinion is against them. This means, on the one hand, that patients' interests are very well protected and on the other that there are sections of medicine whose effectiveness cannot at present be measured and which, *in toto*, probably reduce the overall efficiency of the NHS.

There are other limitations on the general applicability of the RCT. One important area is the group of diseases where improvement or deterioration has to be measured subjectively. It was hoped that the double-blind modification would avoid this trouble, but it has not been very successful in, say, psychiatry. Similarly the assessment of the 'quality of life' in such trials has proved very difficult. A good example is the various forms of treatment attempted for recurrences after operation for carcinoma of the breast. We have so far failed to develop any satisfactory way of measuring quality.

Another very different reason for the relatively slow use of the RCT in measuring effectiveness is illustrated by its geographical distribution. If some such index as the number of RCTs per 1,000 doctors per year for all countries were worked out and a map of the world shaded according to the level of the index (black being the highest), one would see the UK in black, and scattered black patches in Scandinavia, the USA, and a few other countries; the rest would be nearly white. It appears in general it is Catholicism, Communism, and underdevelopment that appear to be against RCTs. In underdeveloped countries this can be understood, but what have Communism and Catholicism against RCTs? Is authoritarianism the common link, or is Communism a Catholic heresy? Whatever the cause this limitation to small areas of the world has certainly slowed down progress in two ways. There are too few doctors doing the work and the load on the few is becoming too great. An RCT is great fun for the co-ordinator but can be very boring for the scattered physicians filling in the forms.

In writing this section in praise of the RCT I do not want to give the impression that it is the only technique of any value in medical research. This would, of course, be entirely untrue. I believe, however, that the problem of evaluation is the first priority of the NHS and that for this purpose the RCT is much the most satisfactory in spite of its snags. The main job of medical administrators is to make choices between alternatives. To enable them to make the correct choices they must have accurate comparable data about the benefit and cost of the alternatives. These can really only be obtained by an adequately costed RCT.

If anyone had any doubts about the need for doing RCTs to evaluate therapy, recent publications using this technique have given ample warning of how dangerous it is to assume that well-established therapies which have not been tested are always effective. Possibly the most striking result is Dr Mather's RCT in Bristol[1] in which hospital treatment (including a variable time in a coronary care unit) was compared with treatment at home for acute ischaemic heart disease. The results do not suggest that there is any medical gain in admission to hospital with coronary care units compared with treatment at home. Equally striking are the results of the multi-centre American trial on the value of oral anti-diabetic therapy, insulin, and diet in the treatment of mature diabetics.[2,3] They suggest that giving tolbutamide and phenformin is definitely disadvantageous, and that there is no advantage in giving insulin compared with diet. Dr Elwood, in my unit, has demonstrated very beautifully how ill-founded was the general view of the value of iron in pregnant women with haemoglobin levels between 9 g and 12 g per 100 ml in curing the classical symptoms of anaemia.[4]

I have neither the ability, knowledge, time, or space to classify all present-day therapies. All I feel capable of is a rough classification:

1. Those therapies, with no backing from RCTs, which are justified by their immediate and obvious effect, for example, insulin for acute juvenile diabetes, vitamin B_{12} for pernicious anaemia, penicillin for certain infections, etc.

2. Those therapies backed by RCTs. The best example is the drug therapy of tuberculosis, but there are, of course, many others.

3. Those where there is good experimental evidence of some effect, but no evidence from RCTs, of doing more good than harm to the patient, particularly in the long-term. A good example, mentioned above, is the effect of iron on raising haemoglobin levels. This rise is very simply demonstrated, and there was a general belief that raising the haemoglobin level cured all the symptoms traditionally associated with low levels, until Dr Elwood published his results.

4. Those therapies which were well established before the advent of RCTs whose effectiveness cannot be assessed because of the ethical situation, but where there is some real doubt about the effectiveness, for example treatment for carcinoma of the bronchus and of the breast.

5. Those therapies where the evidence from RCTs is equivocal. The best example is tonsillectomy.

6. Those therapies under-investigated by RCT, although there are no ethical constraints, which are over-ripe for them. Psychotherapy and physiotherapy are probably the most important members of this group.

If effectiveness has been rather under-investigated, efficiency has hardly been investigated at all.

1. The most important type of inefficiency is really a combination of two separate groups, the use of ineffective therapies and the use of effective therapies at the wrong time. They are closely connected; for instance I should, without thinking, have classified tonics as ineffective but many of them contain medicaments which could be effective in some circumstances. Iron and the vitamins, which are common ingredients of tonics, can, of course, on occasions be very effective. It is important to distinguish the very respectable, conscious use of placebos. The effect of placebos has been shown by RCTs to be very large. Their use in the correct place is to be encouraged. What is inefficient is the use of relatively expensive drugs as placebos.

At the other end of the scale are the therapies for which there is no evidence of effectiveness, but where something has to be done. Simply mastectomy is a case in point for carcinoma of the breast. This I do not consider inefficient, but on present evidence I would not classify the use of radical mastectomy as efficient.

2. The incorrect place of treatment. This is possibly the least-recognized type of inefficiency, but it seems probable that the increasing cost of hospitalization will force attention to it. There are in general five places where treatment can be given: at the GP's surgery, at home, at the out-patient department, in hospital, or more recently in a 'community' hospital. Traditions have grown up as to the correct place for treatment for particular diseases, and until very recently no one has treated these traditional decisions as hypotheses which should be tested. I have already mentioned Dr Mather's comparison of the treatment of

acute ischaemic heart disease at home and in a hospital with a coronary care unit. Weddell has compared the treatment of varicose veins in hospital and in the out-patient department using the RCT technique.[5] No evidence was found of any advantage associated with hospitalization for those cases without skin damage. It is to be hoped that such demonstrations that RCTs are possible and ethical will encourage others to follow suit in this new sphere.

   3. Incorrect length of stay in hospital. It is not surprising, given the economic and psychological facts of the NHS, that the average length of stay in hospital in this country is higher than in some other countries. In addition, evidence has been accumulating of

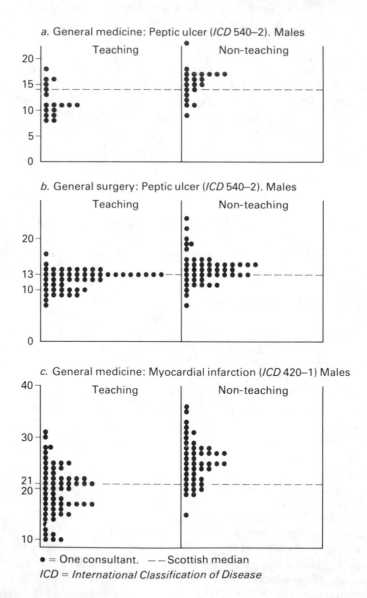

a. General medicine: Peptic ulcer (*ICD* 540–2). Males

b. General surgery: Peptic ulcer (*ICD* 540–2). Males

c. General medicine: Myocardial infarction (*ICD* 420–1) Males

● = One consultant.   − − Scottish median
ICD = International Classification of Disease

Figure 1 Median duration of stay in days for two diagnoses for individual consultants in Scotland (data for 1967)

large differences in length of stay between regions and between different consultants when treating the same disease. The most striking evidence (and the most accurate) comes from Heasman and Carstairs[6] from whose paper Figure 1 is taken. The extent of the differences is really surprising when hospitalization in a district general hospital is one of the costliest treatments that can be prescribed, and that the majority of patients wish to leave hospital as soon as possible. The only condition in which length of stay has been much investigated is again hernia. One group were discharged on the first day post-operatively. [No] serious disadvantages of early discharge [were] noted, but early discharge of herniorrhaphies has hardly become routine. The mean length of stay for hernia in England and Wales in 1967 was 9.1 days for males.

Unfortunately this observational evidence does not take us very far. All the consultants cannot be right, but this does not help us to determine the optimum length of stay. This can again be best approached by RCTs, but it will not be easy. The main index will have to be the incidence of complications and as these will in general not be high, very large populations are required to establish an optimum.

I am conscious that I have only scratched the surface of inefficiency. I could have stressed the rising percentage of hospital admissions for iatrogenic diseases; I could have stirred the dirty waters of medical administration, but I think for my limited purposes I have done enough.

An illustrative example: pulmonary tuberculosis

The change in the tuberculosis world between 1944 when I was burying my POW tuberculosis patients in Germany and the present day when TB deaths are the subject of a special investigation, as in theory they should not happen, is one of the most cheering things I have experienced in my life. The way in which the new treatments and preventive measures were introduced can also serve as a model for the introduction of all new treatments in the future. RCTs were used from the very beginning, and through this the correct dosages and combinations of drugs were quickly established; 'resistance to drugs' was quickly identified and means found of preventing it; each new drug was carefully assessed as it came on the market. The result is that there now are effective methods of treatment and prevention for TB. The speed of its development is very much to the credit of the MRC, WHO, and the British Tuberculosis Association, but it would have been impossible without the technique of the RCT.

On the efficiency side there is also a great deal to the credit of this branch of medicine. 'Place of treatment' was first investigated by an RCT when hospital and home care for the tuberculous were compared in Madras[7] and various studies in this country and the USA have confirmed the Madras finding that bed rest was unimportant.[8,9,10]

In spite of the striking evidence about the unimportance of bed rest, it is surprising to find how slowly the mean length of stay in hospitals in England and Wales is falling (Figure 2), and how much the variation in length of stay seems to depend on individual consultants (Figure 3). The real problem is how to ensure that patients take their chemotherapy after leaving hospital. Some doctors react by keeping their patients longer in hospital, others try biweekly supervised chemotherapy. The correct solution is still unknown, and until it is the treatment will not be completely efficient.

There are other details which need tidying up. There are remarkable differences for instance in radiographic routine. In an unpublished study of a twelve-month follow-up of all cases admitted during one year the type of case admitted to three hospitals were reasonably comparable, but in one hospital only 10 per cent, in another 52 per cent, and in the

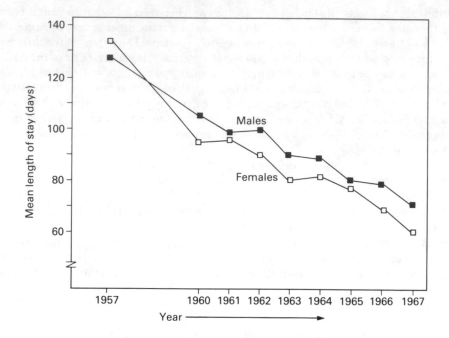

Figure 2 Mean length of hospital stay (days) for patients with respiratory tuberculosis (*ICD*, 7th revision, causes 001–008) in England and Wales, 1957–67

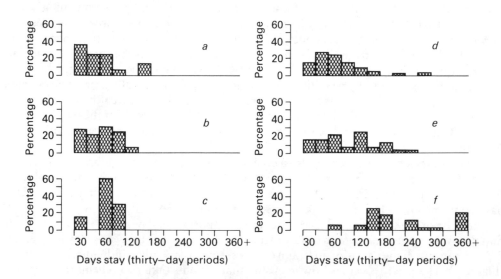

Figure 3 Length of hospital stay in thirty-day periods for male patients with pulmonary tuberculosis (*ICD*, 8th revision, cause 011) before discharge home from six selected chest hospitals in 1969

third 85% had at least one tomogram.

Some one, rather sardonically, asked me once how far I was prepared to take this randomizing game'. I answered, without thinking, 'You should randomize until it hurts (the clinicians).' In spite of my great admiration for the effective therapy and the efficiency with which it has been applied in this field I still think there is room for improvement. The TB world has not randomized until it hurts.

References

1. Mather, H. G., Pearson, W. G., Read, K. L. Q., Shaw, D. B., Steed, G. R., Thorne, M. G., Jones, S., Guerrier, C. J., Eraut, C. D., McHugh, P. M., Chowdhury, N. R., Jafary, M. H., and Wallace, T. J. 'Acute myocardial infarction: Home and hospital treatment', *Br. med. J.* 3, 334 (1971).
2. Universities Group Diabetes Program 'A study of the effects of hypoglycemic agents on vascular complications in patients with adult-onset diabetes. II, Mortality results', *Diabetes,* 19, suppl. 2 (1970).
3. Knatterud, G. L., Meinhert, C. L., Klimit, C. R., Osborne, R. K., and Martin, D. B. 'Effects of hypoglycemic agents on vascular complications in patients with adult onset diabetes', *J. Am. med. Ass.* 217, 6, 777 (1971).
4. Elwood, P. C., Waters, W. E., Green, W. J., and Wood, M. M. 'Evaluation of a screening survey for anaemia in adult non-pregnant women', *Br. med. J.* 4, 714 (1967).
5. Piachaud, D. and Weddell, J. M. 'The economics of treating varicose veins', *International J. Epid.* 1(3), 287–294 (1972).
6. Heasman, M. A., and Carstairs, V. 'Inpatient management variations in some aspects of practice in Scotland', ibid. 1, 495 (1971).
7. Dawson, J. J. Y., Devadatta, S., Fox, W., Radharkrishna, S., Ramakrishnan, C. V., Somasundarah, P. R., Stott, H., Tripathy, S. P., and Velu, S. Tuberculosis Chemotherapy Centre, Madras 'A five year study of patients with pulmonary tuberculosis— a current comparison of home and sanatorium treatment for 1 year with isoniazid plus P.A.S.', *Bull. Wld Hlth Org.* 34, 533 (1966).
8. Tuberculosis Society of Scotland 'The treatment of pulmonary tuberculosis at work: a controlled trial', *Tubercle. Lond.* 41, 161 (1960).
9. Spriggs, E. A., Bruce, A. A., and Jones, M. 'Rest and exercise in pulmonary tuberculosis: A controlled study', ibid. 42, 267 (1961).
10. Tyrell, W. F. 'Bed rest in the treatment of pulmonary tuberculosis', *Lancet,* i, 821 (1956).

A. L. (Archie) Cochrane was Director of the Medical Research Council's Epidemiology Unit in Cardiff before his retirement. These extracts are taken from his book, *Effectiveness and Efficiency; random reflections on health services,* produced for the 1971 Rock Carling Fellowship, published by Nuffield Provincial Hospital Trust.

3.3

Changes in Medical Therapy During the Past Half Century

Paul B. Beeson

Introduction

During the second and third quarters of the present century, there has been an unprecedented endeavour in biochemical research. Although physicians in general are convinced that medical therapy has substantially improved during that period, many members of the general public have become skeptical about the extent of our 'progress', especially considering the massive financial support they have provided. This disenchantment began in the 1960s, partly because of the great increase in the cost of medical care, and also because some major causes of disability and death have as yet been little affected. There have been calls for a shift in health care policy, with less money and effort allocated to biomedical research and hospital care and greater emphasis given to preventive medicine and health education. New appraisers of the medical scene—social workers, politicians, and physicians primarily interested in public health or preventive medicine—have tended to support this view. They stress the (indubitable) evidence that the improvements observed in morbidity and morality statistics during the past century are mainly from better nutrition and living conditions, and they argue that interventions of personal-service physicians have had a comparatively minor effect.[1,2] Suggestions are now being heard that we should re-direct our efforts, searching for 'alternative strategies of medical care'.

McDermott has answered some of these criticisms, emphasizing the difficulties in evaluating the efficacy of medical practice simply by inspection of mortality statistics, and has shown that some of the figures cited create a false impression.[3] Thomas has argued that real advances in the control of disease, such as the prevention of poliomyelitis, while never specifically predictable, are certain to occur if the present broad effort in basic science research is permitted to continue.[4] In contrast to McKeown and some of the others, Thomas pleads for an expansion, rather than a contraction of support for biomedical research, and predicts that the prevention and treatment of disease will be far less costly when we know more about the fundamental mechanisms of life processes.

Although most clinicians do not doubt that there has been substantial improvement in the treatment of disease during the past few decades, it is difficult to assess the dimensions because changes occur so continually. For that reason, I have attempted to obtain some objective information on our progress by comparing treatments recommended in the

1st (1927) and 14th (1975) editions of a multi-authored textbook of medicine.[5,6] It seems reasonable to assume that the therapy advocated by respected specialists at those two time-periods is fairly indicative of the conventional wisdom and the effectiveness of treatment at the beginning and end of the half century surveyed.

Limitations of This Survey

Judgment of the worth of a given treatment must be somewhat subjective and is more likely to be faulty with regard to the present than when aided by retrospection after a half century. Having served as co-editor of two American textbooks of medicine since 1947, I have had ample opportunity to observe that views about therapy constantly change. Unquestionably, forms of treatment strongly advocated currently will soon be supplemented by even better and perhaps simpler methods. Indeed, some may later be considered useless or harmful, as some of the treatments recommended in 1927 are now.

This comparison is necessarily incomplete because so many 'new' diseases and syndromes have been identified in the last fifty years. Some clinical entities that we now consider familiar—Crohn's disease, disseminated lupus erythematosus, sarcoidosis, and hyperparathyroidism—were not included in the 1st edition. Scores of viruses which cause disease in man, for example 90 different rhinoviruses, have been discovered since that time. In 1927 it was not known that sickle cell anemia is caused by an abnormal hemoglobin, whereas by 1975, 180 different hemoglobinopathies had been discovered. Furthermore, many disorders regarded as discrete entities in 1927 have since been shown to comprise groups of conditions for which there are now new names and differing forms of therapy.

Conversely, some subjects discussed in the 1st edition, for example 'milk sickness', are not found in the most recent one. In the section on diseases of the digestive tract, there were articles about 'primary dyspepsia', 'hyperesthesia of the gastric mucosa', 'gastroptosis', 'atonic dilatation of the stomach', 'visceroptosis', 'intestinal sand', and 'chronic appendicitis'.

Explanation of Rating System

1. *Recommended Treatment Now Regarded as Valueless.* Certain therapeutic recommendations in the 1927 edition can now be designated ineffective. Fowler's solution (arsenic trioxide), for example, was recommended for at least forty diseases, including tuberculosis, pellagra, gastroptosis, and Sydenham's chorea. It should be noted too that some of the treatments given a rating of 1 appear now not only to have been valueless, but very likely harmful.

2. *No Effective Treatment Available.* In the 1st edition this was said of mercury poisoning, and in the current edition it still pertains to such disorders as pneumoconiosis.

3. *Treatment Only Marginally Helpful, at Best.* At the time of the 1st edition antisera were used in treating several specific infections, such as meningococcal meningitis and erysipelas. The authors of those chapters were convinced that the treatment conferred some benefit, and I find it impossible now to evaluate the worth of those recommendations. In modern practice anticoagulant therapy in myocardial infarction and vascular shunts to prevent bleeding from esophageal varices seem to belong in this unsettled category.

4. *Measures for Relief of Symptoms.* This designation is applied to nonspecific treatments that make the patient more comfortable and perhaps hasten recovery, such as bed

rest, appropriate fluids, analgesics, good nursing care, and reassurance.

5. *Treatment Undoubtedly Effective, but in Limited Circumstances*. In 1927 the management of tuberculosis by prolonged rest in a sanatorium and the occasional use of pneumothorax or thoracoplasty was undoubtedly helpful in some cases, but these cumbersome kinds of treatment were only partial aids to recovery. The same was true of fever therapy for central nervous system syphilis. Today, examples suited to this code number are surgical treatment of lung cancer and our methods of dealing with obesity and drug abuse.

6. *Effective Preventive Measures, in Limited Circumstances*. This code number is for preventive measures where the protection is incomplete or short-lived. Examples in 1927 are typhoid or cholera vaccine and avoidance of insect vectors; today they include influenza vaccine and avoidance of industrial exposure to harmful chemicals.

7. *Treatment Suppresses or Controls Disease, but Must be Maintained Indefinitely*. In 1927 this applied to the liver diet for pernicious anemia (and likewise today for the simpler vitamin B^{12}), and anticonvulsant drugs for epilepsy. Other examples in modern therapy are allopurinol for gout and levodopa for parkinsonism.

8. *Therapy Substantially Improved and/or Diversified*. This rating describes broad advances in treatment, wherein different therapies acting by different mechanisms can be used, depending on the circumstances, or when one far better treatment is available.

9. *Effective Treatment, in Most Circumstances*. This was applicable in 1927 to the use of arsphenamine for relapsing fever. It applies to penicillin for hemolytic streptococcal infection in 1975 and, in general, characterizes the value of antibiotics for most of the common bacterial infections. It was appropriate for surgery for chronic cholecystitis in 1927, just as it is now.

10. *Effective Preventive Treatment*. This highest number is given to the ideal in all medical management—prevention of a disease. It was appropriate in 1927 for vaccination against smallpox, and in 1975 for poliomyelitis, yellow fever, measles and tetanus. A rating of 10 is used for preventive measures that are considered far superior to those given a rating of 6.

Findings and Discussion

Figure 1 depicts the general trend of changes in therapy over the period covered by this survey. For purposes of simplification, the ten categories have been divided into four groupings. Scores of 4 or less apply where the recommended treatment is nil, harmful, useless, of questionable value, or merely symptomatic. Categories 5 and 6 include curative or preventive measures effective only in limited circumstances. Ratings 7 and 8 describe treatments or preventive measures presently considered to be effective and helpful. Categories 9 and 10 denote highly effective therapy or prevention of disease. The figure provides graphic evidence that there has indeed been a substantial improvement in the management of medical diseases during the period covered in this survey. Whereas treatments falling in categories 7 through 10 were available in only 6 per cent of the 362 diseases in 1927, this rating could be given to 50 per cent by 1975.

Particularly gratifying in this tabulation is that category 1 ratings (useless or harmful) were eliminated in no fewer than 74 instances. This in itself has to be looked upon as a positive achievement. Indeed, perhaps one of the real advances of the past half century has been far greater objectivity in assessment of therapeutic practices. Probably a 'fringe benefit' of our larger biomedical science training for clinicians has been the fostering of a scientific approach to the evaluation of therapy. It is unlikely that we will ever again adopt

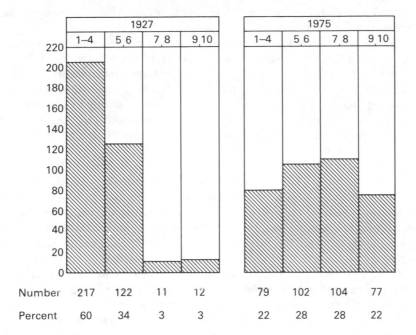

	1927				1975			
	1–4	5 6	7 8	9 10	1–4	5 6	7 8	9 10
Number	217	122	11	12	79	102	104	77
Percent	60	34	3	3	22	28	28	22

Figure 1

so unquestioningly a concept like that of 'focal infection', which led to millions of unnecessary 'ectomies'. Along the same line, I was shocked to see some of the advice given in early editions of the Textbook by physicians I had known and greatly respected: advice such as to roll a small cannon ball about on the abdominal wall for the treatment of gastroptosis. The new academic subspecialty of clinical pharmacology has helped to devise far more acceptable methods for designing and assessing the results of clinical trials. While one cannot claim that we are now free of a tendency to indulge in unwarranted prejudices by reliance on personal experience, we have nevertheless made real progress toward a more scientific assessment of treatment. Although we may look back on some of our present therapy, such as the use of cytotoxic drugs, as most unattractive, there is usually some plausible justification for its employment, and it is never likely to be classed with the bleeding and purging that characterized 18th and early 19th century medical therapy.

The improvement depicted in Figure 1 is not solely based on major advances in any one particular area of internal medicine. Although certain areas stand out, we can assert with assurance that the system of biomedical research in operation during the past few decades has produced important practical benefits, ranging over the entire spectrum of internal medicine. These improvements have resulted from various approaches, including better drugs, better surgery, and new therapies that depend on neither of these agencies.

Advances in pharmacotherapy have been particularly notable in the period under study. In going through the 1st edition of the Textbook, one cannot fail to be impressed by the paucity of available drugs. I have already referred to the popularity of two preparations: Fowler's solution (containing arsenic trioxide) and potassium iodide. These standbys were confidently recommended for the treatment of a dismaying variety of pathologic disorders. I was unable to find much rationale for their use by consulting textbooks of therapeutics published at the same time. Quite a few medicines used in 1927 have simply disappeared, examples being dried extracts of many endocrine organs, strychnine, the anti-treponemal arsenicals [and] oil of chenopodium. Only about 30 drugs mentioned in the 1st edition are still used today.

In the past half century a huge number of new drugs have been made available, amounting to several thousand preparations. We owe the newly introduced drugs almost exclusively to research and development carried on by large pharmaceutical manufacturers. This kind of activity is beyond the capabilities of academic institutions because of the cost, the time required to bring a new drug to the market following its discovery, and the complex restrictive rules of agencies such as the US Food and Drug Administration. I feel it is only proper to express appreciation of the activities of pharmaceutical research workers.

We internists have always depended on surgeons to treat some of the disorders that first come to our attention. The past half century has, of course, witnessed some striking changes in the indications for, and feasibility of, surgical therapy. Sometimes medical measures have lessened the need for operative treatment, e.g. thoracoplasty for tuberculosis, or thyroidectomy for thyrotoxicosis. It is particularly gratifying that we have ceased to ask surgeons to remove suspected 'foci of infection' for diseases like rheumatoid arthritis or multiple sclerosis. Nevertheless, we are now more dependent on surgeons than ever before, for the treatment of such conditions as valvular and congenital heart disease, angina pectoris, aneurysms, various localized pulmonary diseases, Hirschprung's disease, massive hemorrhage from the gastrointestinal tract, and organ transplantation.

In addition to the help of our surgical colleagues and the pharmaceutical industry, internists themselves can take credit for some important advances in therapy. Notable among these is the detection and correction of disordered fluid and electrolyte balance (including calcium, phosphate and magnesium). Renal dialysis (and the care of renal transplant patients) has created a subspecialty of practice. The ability to monitor and treat arrhythmias and early manifestations of heart failure has become another important facet of critical care medicine. The cardiac pacemaker is a combined medical-surgical device. The use of immunostimulation in the treatment of leukemia and certain other neoplastic states is at least a promising avenue to be explored. So, we in clinical medicine can fairly claim to have developed many successful measures.

It is not surprising to find that infectious diseases is the field in which the most spectacular improvements in prevention and treatment have occurred in recent decades. Effective vaccines have been developed for the prevention of diphtheria, whooping cough, and tetanus, as well as for the important viral diseases of poliomyelitis, yellow fever, measles and mumps. The great void in therapy of infections remains among those due to viruses.

The use of antimicrobial therapy has greatly altered the feasibility of many surgical procedures. For example, rupture of the esophagus was considered a uniformly fatal accident in 1927, but can now often be repaired, with reliance on chemotherapy to control mediastinal infection. The great recent advantages in surgery of the heart and lungs, and in some orthopaedic procedures, would have been impossible without antimicrobial agents to control the complicating infections that would be so devastating after many of these procedures.

Gratifying progress during the past quarter century has also occurred in cardiovascular diseases. The mortality from this important group of disorders has decreased more than 30 per cent in the past thirty years, much of that during the last ten years.

Another (success) area is hematology. Progress here might have been predicted because investigators of hematologic disease deal with an organ system that can be sampled repeatedly, with little risk or discomfort to the patient, and in which cell turnover is so rapid that effects of attempted therapy can be readily determined. Consequently, it has been comparatively easy to take advantage of advances in immunology and biochemistry.

Comparable progress has occurred in disorders of the gastrointestinal tract. Better physical and chemical techniques have enabled identification and characterization of many of the enzymes and hormones produced by organs of the digestive system, including the liver and pancreas. Instruments have been devised for the inspection and relatively risk-free biopsy of the cells which line the entire tract.

Even in the area of disorders of the nervous system one finds quite a few improvements. Although many major disorders in neurology and psychiatry remain without effective treatment, especially those of hereditary or congenital origin, when one considers the effect of levodopa in parkinsonism, and the recent discoveries showing that the brain is the site of production of a large number of biologically active chemical products, one can hope that real advances in therapy of diseases now looked on as hopeless—perhaps even 'senile dementia'—may be within reach.

This study has focused on internal medicine and therefore omits the important achievements in other fields of medical practice. Successes have been accomplished in many of the surgical subspecialties, not only of the heart, lungs, and blood vessels, but also in such fields as ophthalmology, otology, urology and orthopedics. Maternal and perinatal mortality rates have fallen steadily during this period, even in hospitals dealing with the same social classes, where there is no reason to believe that factors such as housing or nutrition have greatly changed. Dermatologic therapy has been altered almost unrecognizably by the availability of steroid hormones. The necessity for long-time incarceration of patients with some psychiatric disorders such as schizophrenia has been dramatically reduced by the availability of drugs like the phenothiazine compounds.

Conclusions

A comparison has been made of the therapeutic recommendations in the 1st (1927) and 14th (1975) editions of a multi-authored Textbook of Medicine. While it cannot be denied that we have a long way to go, the findings in this comparative study justify the claim that our recent broadly oriented effort in basic biomedical science has achieved many important practical results that are being applied with benefit in the care of the ill. Substantial advances have been made along the whole frontier of medical treatment. A patient today is likely to be treated more effectively, to be returned to normal activity more quickly, and to have a better chance of survival than fifty years ago. These advances are independent of such factors as better housing, better nutrition, or health education.

If we are given continued support and are allowed to follow the methods already proven, we can confidently expect similar impressive advances during the next few decades, even though we cannot (and should not) make specific promises about just where and when these advances will occur.

References

1. Dixon, B. *Beyond the Magic Bullet,* George Allen & Unwin, Boston, (1978).
2. McKeown, T. *The Role of Medicine,* The Nuffield Provincial Hospitals Trust, London (1976).
3. McDermott, W. 'Medicine: the public good and one's own'. *Perspect. Biol. Med.,* 21, 167 (1978).
4. Thomas L. 'Biomedical science and human health', *Yale J. Biol. Med.,* 51, 133 (1978).
5. Beeson, P. B. and McDermott, W. (eds) *Textbook of Medicine,* 14th Ed., W. B. Saunders Co., Philadelphia (1975).

6. Cecil, R. L. (ed.) *A Textbook of Medicine*, 1st Ed., W. B. Saunders Co., Philadelphia (1927).

Paul Beeson is a leading physician who recently retired from the Veterans' Administration Medical Center, University of Washington. This article is an edited version of an article that appeared in *Medicine* 59(2), 79–85 (1980).

3.4

A New Kind of Doctor

Julian Tudor Hart

In 1971 Cochrane published the first and best of a series of papers by various authors presenting fundamental criticisms of the theory, practice and profession of contemporary medicine, which I shall call the 'radical critique'. Common to all of them are the following beliefs: (1) That medical care has contributed little to improvements in health or expectation of life, compared with the contributions of nutrition, education, and conditions of life and work. (2) That we have expected too much from attempts to restore health by surgical or biochemical excision or substitution, which now incur increasing costs for diminishing returns. (3) That personal medical care should therefore return to a more modest role in curing seldom, relieving often, and comforting always. The authors differ in their assessment of the potential medical role in prevention, but none appear to see this as a substantial alternative employment for medical workers.

The radical critique is based on a large body of empirical evidence developed within medical science itself, derived particularly from epidemiology. Unlike the views of such illustrious predecessors as George Bernard Shaw, it shows little respect for fringe-medicine or faddism, and must be taken seriously. It cannot be dismissed merely because of the showmanship of Illich, or the mediocrity of the 1980 Reith lectures.[1] At its best[2–7] it poses questions which, if not effectively answered, may discourage support for public medical services, and encourage reversion to unplanned medical care in an open market, fuelled by greed and fear. This was certainly not the intention of its authors, all of whom, except Illich, have been supporters of a National Health Service (NHS) and opponents of marketed medical care; but, because they have not given us any new social policy, the radical critique has led to abdication, disarming those who might best have defended our Health Service had they retained more confidence in the value of their own work.

Authors of the radical critique have one failure in common; not one of them has been in clinical practice during the last twenty years. This remoteness may have assisted their objectivity, but it has made them less aware of the possibilities latent in our present everyday practice.

The limits of professionalism

If positive answers to the radical critique are to be found only beyond the present limits of professionalism, we should look at what those limits are. Traditionally the central task of doctors has been to respond to the complaints of individual patients suffering from disease, or the fear of disease. The profession has a minority of doctors who seek to conserve health in populations rather than restore it in sick individuals; but they are at the periphery, and have never been encouraged to combine the functions of prevention and cure. Doctors think of themselves as practical men who pretend no philosophy but common sense, but in fact their acceptance of this essentially passive social role has led and is still leading to failure to apply the effective medical science we already have to a large part of the sick population, to say nothing of those who are well.

McKeown (1979) refers to diphtheria death rates without apparently appreciating the chief significance of the evidence he cites. [Figure 5 in the article by McKeown] shows deaths from diphtheria from 1875 to 1960, indicating three turning points in the history of this disease: identification of the causal organism in 1883, introduction of antitoxin for treatment in 1895, and the beginning of the national immunization campaign in 1942.

McKeown does not refer to the discovery of effective immunization by von Behring in 1913, advocated for universal use by the Chief Medical Officer of the Ministry of Health in his report of 1922, and again advocated in a report by the Medical Research Council in 1927. The MRC concluded that diphtheria toxoid was effective beyond reasonable doubt, that no further evidence was required, and urged all Local Authorities to start mass immunization campaigns. Rhetoric continued throughout the 1920s and 1930s, but few such campaigns were undertaken. From 1922 to 1940 about 3,000 children a year continued to die from this wholly preventable disease, because the main thrust of medical effort was directed to individually presented symptoms: early diagnosis by throat swabs, treatment with antitoxin, admission to diphtheria wards of hospitals, and emergency tracheostomy. By heroic cures, our profession distracted both its own and the public's attention from its failure to prevent, while at the same time claiming that immunization was a medical procedure, and therefore the concern only of our autonomous profession. Not for the last time, we claimed as our own, territory we were unable or unwilling to occupy.

Medical science un-applied: the rule of halves

Since the Second World War, chronic disease has replaced acute illness as the main content of care. Population-based data are available for several major chronic conditions, from which we may estimate the extent to which what is known is actually applied. I take my evidence from three examples: hypertension, diabetes, and lower respiratory tract disease.

Hypertension

Since the reports of the Veterans Administration in 1967, it has been known that at diastolic pressures sustained ≥ 105 mmHg (Phase 5), and at systolic pressures sustained ≥ 180 mmHg, control of high blood pressure saves lives and must be regarded as mandatory. Table 1 shows the proportion of hypertensives above these thresholds in three populations, who have actually had any treatment; in nearly every case it is less, and in most very much less, than half of those in need.

This is what has come to be known as the Rule of Halves; half of those with blood pressure in the range mandatory for treatment are not known, half of those known are not treated, and half of those treated are not controlled. If we are serious about controlling hypertension, or any other chronic condition in which needs correlate poorly with symptoms, on the mass scale required, we must move decisively from our traditional role as shopkeepers passively responding to sick customers, to become active guardians of the health of our registered populations.

Diabetes

For diabetes, there are few studies on valid samples of the general population to give us evidence of the extent to which people cope without medical assistance, beyond repeat prescriptions, usually obtained from a receptionist. Those with supervision did not differ from those without, in the severity of their diabetes. Studies of populations totalling 21,000 in Central London[8] showed that 46 per cent of the known diabetics were attending hospitals. There was no information on the quantity or quality of primary care, but 40 per cent of all diabetics had had no retinal examinations during the previous two years, and over half had evidence of blood glucose levels sustained above the threshold for microvascular complications.

Table 1 Proportions of hypertensives ever treated, in three randomly sampled populations

Hypertension defined as:	Source	Proportion of cases ever treated		Age group
Diastolic pressure $\geqslant 110$ mmHg	South Wales 1971 (Miall & Chinn 1974)	Men	25%	35–64
		Women	44%	
	Australia 1971–72 (Lovell & Prineas 1974)	Men & Women }	11%	50–59
Systolic pressure $\geqslant 200$ mmHg	Framingham, USA 1975 (Kannel 1976)	Men	40%	35–44
		Women	63%	
		Men	28%	45–54
		Women	53%	
		Men	37%	55–64
		Women	40%	

Chiefly through its accelerating effect on coronary disease, diabetes of all grades is a major cause of death. In these terms, it is grossly under-diagnosed, and even for insulin-dependent cases, which are fully known, control and supervision probably reach no more than 50 per cent of requirement.

Lower respiratory tract disease

Management of lower respiratory tract disease is perhaps the worst example of medical custom unrelated to medical science. Death rates from bronchitis and emphysema are directly proportional to the number of cigarettes smoked, and reduced pollution since the Clean Air Act now leaves this as the principal initiating and continuing cause of chronic bronchitis, and the sole cause of severe disability in nearly all cases of emphysema.[9] Antibiotics, either continuously or for acute exacerbations, have no effect on the rate of deterioration of lung function,[10] expectorant medicines have no measurable effects of any kind, and bronchodilators are effective only in cases with underlying asthma; yet such prescriptions have been the chief therapeutic activity of GPs for this common and eventually disabling condition. Smoking is the principal cause, stopping smoking the only way of halting its progression, and action on smoking is clearly the most useful task we can undertake.

There is little evidence on the extent to which GPs record smoking habits, either qualitatively or quantitatively, and none at all on how much time they devote to counselling smokers. Audits of records from 38 practices[11] showed that information on smoking habits over the previous ten years was available in only 23 per cent of sampled medical records for patients aged 20–59. Absence of a written record does not necessarily mean that no advice has been given, but considering the evidence we have had for many years that cigarette smoking is the greatest single avoidable cause of impairment and early death, the extent to which this has penetrated clinical behaviour is astonishingly small.

All these are failures to apply knowledge we already have. I suggest that the principal reasons for this are the ambiguous division of responsibilities between primary and referred care, often leading to lapse from any effective help or supervision, and the reliance of GPs on passive response to individually pressed complaint, rather than active, systematic search and follow up. Neither GPs nor specialists are making and maintaining effective contact with the population at risk.

The shopkeeping inheritance

Like it or not, the working tradition from which general practice stems is the local sick shop, wherein the doctor, thinly disguised as a scientific gentleman, remains a shopkeeper. His contact with the population at risk is limited to occasions of health breakdown. The generally miserable, threadbare 'surgeries', far from inviting customers, silently reproach them for bothering their overworked and under-equipped doctors. All this is the polar opposite of the hard-selling, extravagantly procedural medicine of Continental Europe and the United States, where each consultation and every medical activity (except teaching and listening) sets the till ringing. Clinical activism in Continental Europe and America generates fees; in the UK it generates taxes. Perhaps this underlies our national tradition of sceptical passivity, compared with the uncritical enthusiasm of the world medical market.

We need the scepticism but we should discard the passivity. Medical science, and the clinical medicine derived from it, have not failed: they have simply never been applied rationally. This failure cannot be overcome by putting more people and more money into the social machinery we already have. We need a new kind of doctor, with new functions, within a new structure.

Where we are, and the people we have

Well, where are we, and whom do we have? If we want to control arterial disease, few across-the-board preventive measures are as yet justified on firm present evidence. In order of priority, these are: abolition of cigarette smoking: control of blood pressure sustained 180/105 by drugs, and $\geqslant$160/95 by weight control; maintenance of optimal body weight (metric weight not more than 25 times metric height squared) and, on a nice balance of evidence, physical exercise. Evidence that reduction in dietary animal fat can reduce coronary risk is convincing, but since attainment of ideal weight is rarely sought with a high fat diet, complex dietary advice beyond calorie restriction is probably not an effective additional preventive task. Claims for the effectiveness of small reductions in dietary sodium that might be readily attainable are frankly speculative; present evidence certainly does not justify either mass or personal intervention except on a pilot scale. If we take responsibility for preventive work only of proven value, we shall have our hands full enough, and perhaps avoid the absurd swings of fashion which have discredited doctors' orders in the past.

Any preventive work we do must be added to the ordinary patient-demand facing us each day, which is not only unavoidable, but can also be our chief means of access to the population for preventive and educational work. As health improves, primary consultations contain less gross pathology, and more minor deviations from health. Roughly two-thirds of any population consult a primary doctor at least once a year; this appears to be a constant proportion in industrialized cultures, regardless of care system,[12] and may persist as custom, despite diminishing gross disease. Doctors have a choice of two strategies: to retain the Oslerian model by delegating to intermediate personnel the decision of first contact, so that they can concentrate on the gross pathology appropriate to their skills; or they can retain responsibility for first contact, and accept inevitably increasing minor presenting pathology as a means of contact with people at risk, whose wants are a poor guide to their needs. In this second strategy, paramedical staff would be used to implement the extended, labour-intensive monitoring tasks required for preventive and anticipatory care. GPs and community nurses have authority and accessibility which could make them effective teachers as well as care providers for local populations. By derivation, the word 'doctor' means 'teacher'. The Oslerian doctor is fascinated by the processes but not, as a rule, by the causes of disease; he is bored by health, and communicates with his peers rather than his public. The new doctors we need must reverse each of these features. They must hate the processes of disease, with an informed, precise, and effective hatred, that can motivate large investments of time and work, in organization as well as face-to-face consultation, for small returns.

Rose[13] calculated that, in a screened population aged 35–64, a GP would have to devote 35 patient-years to the control of high blood pressure to prevent one stroke. If that sounds discouraging, try expressing it as the care of 35 patients for one year; either way, it may appear to offer fewer instant satisfactions than the management of acute potentially lethal disease, perhaps because it demands skills that have hitherto had to be self-taught, and leaves unused many of the skills imparted by our present medical schools. But are we not glad to be dealing with a less sick population? Real conservation of health will require more work, more listening and teaching, more patience, more friendliness, more devoted work within communities. These skills and attitudes can be learned and taught, and are beginning to penetrate our medical schools, but they are not central to teaching because they are not imagined as central to the future work of doctors. Simply to make a start, we have most of the health workers we need for mass prevention and anticipatory care already working in the community, but without planning, organization, or encouragement. Community physicians can elaborate strategies to their hearts' content but cannot apply them in combat: and our GPs and community nurses, immersed in lifetimes of exhausting hand-to-hand combat, organize themselves chiefly for coping with demand rather than for altering the content of supply. Between the important strategies of community medicine, and the cynical and exhausted infantry of primary care, stand the hospitals, citadels of Oslerian professionalism, by definition concerned with salvage more than maintenance or prevention. Trained in a hospital ideology unrelated to their needs, and never having worked together, strategists and combatants have little confidence in themselves and less in one another. Both need new ways of thinking which can develop only through new ways of working, requiring not a change of heart, but a change of structure.

A new structure for primary care

The change I propose is to make GP groups responsible for the general public health of their neighbourhoods as well as for personal care. By public health I do not mean environmental control or drains, but the health of the public. The primary care team, as well as retaining responsibility for response to presented symptoms, would be involved in active search for unmet need, in screening for preventable disease, in planning the continuing care of chronic disease, and in both collecting local morbidity, mortality, and risk factor data and making these available in intelligible form to the local population on an annual basis.

The tasks of prevention, data collection, and to a large extent of continuing care of chronic disease, are predictable and limitable, unlike the unplanned response to contingencies hitherto regarded as the main content of the general practice. These tasks could therefore be delegated to an expanded team, including people with social rather than technical skills, as in the present home-help service. Medical care in the community is and will remain labour-intensive. GPs and community nurses know their local populations well, and know where to find unused motivation, integrity and intelligence. To return to anything approaching full employment, our country must create about five million jobs during the next five years. Many of these could be in these expanded primary care teams.

Public investment in general practice implies public accountability. We have to be answerable to someone: why not to our patients?[14] The GP's list consists of names and addresses on a Family Practitioner Committee computer file. It could serve as a list for circulation of an annual report on neighbourhood health, and as a list of voters at an annual patients' meeting. Experience of patient participation groups[15] shows that they release constructive initiative rather than destructive criticism.

Would GPs take up the challenge of neighbourhood public health? If the structure were there, some would and some would not; without it nobody can. We already have a situation in which some practices offer 24-hour care, others do not; some offer comprehensive contraceptive support, others do not; some undertake their own antenatal and well-baby clinics, others do not; some teach, others do not. With realistic payment for time spent, the options are there, and rising public expectations ensure that increasingly they will be adopted. The neighbourhood public health function could be developed in the same way, starting from where we are with the people we have.

Of course there are difficulties. Practices would need to become less dispersed, more neighbourhood-centred; salaried service, though probably not essential, would make it easier to integrate the whole primary care team in these new responsibilities; and the ways in which Community Physicians would relate to the neighbourhood teams could, I suspect, be discovered only in practice. But the important thing is to make a start, with confidence that we are entering times that will become right for a bold turn outward, to a public we have hitherto recognized only as patients, who are our only dependable allies in struggle for a health service capable of implementing medical science on a mass rather than a token scale. Times of crisis become times of legislative change. A century ago we achieved status with one social alliance and the social perceptions it implied: it has impeded medical science ever since. With a different alliance, and a different perception, we could now achieve effectiveness: the choice is ours.

References

1. Kennedy, I. *The Unmasking of Medicine, BBC Reith Lectures, 1980,* Allen & Unwin, London (1981).
2. Cochrane, A. L. *Effectiveness and Efficiency,* Nuffield Provincial Hospitals Trust, London (1971).
3. Cochrane, A. L. *Journal of Epidemiology and Community Health* **32**, 200–205 (1978).
4. Cochrane, A. L. In: *Medicines for the Year 2000,* Teeling-Smith, G. and Wells, N. E. J. (eds), Office of Health Economics, London, pp. 1–11 (1979).
5. McKeown, T. *The Role of Medicine,* Blackwell, Oxford (1979).
6. Powles, J. *Science, Medicine and Man* **1**, 1–30 (1973).

7. Fuchs, V. R. *Who Shall Live?*, Basic Books, New York (1974).
8. Yudkin, J. S., Boucher, B. J., Schopflin, K. E., Harris, B. T., Claff, H. R. *et al. Journal of Epidemiology and Community Health* **34**, 277–280 (1980).
9. Royal College of Physicians *Smoking and Health,* Pitman Medical, London (1977).
10. Medical Research Council Working Party *British Medical Journal* **i**, 1317 (1966).
11. Fleming, D. M. and Laurence, M. S. T. A. *Journal of the Royal College of General Practitioners* **31**, 615–620 (1981).
12. Anderson, O. W. *Health Care: Can there be Equity?* John Wiley, New York (1972).
13. Rose, G. Report to the Department of Health and Social Security of a Working Party on Screening for Hypertension, DHSS, London (1978).
14. Wilson. A. T. M. *British Medical Journal* **i**, 398 (1977).

Julian Tudor Hart is a general practitioner working in a small Welsh community, Glyncorrwg. This article is a substantially edited version of one that appeared in the *Journal of the Royal Society of Medicine* **74**, 871–883 (1981).

3.5

The Economics of Treating Varicose Veins

David Piachaud and Jean M. Weddell

The results at three years after the treatment show no difference between the two methods of treatment. The estimates of costs to the Health Service and the community are greater for surgical treatment than injection-compression scleropathy. On the basis of these results it would benefit the patient, the Health Service and the community if the majority of patients were treated in out-patients by injection-compression scleropathy.

Introduction

At present the treatment of varicose veins is by their removal, either by means of surgery or injection-compression scleropathy; the underlying cause or causes of the development of the condition is not known. The results of treatment are variable, and as the condition is progressive patients may need further treatment. The method of choice should be one that leads to as good clinical results as any other and should be the method most economical of man-power, money and resources.

32.6 beds per million of the population are occupied daily by patients with varicose veins—more than are used for appendicitis.[1] While the mortality of untreated appendicitis is high, the reverse is true of varicose veins. In this condition the mortality is very low, and largely results from the treatment and not from the disease. It is important that the method of treatment should carry a low morbidity and mortality. The combined findings of reported series show that injection-compression scleropathy and surgery carry similar risks, one death in 4,500 after surgery compared with one in 7,000 after injection-compression scleropathy.[2–6]

A randomized controlled trial has been designed to compare the clinical results and cost of routine surgery for varicose veins with injection-compression scleropathy. A total of 339 patients were seen at the varicose vein clinic between February 1967 and February 1968. The patients accepted into the trial were allocated at random to the two forms of treatment, they were under the age of 60, had not previously had treatment for varicose veins and had no medical or social contraindications to treatment by either method. Ninety patients who did not conform to these requirements were excluded (Figure 1).

All patients accepted into the trial were seen by the surgeon and the epidemiologist, a standard questionnaire was administered, and the patient's legs were examined from the front and the back with the patient standing up in a good light.

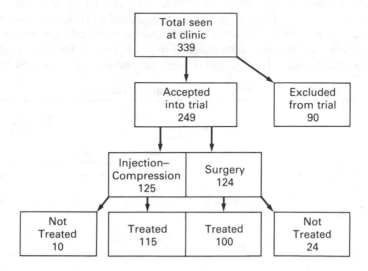

Figure 1

A total of 215 were treated, 47 men and 168 women; 115 had injection-compression scleropathy and 100 had surgery. The men and women in the two groups did not differ significantly in age, height and weight. The parity of the women in the two groups was similar. Thus, any difference found at follow-up is probably due to the treatment given to the patients, and not to any other cause.

The validity of the questionnaire has been established by a series of inter- and intra-observer error studies. These studies showed that 85 per cent or more agreement was reached over age, civil state, height, weight and parity, but that detailed recording of symptoms, the distribution of varicose veins and the skin signs of venous insufficiency were poorly reproducible, agreement being reached in 50 per cent to 70 per cent.

Results

The patients are seen six months, one, two, three, four and five years after treatment. The three-year follow-up is now complete. All the follow-up examinations are carried out by one observer (JMW). At each attendance the address, age, civil state, occupation and, in the case of women, parity are checked; the patients are weighed, they are examined in the same way as at their first attendance, and the symptoms and signs are recorded in a similar manner.

The principal aims of treatment are to relieve symptoms (which include the presence of varicosities), and to treat or prevent oedema, eczema and ulceration. The effectiveness of treatment is estimated by its success or failure in meeting these aims, in terms of the patients' need for further medical care.

The patients have been classified as those who have and have not had any further treatment, in the form of surgery, injection-compression scleropathy therapy or support stocking.

The observer acted as agent for those patients who wished further treatment, and

prescribed support stockings or referred the patient to the surgeon for more active treatment. Some of the surgical incisions were still visible at the time of follow-up, so in some instances the observer knew which form of treatment had been given. While this will not have influenced the classification of patients as improved or those who have had further active treatment, it may have influenced the numbers prescribed support stockings.
Table 1 gives the results of the two methods of treatment used. There is no significant difference at three years between surgery and injection-compression scleropathy.

Table 1 Three-year follow-up, men and women

	Surgery		Injection compression	
	No.	% seen	No.	% seen
No further treatment	77	86	86	78
Prescribed support stockings	10	11	10	9
Given further treatment	3	3	14	13
		% treated		% treated
Total seen	90	90	110	96
Not seen	10	10	5	4
Total treated	100	100	115	100

Thirty-four patients admitted to the trial were not treated. Eight had moved from the area or developed medical contraindications to one form of treatment after their acceptance into the trial and these are not considered further. The other 26 were those who failed to attend for treatment, 18 for surgery and 8 for injection-compression scleropathy. These patients must be considered as needing further treatment, in addition to those who had been given further treatment when they were seen at three years. Thus the total who needed further treatment in the surgical group was 31 and in the injection-compression group was 32, 25 per cent and 27 per cent respectively of the total of those asked to attend for treatment in the two groups.

Immediate Complications

The complications in the injection-compression group were limited to the occasional development of blue staining over the site of injection which has persisted. In addition to this 5 men and 20 women developed superficial phlebitis during the course of treatment; this required no additional treatment other than compression bandaging and walking which was already part of the routine.

Fifteen surgical patients developed complications, mainly stitch abscesses and wound infections, which were treated in out-patients, three developed localized neuritis and phlebitis. Ninety-seven patients in the surgical group made 216 attendances to out-patients after discharge from hospital for removal of stitches and for treatment of local infections.

Discussion of Results

The clinical results show no significant difference between the two forms of treatment. The medical care given in the follow-up period may be influenced by factors other than the clinical condition of the patients. The symptoms complained of at the time of follow-up may be a reflection of the severity of the symptoms or of the patient's temporary need to be ill.[7] Those who wear support stockings may or may not represent the numbers who could get relief in this way from aching, swollen legs. The number of patients given further active treatment will be influenced by their willingness to be referred again to the surgeon, the surgeon's decision to give that patient more treatment, and the acceptance of treatment by the patient. The small numbers of those in the surgical group given further active treatment may reflect the unwillingness of patients or the surgeon to receive or give further treatment, or it may reflect the effectiveness of the original treatment. There are at present no objective measures of the severity of either symptoms or signs, the limitations of the present methods of assessment are considerable and have to be recognized.

Both surgery and injection-compression need considerable care and skill to give good results. Injection-compression scleropathy demands a high level of concentration and application; it is important that all working in such clinics should be very carefully trained and that the clinics be supervised by a senior member of staff.

Costs

The costs of the two forms of treatment, both to the health service and to the patient, will now be compared, and the methods of costing will be discussed. All the costs refer to the period 1967–68 when the trial was conducted. For neither form of treatment was it feasible to estimate the capital cost of the facilities utilized so that the estimates of cost only relate to running costs.

1. Injection-compression treatment

These costs were derived from the costs of each session. The salaries for each of the staff taking part in a typical clinic were assessed. The cleaning, building maintenance and heating were all included under the cost of waiting and treatment rooms and were based on the size of the rooms used for the clinic. The secretarial costs covered the cost of medical records. These patients did not have any other investigations so there are no costs of X-rays, pathology or special investigations such as ECG. The average cost of an outpatient session was £41.50. The average number of patients treated per session was 31; the average number of clinic attendances per patient was 7.3. Thus the average total cost per patient of out-patient injection-compression treatment was £9.77. The break-down of this cost is given in Table 2.

Table 2 Injection-compression treatment

Medical staff	£2.88
Nursing staff	£1.12
Secretarial costs and medical records	£1.04
Cost of rooms	£0.03
Materials for treatment	£4.70
Total	£9.77

2. Surgical treatment

The construction *ab initio* of a complete system to cost the surgical treatment of varicose veins would, if it were to cover the full range of hospital costs, be a vast undertaking. The costs of catering, administration, cleaning, etc., would all have to be measured and a proportion of these costs allocated to varicose vein treatment.

Existing information is, however, quite adequate to estimate most of the costs. The most detailed source of information is the Hospital Costing Return which is prepared for each major hospital; this provides average costs per in-patient week for each of a number of categories of expenditure and unit costs for most of the major departments.

A number of categories of expenditure may be assumed to be 'shared' equally by all in-patients; the cost of these categories to varicose vein cases may be used on the length of stay of varicose vein cases and the average cost per in-patient week for each of these categories of expenditure. The categories of expenditure which may reasonably be assumed to be 'shared', and have been treated in this way are: Domestic Staff, Catering, Staff Residence, Laundry, Power, Light and Heat, Building and Engineering Maintenance, General Administration, General Portering, General Cleaning, Maintenance of Grounds, Transport, Other Services (e.g. staff uniform, cleaning materials), Equipment. The inclusion of the last category—equipment—needs some explanation; while certain items of equipment may rarely, or never, be used on varicose vein patients, it is virtually impossible to say that certain items of equipment are essential for varicose vein patients and that others are not, given the countless contingencies for which a hospital must be prepared. Further, the use of an operating theatre for varicose vein surgery precludes its use for other types of surgery and therefore any equipment primarily for these other types of surgery must necessarily lie idle.

The sum of these 'shared costs' was £29.09 per in-patient week or £15.38 for the average varicose vein patients' stay of 3.7 days.

The cost of nursing and medical staff cannot be assumed to be shared equally by all patients.

On the basis of a small survey of nurses it was estimated that one-quarter of all nursing time (including nursing administrators) was spent on 'general' activities (meals, washing, ward notes, etc.). It was estimated that the time spent on particular nursing activities associated with varicose vein patients averaged $1\frac{1}{2}$ hours during the in-patient stay; in addition approximately half an hour of nursing time was required for out-patient attendances subsequent to discharge. The cost of this particular nursing was therefore some £0.70 per patient; the 'general' nursing for 3.7 days cost £1.32 per patient making a total nursing cost of £2.02 per patient.

A similar method was used to esimate the medical staff cost. About one-eighth of medical staff time was spent on general activities (administration, ward rounds, etc.); for 3.7 days this gives a cost of £0.51. The number of medical staff hours devoted particularly to varicose vein patients averaged one hour per patient at a cost of some £1.50. This gives a total medical staff cost of £2.01 per patient.

The average cost per operation for the use of the operating theatre (drugs, dressings, equipment and staff employed on theatre duties, etc.) was £13.71. A large proportion of the costs of operations are common to all types of operation: for example the costs of preparing the patient, of the recovery room and of theatre cleaning do not differ substantially between operations. The average cost per operation is a reasonable approximation for the cost of varicose vein operation.

The total cost of in-patient surgical treatment was estimated to be £44.22 on the basis of the methods and assumptions described. The breakdown of this cost is shown in Table 3.

3. Costs to patients

A follow-up survey of patients normally in full-time employment who received surgical and injection-compression treatment was conducted including 35 of those treated surgically and 38 treated by injection-compression. The mean number of days taken off work

Table 3 Surgical treatment

Average cost per patient treated	
'Shared' costs	£15.38
Medical staff	£2.02
Nursing staff	£2.02
Operating theatre	£13.71
Pathology	£1.19
X-ray	£5.80
Drugs and pharmacy	£0.26
Dressings	£1.08
Medical records	£2.76
Total	£44.22

at the time of treatment and for convalescence was 6.4 days for those treated by injection-compression, compared with 31.3 days for those treated surgically.

To assess the economic effects on patients—and thus the community—the loss of earnings has been calculated for those receiving surgical treatment and those receiving injection-compression treatment on the basis of the number of days off work and average earnings taking account of differences in earnings between men and women and manual and non-manual occupations.

The average loss of earnings of those in full-time employment receiving surgical treatment was £118 and of those receiving injection-compression treatment was £29. Injection-compression treatment therefore saved £89 per patient in lost earnings compared with surgical treatment.

Those patients who had surgery spent a mean of 3.7 days in hospital; after discharge these patients made a mean of 2.2 out-patient attendances for the removal of sutures, and the renewal of dressings and pressure bandages. The patients in the injection-compression scleropathy group attended the clinic on average seven times; at the most the patients could spend two hours at the clinic. If two hours is allowed for travelling time, then injection-compression scleropathy would involve a maximum of 30 hours of the patient's time, compared with 100 hours taken up by surgery.

Discussion of Costs

On the basis of the most realistic assumptions possible, the cost of injection-compression treatment was found to be slightly less than £10 per case and of surgical treatment £44 per case.

The two principal determinants of the cost of in-patient surgical treatment were the length of stay and, as already mentioned, the cost of the operation. It is interesting to consider how the cost would have been affected by a shorter stay or if the treatment had been performed outside a large district general hospital.

The 'shared' costs based on length of stay were the largest item in the in-patient costs—£15.38. The mean length of stay of 3.7 days for the patients in this study was very much less than the mean national length of stay for varicose vein cases of 11.7 days which ranges between regions from 7.5 to 15.7 days;[1] the 'shared' costs in this study are thus well below the national average. The length of stay might, however, be reduced. If varicose vein patients were admitted to a day ward for surgery this would reduce the total 'shared' costs for surgery by over two-thirds to about £5. The 'shared' costs could be further reduced if the patient was admitted to a typical cottage hospital, where the cost for 3.7 days would be about £9 and for one day would be £2.50. A day admission would also lead to small reductions in the nursing and medical costs, possibly of up to £1. Notwithstanding, the cost of the injection-compression treatment is lower than the hypothetical minimum cost of surgical treatment.

In costing the two treatments no attempt was made to estimate the capital cost of the buildings and equipment utilized. The major obstacle was the virtual impossibility of identifying that proportion of the total hospital facilities which were necessary for surgical treatment.

No estimates are available of the national cost of in-patient treatment of varicose vein cases but it might reasonably be assumed that the substitution of injection-compression scleropathy would reduce the average cost of treatment by about £35. The total annual saving to the Health Service resulting from replacing surgical treatment by injection-compression would be well over £1 million per annum.

Costs to the community have been calculated on the basis of the loss of earnings of those in full-time employment. These results make no attempt at a complete assessment of loss of income of those normally in full-time employment, as no account has been taken of sickness benefits, pensions or other sources of income. In this series, 73 out of 215 were in full-time employment—only 34 per cent of the total treated.

The most serious omission in calculating the costs to the community in the manner described is that it fails to take account of those not employed but who are nevertheless productive and provide valuable services, the most obvious example being, of course, housewives. No attempt is made here to place a value on such services but an indication of the comparative cost to the community of the two treatments in terms of the loss of these services may be obtained from the length of time each treatment took. It was estimated that injection-compression treatment would involve a maximum of 30 hours of the patient's time (including travelling time), compared with 100 hours for surgery. It seems reasonable to assume that housewives and mothers—the majority of all patients—find seven out-patient attendances each taking at most four hours of their time more acceptable than the reorganization of the household that is necessary for admission to hospital that will probably last three or four days, but may last longer. Thus it is clear that injection-compression treatment involves substantially lower costs to the community than surgical treatment.

References

1. Ministry of Health and General Register Office: Report on Hospital In-Patient Enquiry for the Year 1966. Part 1. Tables. London, H.M.S.O., 1968.
2. Payne, R. T. 'The ambulatory treatment of varicose veins. Reactions, complications and results', Lancet, 1, 240 (1928).
3. Sigg, K. 'The treatment of varicosities and accompanying complications', Angiology, 3, 355 (1952).
4. Saarenmaa, E. 'Varices of the lower limbs', Acta Chir. Scand. 125, 411 (1963).
5. Natali, J. 'Surgical treatment of varices: Enquiry into 87,000 cases', J. Cardiovasc. Surg. (Torino), 5, 713, (1964).
6. Jones, H. O., Townsend, J. C., and Roberts, J. T. 'Varicose veins, oral contraceptives, and thromboembolism', Brit. Med. J., 2, 637 (1967).
7. Holmes, J. 'Varicose veins, an optional illness', Practitioner, 204, 549 (1970).

Postscript

Varicose Veins: A Comparison of Surgery and Injection/Compression Scleropathy

Five-year Follow-up
S. A. A. Beresford, A. D. B. Chant, H. O. Jones, and D. Piachaud
*Department of Social Science and Administration, London School of Economics
and Political Science*
J. M. Weddell
*Department of Community Medicine, St Thomas' Hospital Medical School,
London SE1 7EH*

Summary: A randomised controlled trial was carried out to compare the clinical outcome 5 years after inpatient surgery and outpatient injection/compression scleropathy. 91.3% of patients originally treated by injection/compression scleropathy and 93.9% of those originally treated surgically were seen at follow-up. 40% of patients treated initially by injection/compression scleropathy and 24.2% of those treated surgically were given further treatment. The probability of having no further treatment is significantly greater for those treated surgically. The improved outcome after surgery increased with age, being most striking in those aged over 45.

David Piachaud is a social policy analyst working in the Department of Social Science and Administration, London School of Economics and Political Science. Jean Weddell is a specialist in community medicine with the North-West Thames Regional Health Authority (though at the time of this paper was in the Department of Community Medicine, St Thomas' Medical School). This article is an edited version of one that appeared in the *International Journal of Epidemiology*, 1 (3), 287–294 (1972).

3.6

Ethical Dilemmas in Evaluation—A Correspondence

The following (edited) article appeared in *The Lancet* on 16 February 1980.

Possible Prevention of Neural-tube Defects by Periconceptional Vitamin Supplementation

R. W. Smithells, S. Sheppard, and C. J. Schorah
Department of Paediatrics and Child Health, University of Leeds

M. J. Seller
Paediatric Research Unit, Guy's Hospital, London

N. C. Nevin
Department of Medical Genetics, Queen's University of Belfast

R. Harris, and A. P. Read
Department of Medical Genetics, University of Manchester

D. W. Fielding
Department of Paediatrics, Chester Hospitals

Summary
Women who had previously given birth to one or more infants with a neural-tube defect (NTD) were recruited into a trial of periconceptional multivitamin supplementation. One of 178 infants/fetuses of fully supplemented mothers (0.6 per cent) had an NTD, compared with 13 of 260 infants/fetuses of unsupplemented mothers (5.0 per cent).

Introduction
The well-known social-class gradient in the incidence of neural-tube defects (NTD) suggests that nutritional factors might be involved in NTD aetiology. A possible link between folate deficiency and NTDs in man was first reported in 1965.[1] More recently, significant social-class differences in dietary intakes in the first trimester,[2] and in first-trimester values for red cell folate, leucocyte ascorbic acid, red-blood-cell riboflavin, and serum vitamin A have been reported,[3] dietary and biochemical values being higher in classes I and II than in classes III, IV, and V. Furthermore, seven mothers, of whom six subsequently gave birth to NTD infants and one to an infant with unexplained microcephaly, had first-trimester mean values for red cell folate and leucocyte ascorbic acid that were significantly lower than those of controls.

These observations are compatible with the hypothesis that subclinical deficiencies of one or more vitamins contribute to the causation of NTDs. We report preliminary results of an intervention study in which mothers at increased risk of having NTD infants were offered periconceptional multivitamin supplements.

Patients and Methods
Women who had one or more NTD infants, were planning a further pregnancy, but were not yet pregnant were admitted to the study. All women referred to the departments involved in the study and who met these criteria were invited to take part. Patients came from Northern Ireland, South-East England, Yorkshire, Lancashire, and Cheshire. One hundred and eighty-five women who received full vitamin supplementation (see below) became pregnant.

The control group comprised women who had had one or more previous NTD infants but were either pregnant when referred to the study centres or declined to take part in the study. Some centres were able to select a control for each supplemented mother, matched for the number of previous NTD births, the estimated date of conception, and, where possible, age. There were 264 control mothers. The numbers of fully supplemented (S) and control (C) mothers in each centre were as follows: Northern Ireland S 37, C 122; South-East England S 70, C 70; Yorkshire S 38, C 35; Lancashire S 31, C 27; Cheshire S 9, C 10.

All mothers in supplemented and control groups were offered amniocentesis. Six mothers in Northern Ireland (three supplemented; three controls) declined amniocentesis and their pregnancies continue. They are not included in the figures above or in the accompanying table. All mothers with raised amniotic-fluid alpha-fetoprotein (AFP) values (one supplemented, eleven controls) accepted termination of pregnancy

Study mothers were given a multivitamin and iron preparation ('Pregnavite Forte F' Bencard), one tablet three times a day for not less than twenty-eight days before conception and continuing at least until the date of the second missed period, i.e. until well after the time of neural-tube closure.

Results
One hundred and eighty-seven control mothers have delivered 192 infants (including five twin pairs) without NTDs, and a further thirty-eight have normal amniotic-fluid AFP values (table). Thirteen mothers have been delivered of NTD infants/fetuses. Seventeen fetuses of a further twenty-six control mothers who aborted spontaneously were examined and had no NTD. The provisional recurrence-rate of NTDs is 5.0 per cent (13 in 260), consistent with those previously reported and widely adopted in genetic counselling.

One hundred and thirty-seven fully supplemented mothers have given birth to 140 babies (including three twin pairs) without NTD, twenty-six have normal amniotic-fluid AFP values and their pregnancies continue, and one has had a further affected infant. Eleven fetuses of twenty-one mothers who aborted spontaneously were examined; none had an NTD. The provisional recurrence-rate in the supplemented group is therefore 0.6 per cent (1 in 178).

Comparison of NTD frequencies in the supplemented and control groups by Fisher's exact test showed significant differences ($p<0.01$) for subtotals (1), (2), and (3) (table).

Discussion
Despite problems with choosing controls, the control women in this study have shown recurrence-rates for NTDs entirely consistent with published data. By contrast the supplemented mothers had a significantly lower recurrence-rate. Possible interpretations of this observation include the following:

Outcome of pregnancy in fully supplemented and control mothers

	Fully supplemented	Controls
Infant/fetus with NTD	1	12
Infant without NTD	140(3)	192(5)
Subtotal (1)	141(3)	204(5)
Normal amniotic AFP	26	38
Subtotal (2)	167(3)	242(5)
Spontaneous abortions		
Examined, NTD	0	1
Examined, no NTD	11	17
Subtotal (3)	178(3)	260(5)
Not examined	10	9
Total	188(3)	269(5)

All numbers relate to infants/fetuses.
Figures in parentheses indicate numbers of twin pairs included.

(1) *A group of women with a naturally low recurrence risk has unwittingly selected itself for supplementation.* Apart from geographic and secular variations there is no evidence to suggest that any particular sub-group within populations, whether by social class or any other division, has a higher or lower recurrence risk. In genetic counselling clinics it is customary to quote the same risk for all mothers after one affected child. We cannot exclude the possibility that women who volunteered and cooperated in the trial might have had a reduced risk of recurrence of NTD.

(2) *Supplemented mothers aborted more NTD fetuses than did controls.* The proportion of pregnancies ending in spontaneous abortion is similar in the two groups (supplemented 11.4 per cent, control 9.6 per cent). If the supplemented mothers have aborted more NTD fetuses, they must have aborted fewer other fetuses or had a lower initial risk of abortion. Eleven of twenty-one abortuses of supplemented mothers have been examined and none had an NTD. Eighteen of twenty-seven had an NTD. An explanation based on selective abortion of fetuses with NTD seems improbable.

(3) *Something other than vitamin supplementation has reduced the incidence of NTDs in the treated group.* This is an almost untestable hypothesis, but if anything has reduced the incidence of NTDs it needs to be identified urgently.

(4) *Vitamin supplementation has prevented some NTD.* This is the most straightforward interpretation and is consistent with the circumstantial evidence linking nutrition with NTDs. If the vitamin tablets are directly responsible, we cannot tell from this study whether they operate via a nutritional or a placebo effect.

We hope that the data presented will encourage others to initiate similar and related studies.

References

1. Hibbard, E. D. and Smithells, R. W. 'Folic acid metabolism and human embryopathy', *Lancet*, i, 1254–56 (1965).
2. Smithells, R. W., Ankers, C., Carver, M. E., Lennon, D., Schorah, C. J. and Sheppard, S. 'Maternal nutrition in early pregnancy', *Br. J. Nutr.* 38, 497–506 (1977).

3. Smithells, R. W., Sheppard, S. and Schorah, C. J. 'Vitamin deficiencies and neural tube defects', *Arch. Dis. Childh.* **51**, 944–50 (1976).

The following letters appeared in *The Lancet* on 22 March 1980.

Possible Prevention of Neural-Tube Defects by Periconceptional Vitamin Supplementation

Sir, Professor Smithells and others believe they have observed a preventive effect of periconceptional vitamin supplementation on the recurrence of neural-tube defect (NTD). Their conclusions are based on the observation that the incidence of NTD in 185 fully supplemented women was significantly lower than that in 264 unsupplemented or control women.

Such an interpretation of the data rests upon the assumption that both the supplemented and the control women were, initially, at equal risk of conceiving a further affected fetus. A geographical analysis of the total sample shows that this was probably not so. In the accompanying table the study subjects are characterised as falling into one of two groups—a 'relatively high risk' group, residing in Northern Ireland, Lancashire, and Cheshire; and a 'relatively low risk' group residing in south-east England and Yorkshire. (The varying geographical risk of NTD is well established.) It is clear that the supplemented sample is as heavily biased towards 'relatively low risk' areas as the control sample is towards 'relatively high risk' areas. The higher incidence of recurrent NTD in the control group is therefore hardly surprising.

Geographical distribution of supplemented and control mothers

	Relatively high risk areas No. (%)	Relatively low risk areas No. (%)	Total No. (%)
Supplemented mothers	77 (41.6)	108 (58.4)	185 (100)
Control mothers	159 (60.2)	105 (39.8)	264 (100

Why, I wonder, did Professor Smithells and his co-workers not evaluate their interesting hypothesis by means of a randomised controlled trial, which would have been eminently practicable, would have minimised selection bias, and would have been more likely to convince the sceptics?

University of Glasgow
Social Paediatric and
Obstetric Research Unit,
Glasgow   David H. Stone

Sir, with the wisdom of hindsight, we should have stated in our preliminary communication that our original intention had been a double-blind controlled study for which placebo tablets had already been prepared, but that the protocol was rejected by three separate hospital research ethics committees, and we had to resort to a less satisfactory design.

The number of fully supplemented (S) and 'control' mothers (C) was almost identical in all centres except Northern Ireland which had an excess of controls (Northern Ireland S 37, C 122; S-E England S 70, C 70; Yorkshire S 38, C 35; Lancashire S 31, C 27; Cheshire S 9, C 10). The recurrence rate of NTDs in the controls was in keeping with earlier reports. The excess of controls in Northern Ireland does not alter the fact that there was only one recurrence among the progeny of 185 fully supplemented mothers.

The geographical variation in the *incidence* of NTD is well recognised. What is relevant to our study is geographical variation in *recurrence* rate, about which little is known.

Dr Stone makes reference to what we 'believe', to our 'conclusions', and to 'an interpretation'. In our paper we subscribe to no belief, reach no conclusions, and offer four possible interpretations, of which the first covers the point Dr Stone raises.

We are not trying 'to convince the sceptics', among whom we count ourselves. We present some observations (which will be fully detailed in a later paper) and would welcome further studies to assist in their interpretation.

R. W. Smithells, S. Sheppard

Sir, Professor Smithells and his colleagues have opened the next chapter in the saga of neural-tube defects. Since a deficiency of some nutrient has been proposed as the source of nearly every ailment since antiquity, why not propose another? An unfortunate effect of this form of communication is that women will be induced to self-administer large quantities of vitamins, some of which may be teratogenic. I hope that future studies will incorporate properly selected controls treated with placebos and that nutritional assessment of the mother, before and during therapy, will be done.

Department of Pediatrics,
Emory University School of Medicine,
Atlanta, Georgia   Paul M. Fernhoff

The following extract is from an editorial which appeared in *The Lancet* on 17 May 1980.

Vitamins, Neural-tube Defects and Ethics Committees

Some years ago Renwick[1] suggested that a specific teratogen present in blighted potatoes might be the causal agent. The plausibility of Renwick's hypothesis did draw attention to the possibility of maternal nutritional factors in the aetiology of neural-tube defects. An investigation reported in *The Lancet* in February suggests that subclinical maternal vitamin deficiency may be one of these factors.

At a time when the reduction in birth incidence of neural-tube defects rests largely on alpha-fetoprotein screening and selective abortion, this is an exciting finding. However, the study by Smithells *et al.* depends critically on the assumption that the vitamin-supplemented group and their controls were equally at risk of conceiving a further affected fetus. On this point there must be some doubt.

The vitamin-supplemented group were recruited on the basis of their ability to adhere to a fairly stringent regimen of tablet-taking while the controls were those who could not or would not adhere to the required protocol. Thus, selection was based on self-motivation and self-discipline, and one suspects that such women will have better-than-average outcome of pregnancy. A randomised control trial would have been more appropriate. But, as Professor Smithells[2] explains, such a study was proposed by the investigators and rejected by three separate hospital research ethics committees. As a result a far less satisfactory design was chosen.

How much does this matter? The results achieved by Smithells *et al.* are so striking that they provide a strong argument for the immediate vitamin supplementation of all mothers who are at risk of bearing a child with a neural-tube defect. If vitamins were completely harmless one could perhaps extend this argument to all mothers. But already there is evidence that at least one of the components of the multivitamin preparation, vitamin A, is a teratogen in rodents.[3,4] Doctors are thus faced with a dilemma; if they ignore the results of the Smithells study they may be allowing the conception of infants with neural-tube defects whose malformations might have been prevented. If they advise vitamin supplementation to all would-be mothers they may be contributing to the induction of a different range of congenital abnormalities whose appearance may not be recognised for some time.

The problem would probably be best resolved by a large randomised controlled trial on a general population of mothers, with vitamins being administered to one group and placebos to the other. But if this design has already been rejected by an ethics committee, it is even less likely to be acceptable now that the results of the Smithells trial are known. This raises the question of accountability. Research workers are quite properly called upon to explain and justify any investigation involving patients, both directly to an ethics committee and indirectly in the publication of their results. Ethics committees are less subject to scrutiny. They may explain their decision to individual workers, but many researchers find these arbitrary and lacking the coherence necessary to stand up to public examination. Perhaps the time has come to devise a system for making those ubiquitous committees more accountable.

References

1. Renwick, J. H. 'Anencephaly and spina bifida are usually preventable by avoidance of a specific unidentified substance present in certain potato tubers', *Br. J. Prev. Soc. Med.*, **26**, 67–88 (1972).
2. Smithells, R. W. and Sheppard S. 'Possible prevention of neural tube defects by periconceptional vitamin supplementation', *Lancet*, **i**, 647 (1980).
3. Seller, M. J., Embury, S., Polani, P. F. and Adinolphi, M. 'Neural tube defects in curly-tail mice. II Effect of maternal administration of vitamin', *Proc. Roy. Soc. Lond. B.*, **206**, 95–107 (1979).
4. Nakamura, H. 'Digital anomalies in the embryonic mouse limb cultured in the presence of excess vitamin A', *Teratology*, **14**, 195–202 (1977).

The following letter appeared in *The Lancet* on 14 June 1980.

Vitamins, Neural Tube Defects, and Ethics Committees

Sir, As a result of the study by Professor Smithells and his colleagues there is now a suggestion that periconceptional multivitamin supplementation may reduce the incidence of fetal neural tube defect (NTD). This possibility is of great interest in Ireland where the incidence of NTD is high.

Some of the shortcomings of the research design used by Smithells *et al.* have been discussed in your editorial and in your correspondence columns. The essential problem is the lack of comparability of the supplemented and non-supplemented mothers: we do not know whether the favourable outcome in the fully supplemented mothers is greater than might be expected for such a highly selected group.

You emphasise, as do your correspondents, the need for a randomised controlled trial but suggest that such a design is even less likely to be acceptable to research ethics committees now in the light of the Smithells study. If this is so, then it is a matter for concern. Perhaps the most serious consequence of not testing this hypothesis with the most appropriate research design is the possibility that millions of mothers-to-be may take multivitamin preparations around the time of conception in the as yet unproven belief that to do so significantly reduces the risk of having a baby with NTD. Furthermore there is the important question of possible teratogenic effects. How certain are we that the ingestion by mothers of considerable qualities of this multivitamin, iron, and calcium preparation ('Pregnative Forte F') during the period of most rapid fetal organogenesis is safe? By rejecting randomised controlled trials, ethics committees are sanctioning what amounts to a situation of uncontrolled experimentation on mothers and their babies. In so doing can they be said to be carrying out their function of protecting the welfare of patients?

The weight of medical scientific opinion is that only a large randomised controlled trial will permit us to say with confidence whether periconceptional multivitamin supplementation reduces the incidence of NTD, and whether such regimes are free from teratogenic effects. Our professional duty would seem to be clear—to conduct such a trial as soon as possible.

Medico-Social Research Board,
Dublin, Ireland   Peadar N. Kirke

The following (edited) article appeared in *British Medical Journal* on 9 May 1981.

Double-blind randomised controlled trial of folate treatment before conception to prevent recurrence of neural-tube defects

Department of Child Health, Welsh National School of Medicine, Cardiff CF4 4XN
K. M. Laurence, DSC, FRCP(E), professor of paediatric research and clinical geneticist
Nansi James, MB, MRCP, fieldworker
Mary H. Miller, MB, DCH, fieldworker
Department of Haematology, Welsh National School of Medicine
G. B. Tennant, MSC, senior scientific officer
Department of Medical Stastistics, Welsh National School of Medicine
H. Campbell, FRCP, FRSS, professor

Abstract
A randomised controlled double-blind trial was undertaken in South Wales to prevent the recurrence of neural-tube defects in women who had had one child with a neural-tube

defect. Sixty women were allocated before conception to take 4 mg of folic acid a day before and during early pregnancy and 44 complied with these instructions. Fifty-one women were allocated to placebo treatment. There were no recurrences among the compliant mothers but two among the non-compliers and four among the women in the placebo group. Thus there were no recurrences among those who received supplementation and six among those who did not; this difference is significant (p=0.04).

It is concluded that folic acid supplementation might be a cheap, safe, and effective method of primary prevention of neural-tube defects but that this must be confirmed in a large, multicentre trial.

Subjects and methods
Women resident in Glamorgan and Gwent who had had a pregnancy complicated by a fetal neural-tube defect (anencephaly, encephalocele, and spina bifida cystica) between 1954 and 1969 were traced. Those under 35 years of age at the time of study were visited in their homes by medically qualified fieldworkers.

During the home visit a questionnaire was completed giving details of the women's diet during the interpregnancy period and during her previous pregnancies. A simple diet sheet was used that provided a general pattern for meals and a check list showing the amount of food consumed during the average week and listing first-class proteins, dairy products, fresh vegetables and salads, cereals, and refined carbohydrates, paying special attention to those items rich in folic acid. Diets were judged as good, fair, or inadequate, those that were poor or fair but deranged by an excessive amount of fat and refined carbohydrates being judged as inadequate.[1] A sample of blood was taken from all women who were planning to have further children for estimation of serum and red-cell folic acid concentrations. Those willing to cooperate were asked to take twice a day a tablet containing either 2 mg of folic acid or placebo starting from the time contraceptive precautions were stopped. Women were allocated to receive treatment or placebo by random numbers and did not know the content of the tablets; we were also unaware of the treatment prescribed. Women were instructed to report to us within six weeks of a missed period and were revisited as soon as possible thereafter. Inquiries were made about the quality of the diet during the current pregnancy and about any anorexia or vomiting, drugs, or illness, and a further sample was taken for folate estimation and other investigations. The women were revisited at six months and again at the end of pregnancy, when details of the outcome of the pregnancy were available.

Results
Altogether 905 women who had had a child with a neural-tube defect were seen by the fieldworkers, of whom 111 (12.3 per cent) agreed to take part in the prophylactic randomised controlled trial and achieved a subsequent pregnancy. Of these, 60 had been randomised to receive folate supplementation and 51 placebo.

Compliance in taking the folate tablets was monitored at the sixth to ninth week of estimated gestation; if the serum folate concentration at this stage was higher than 10 μg/l the woman's account of taking the tablets during the earlier part of the pregnancy could be accepted as valid. If the serum folate concentration was below 10 μg/l the woman was classified as a non-complier. None of the placebo group had a serum folate concentration above 12 μg/l. There were 16 non-compliers (27 per cent) among the 60 women allocated to receive folate treatment (Table 1). Compliance was not tested among the controls.

Six pregnancies resulted in a fetus with a neural-tube defect (Table 1): none in the compliers, two in the non-compliers, and four in the placebo group.

Table 2 shows the number of women taking a good, fair, or inadequate diet classified by outcome of pregnancy and whether they had received folate treatment. The proportion of women with inadequate diets was similar in the two treatment groups: 10 out of the 44 compliers and 17 out of the 67 non-compliers and women in the placebo group. All six of the recurrences of fetal neural-tube defects occurred in women taking an inadequate diet.

Table 1 Outcome of pregnancy by treatment group

Outcome of pregnancy	Folate groups		Placebo group
	Compliers	Non-compliers	
Normal fetus	44	14	47
Fetus with neural-tube defect	0	2	4
All cases	44	16	51

Table 2 Numbers of women taking good, fair, or inadequate diets classified according to whether they received folate treatment and whether fetus was normal or had a neural-tube defect

Diet	Received folate		Did not receive folate		All cases
	Normal	Neural-tube defect	Normal	Neural-tube defect	
Good	17	0	26	0	43
Fair	17	0	24	0	41
Inadequate	10	0	11	6	27
All cases	44	0	61	6	111

Table 3 shows the mean red-cell folate concentration in each treatment group by the adequacy of the diet. In each dietary group the compliers had a mean concentration at least twice that in the placebo group, and these differences were significantly different $(p<0.001)$.

Table 3 Mean $\pm$SD red-cell folate concentration (μg/l red blood cells) by treatment group and quality of diet

Diet	Folate groups		Placebo group
	Compliers	Non-compliers	
Good	618±60 (n=17)	277±44 (n=5)	278±25 (n=21)
Fair	847±60 (n=17)	292±23 (n=6)	298±34 (n=18)
Inadequate	761±85 (n=10)	193±34 (n=5)	250±26 (n=12)
All cases	738±42 (n=44)	256±22 (n=16)	278±16 (n=51)

Discussion

None of the 44 women who received treatment had a recurrence, whereas there were six recurrences among 67 untreated cases. The probability of such a distribution, using Fisher's exact test with a single tail, was p=0.04.

The specific effect of folate has to be separated from the non-specific effect of diet. There were no recurrences among the 84 women who received good or fair diets, but there were six recurrences among the 27 women receiving a poor diet (p<0.0001, Fisher's exact test). As we have shown, [2] women who take poor diets are at an extremely high risk of a recurrence of fetal neural-tube defects. Within this high-risk group of women, however, there were no recurrences in the 10 who had taken folate supplementation but six recurrences in the 17 who had not taken supplementation (p=0.04, Fisher's exact test). Thus although there may have been some bias owing to women who were receiving an inadequate diet also failing to comply, yet within this group receiving an inadequate diet the preventive effect could still be detected. We conclude that women receiving a poor diet who are at high risk of a recurrence of fetal neural-tube defects can reduce their risk either by improving their diet or by taking folate supplements.

The use of folate as an effective prophylactic regimen to prevent neural-tube defects in high-risk groups, communities with a high incidence of such defects, or even all women at risk of pregnancy should be further tested in a larger controlled trial conducted at several centres. Such a trial would be ethical as we found a probably biological beneficial effect, but the problem might be to consider an alternative regimen. A placebo could be justified by the argument that it is not normal practice to begin supplementation before conception is confirmed. As a result of the study by Smithells *et al.*[3] Pregnative Forte F without folate would seem to be a suitable alternative. With an expensive blunderbuss preparation of that type, which includes several agents in addition to folate, the specific beneficial agent and the hazards that might arise from the other constituents should be identified.

References

1. Laurence, K. M., James, N., Miller, M. and Campbell, H. 'The increased risk of recurrence of neural tube defect to mothers on poor diets and the possible benefit of dietary counselling', *Br. Med. J.*, **281**, 1542–4, (1980).
2. Tennant, G. B. and Withey, J. L. 'An assessment of work simplified procedures for the microbiological array of serum vitamin B12 and serum folate', *Medical Laboratory Technology*, **29**, 171–81 (1972).
3. Smithells, R. W., Sheppard, S., Schorah, C. J. *et al.* 'Possible prevention of neural tube defects by preconceptional vitamin supplementation', *Lancet*, i, 339–40 (1980).

The following (edited) letter appeared in *British Medical Journal* on 30 May 1981.

Trial of folate treatment to prevent recurrence of neural tube defects

Sir, We have been extremely interested to read the recent papers by Dr K. M. Laurence and others. We are puzzled by their use of the term 'double-blind' in their more recent paper, which can only have applied until six to nine weeks of gestation, when blood folate levels were estimated and 'non-compliers' were identified. The high rate of non-compliance must also have disappointed the authors. We entirely endorse their view that further studies are needed, directed towards the following ends:

(1) To provide further confirmation that vitamin prophylaxis is effective.
(2) To define further the role of folic acid and other vitamins.

(3) To study carefully mothers who are enrolled for supplementation but who comply only in part.

There is considerable urgency. The medical correspondent of *The Times* has advocated (8 May) vitamin supplementation on the basis of our series and those of the Cardiff group. It can no longer be assumed that mothers not given vitamin supplements by research workers necessarily have none. There is also a danger of 'do-it-yourself' supplementation by mothers obtaining over-the-counter vitamin preparations, none of which contains folic acid.

R. W. Smithells
Sheila Sheppard
C. J. Schorah
N. C. Nevin
Mary J. Seller

The following (edited) article appeared in *The Guardian* on 10 December 1982.

Specialists voice fear that some doctors and patients will boycott scheme to test vitamin theory

Women to act as guinea-pigs in spina bifida trials,
by Andrew Veitch

The controversial plan to find out whether vitamin supplements prevent mothers from having spina bifida babies is to go ahead, the Medical Research Council said yesterday. It involves denying the vitamins to hundreds of mothers known to be at risk.

Specialists said yesterday that it might be doomed from the start because not enough women or doctors would volunteer to take part.

The public controversy about the proposals—which reached a peak two weeks ago when the MRC secretary, Sir James Gowans, was accused of suppressing debate—and the mass of evidence of the merits of folic acid which had accumulated in the past two years, meant that few mothers would be prepared to volunteer for a trial in which they faced a one-in-two chance of not having folic acid and a one-in-four chance of receiving no vitamins at all.

Medical teams in Manchester, Leeds and Belfast have declined to take part in the trial. Teams in Liverpool and Chester are thought likely to follow suit. So the area with the highest incidence of spina bifida—the North-west—will not be represented.

Professor Norman Nevin, head of medical genetics at Queen's University Belfast, said that the MRC was not justified in giving some women a placebo. The trial was also condemned yesterday by the National Childbirth Trust. 'It is not ethical to withhold vitamins from some women', said the Trust's secretary, Ms. Hanna Corbishley.

The following (edited) article appeared in *The Guardian* on 13 December 1982.

Wasted years, damaged lives

After two years of dithering the Medical Research Council has finally decided to go ahead with its plan to establish conclusively whether vitamin supplements prevent spina bifida in babies. In view of the large controversy these trials have generated, however, it is hard to see how they can now produce any evidence worth having. Medical teams in Manchester, Leeds and Belfast are refusing to take part, and it seems likely that Liverpool and Chester will follow suit. Moreover, it is hard to see how any woman would want to take part in these trials in the first place. Surely, any woman who has already had a spina bifida baby will reply that if there is even a slim chance that vitamins and folic acid will reduce the likelihood of another damaged child—and such supplements have no known toxic effects—then she would very much like to have them, please, and no, she wouldn't be prepared to run the slightest extra risk.

It is said that the Department of Health is reluctant to fund a national programme of vitamin and folic acid supplements until conclusive proof is provided. This means that, for the next five years, these supplements will not be available automatically to women at risk of producing a spina bifida baby—because of a trial whose conclusions are likely to be as dubious as its ethics.

The following (edited) letter appeared in *The Guardian* on 14 December 1982.

Spina bifida: a new trial

Sir, I oppose the proposed trial both on ethical and practical grounds, and consider that it is unlikely to produce a more conclusive answer than is already available from the admittedly imperfect trials conducted by Professor Smithells and his colleagues.

Nevertheless, the results are so promising that to deprive women of a totally harmless vitamin cocktail seems unethical. I would find it difficult to persuade the mothers of any of my patients to have a placebo, when they could have something which is likely to be helpful.

It is true that we do not know which vitamins, or which combination of them, is likely to decrease the incidence of neural-tube defects, but I see no evidence that folic acid alone has shown itself to be of benefit. The data relating to this are based on very few pregnancies.

There is, however, an alternative and totally ethical way in which the question could be settled without difficulty. It is known that the incidence of neural-tube defects is 5 per cent after the birth of a baby with spina bifida or anencephaly. If, therefore, all women at risk are offered vitamin supplementation starting some three months before pregnancy is contemplated, within a very short time it will be apparent whether vitamin supplementation is helpful or not. It does not really matter which of the vitamins or their combination is helpful.

John Lorber
(Emeritus Professor of Paediatrics), Sheffield

3.7

The Epidemics of Modern Medicine

Ivan Illich

During the past three generations the diseases afflicting Western societies have undergone dramatic changes. Polio, diphtheria, and tuberculosis are vanishing; one shot of an antibiotic often cures pneumonia or syphilis; and so many mass killers have come under control that two-thirds of all deaths are now associated with the diseases of old age. Those who die young are more often than not victims of accidents, violence, or suicide.

These changes in health status are generally equated with a decrease in suffering and attributed to more or to better medical care. Although almost everyone believes that at least one of his friends would not be alive and well except for the skill of a doctor, there is in fact no evidence of any direct relationship between this mutation of sickness and the so-called progress of medicine. The changes are dependent variables of political and technological transformations, which in turn are reflected in what doctors do and say; they are not significantly related to the activities that require the preparation, status, and costly equipment in which the health professions take pride. In addition, an expanding proportion of the *new* burden of disease of the last fifteen years is itself the result of medical intervention in favor of people who are or might become sick. It is doctor-made, or *iatrogenic*.

After a century of pursuit of medical utopia, and contrary to current conventional wisdom, medical services have not been important in producing the changes in life expectancy that have occurred. A vast amount of contemporary clinical care is incidental to the curing of disease, but the damage done by medicine to the health of individuals and populations is very significant. These facts are obvious, well documented, and well repressed.

Doctors' Effectiveness—An Illusion

The study of the evolution of disease patterns provides evidence that during the last century doctors have affected epidemics no more profoundly than did priests during earlier times. Epidemics came and went, imprecated by both but touched by neither. They are not modified any more decisively by the rituals performed in medical clinics than by those customary at religious shrines. Discussion of the future of health care might usefully begin with the recognition of this fact.

The infections that prevailed at the outset of the industrial age illustrate how medicine came by its reputation. Tuberculosis, for instance, reached a peak over two generations. In New York in 1812, the death rate was estimated to be higher than 700 per 10,000; by 1882, when Koch first isolated and cultured the bacillus, it had already declined to 370 per 10,000. The rate was down to 180 when the first sanatorium was opened in 1910, even though 'consumption' still held second place in the mortality tables. After World War II, but before antibiotics became routine, it had slipped into eleventh place with a rate of 48. Cholera, dysentry, and typhoid similarly peaked and dwindled outside the physician's control. By the time their etiology was understood and their therapy had become specific, these diseases had lost much of their virulence and hence their social importance. The combined death rate from scarlet fever, diphtheria, whooping cough, and measles among children up to fifteen shows that nearly 90 per cent of the total decline in mortality between 1860 and 1965 had occurred before the introduction of antibiotics and widespread immunization. In part this recession may be attributed to improved housing and to a decrease in the virulence of micro-organisms, but by far the most important factor was a higher host-resistance due to better nutrition. In poor countries today, diarrhoea and upper-respiratory tract infections occur more frequently, last longer, and lead to higher mortality where nutrition is poor, no matter how much or how little medical care is available. In England, by the middle of the nineteenth century, infectious epidemics had been replaced by major malnutrition syndromes, such as rickets and pellagra. These in turn peaked and vanished, to be replaced by the diseases of early childhood and, somewhat later, by an increase in duodenal ulcers in young men. When these declined, the modern epidemics took over: coronary heart disease, emphysema, bronchitis, obesity, hypertension, cancer (especially of the lungs), arthritis, diabetes, and so-called mental disorders. Despite intensive research, we have no complete explanation for the genesis of these changes. But two things are certain: the professional practice of physicians cannot be credited with the elimination of old forms of mortality or morbidity, nor should it be blamed for the increased expectancy of life spent in suffering from the new diseases. For more than a century, analysis of disease trends has shown that the environment is the primary determinant of the state of general health of any population. Medical geography, the history of diseases, medical anthropology, and the social history of attitudes towards illness have shown that food, water, and air, in correlation with the level of sociopolitical equality and the cultural mechanisms that make it possible to keep the population stable, play the decisive role in determining how healthy grown-ups feel and at what age adults tend to die. As the older causes of disease recede, a new kind of malnutrition is becoming the most rapidly expanding modern epidemic. One-third of humanity survives on a level of undernourishment which would formerly have been lethal, while more and more rich people absorb ever greater amounts of poisons and mutagens in their food.

Some modern techniques, often developed with the help of doctors, and optimally effective when they become part of the culture and environment or when they are applied independently of professional delivery, have also effected changes in general health, but to a lesser degree. Among these can be included contraception, smallpox vaccination of infants, and such nonmedical health measures as the treatment of water and sewage, the use of soap and scissors by midwives, and some antibacterial and insecticidal procedures. The importance of many of these practices was first recognized and stated by doctors— often courageous dissidents who suffered for their recommendations—but does not consign soap, pincers, vaccination needles, delousing preparations, or condoms to the category of 'medical equipment'. The most recent shifts in mortality from younger to older groups can be explained by the incorporation of these procedures and devices into the layman's culture.

In contrast to environmental improvements and modern nonprofessional health measures, the specifically medical treatment of people is never significantly related to a decline in the compound disease burden or to a rise in life expectancy. Neither the proportion of doctors in a population nor the clinical tools at their disposal nor the number of hospital beds is a causal factor in the striking changes in over-all patterns of disease. The new techniques for recognizing and treating such conditions as pernicious anemia and hypertension, or for correcting congenital malformations by surgical intervention, redefine but do not reduce morbidity. The fact that the doctor population is higher where certain diseases have become rare has little to do with the doctors' ability to control or eliminate them. It simply means that doctors deploy themselves as they like, more so than other professionals, and that they tend to gather where the climate is healthy, where the water is clean, and where people are employed and can pay for their services.

Useless Medical Treatment

Awe-inspiring medical technology has combined with egalitarian rhetoric to create the impression that contemporary medicine is highly effective. Undoubtedly, during the last generation, a limited number of specific procedures have become extremely useful. But where they are not monopolized by professionals as tools of their trade, those which are applicable to widespread diseases are usually very inexpensive and require a minimum of personal skills, materials and custodial services from hospitals. In contrast, most of today's skyrocketing medical expenditures are destined for the kind of diagnosis and treatment whose effectiveness at best is doubtful. To make this point I will distinguish between infectious and noninfectious diseases.

In the case of infectious diseases, chemotherapy has played a significant role in the control of pneumonia, gonorrhea, and syphilis. Death from pneumonia, once the 'old man's friend', declined yearly by 5 to 8 per cent after sulphonamides and antibiotics came on the market. Syphilis, yaws, and many cases of malaria and typhoid can be cured quickly and easily. The rising rate of venereal disease is due to new mores, not to ineffectual medicine. The reappearance of malaria is due to the development of pesticide-resistant mosquitoes and not to any lack of new antimalarial drugs. Immunization has almost wiped out paralytic poliomyelitis, a disease of developed countries, and vaccines have certainly contributed to the decline of whooping cough and measles, thus seeming to confirm the popular belief in 'medical progress'. But for most other infections, medicine can show no comparable results. Drug treatment has helped to reduce mortality from tuberculosis, tetanus, diphtheria, and scarlet fever, but in the total decline of mortality or morbidity from these diseases, chemotherapy played a minor and possibly insignificant role. Malaria, leishmaniasis, and sleeping sickness indeed receded for a time under the onslaught of chemical attack, but are now on the rise again.

The effectiveness of medical intervention in combatting noninfectious diseases is even more questionable. In some situations and for some conditions, effective progress has indeed been demonstrated: the partial prevention of caries through fluoridation of water is possible, though at a cost not fully understood. Replacement therapy lessens the direct impact of diabetes, though only in the short run. Through intravenous feeding, blood transfusions, and surgical techniques, more of those who get to the hospital survive trauma, but survival rates for the most common types of cancer—those which make up 90 per cent of the cases—have remained virtually unchanged over the last twenty-five years. This fact has consistently been clouded by announcements from the American Cancer Society reminiscent of General Westmoreland's proclamations from Vietnam. On the other hand, the diagnostic value of the Papanicolaou vaginal smear test has been proved: if the tests are given four times a year, early intervention for cervical cancer demonstrably increases the five-year survival rate. Some skin-cancer treatment is highly effective. But there is little evidence of effective treatment of most other cancers. The five year survival rate in breast-cancer cases is 50 per cent, regardless of the frequency of medical check-ups and regardless of the treatment used. Nor is there evidence that the rate differs from that among untreated women. Although practicing doctors and the publicists of the medical establishment stress the importance of early detection and treatment of this and several other types of cancer, epidemiologists have begun to doubt that early intervention can alter the rate of survival. Surgery and chemotherapy for rare congenital and rheumatic heart disease have increased the chances for an active life for some of those who suffer from degenerative conditions. The medical treatment of common cardiovascular disease and the intensive treatment of heart disease, however, are effective only when rather exceptional circumstances combine that are outside the physician's control. The drug treatment of high blood pressure is effective and warrants the risk of side-effects in the few in whom it is a malignant condition; it represents a considerable risk of serious harm, far outweighing any proven benefit, for the 10 or 20 million Americans on whom rash artery-plumbers are trying to foist it.

Doctor-Inflicted Injuries

Unfortunately, futile but otherwise harmless medical care is the least important of the damages a proliferating medical enterprise inflicts on contemporary society. The pain, dysfunction, disability, and anguish resulting from technical medical intervention now rival the morbidity due to traffic and industrial accidents and even war-related activities, and make the impact of medicine one of the most rapidly spreading epidemics of our time. Among murderous institutional torts, only modern malnutrition injures more people than iatrogenic disease in its various manifestations. In the most narrow sense, iatrogenic disease includes only illnesses that would not have come about if sound and professionally recommended treatment had *not* been applied. Within this definition, a patient could sue his therapist if the latter, in the course of his management, failed to apply a recommended treatment that, in the physician's opinion, would have risked making him sick. In a more general and more widely accepted sense, clinical iatrogenic disease comprises all clinical conditions for which remedies, physicians, or hospitals are the pathogens, or 'sickening' agents. I will call this plethora of therapeutic side-effects *clinical iatrogenesis*. They are as old as medicine itself, and have always been a subject of medical studies.

Medicines have always been potentially poisonous, but their unwanted side-effects have increased with their power and widespread use. Every twenty-four to thirty-six hours, from 50 to 80 per cent of adults in the United States and the United Kingdom swallow a medically prescribed chemical. Some take the wrong drug; others get an old or a contaminated batch, and others a counterfeit; others take several drugs in dangerous combinations, and still others receive injections with improperly sterilized syringes. Some drugs are addictive, others mutilating, and others mutagenic, although perhaps only in combination with food coloring or insecticides. In some patients, antibiotics alter the normal bacterial flora and induce a superinfection, permitting more resistant organisms to proliferate and invade the host. Other drugs contribute to the breeding of drug-resistant strains of bacteria. Subtle kinds of poisoning thus have spread even faster than the bewildering variety and ubiquity of nostrums. Unnecessary surgery is a standard procedure. *Disabling nondiseases* result from the medical treatment of nonexistent diseases and are on the increase: the number of children disabled in Massachusetts through the treatment of cardiac nondisease exceeds the number of children under effective treatment for real cardiac disease.

Doctor-inflicted pain and infirmity have always been a part of medical practice. Professional callousness, negligence, and sheer incompetence are age-old forms of malpractice. With the transformation of the doctor from an artisan exercising a skill on personally known individuals into a technician applying scientific rules to classes of patients, malpractice acquired an anonymous, almost respectable status. What had formerly been considered an abuse of confidence and a moral fault can now be rationalized into the occasional breakdown of equipment and operators. In a complex technological hospital, negligence becomes 'random human error' or 'system breakdown', callousness becomes 'scientific detachment', and incompetence becomes 'a lack of specialized equipment'. The depersonalization of diagnosis and therapy has changed malpractice from an ethical into a technical problem.

In 1971, between 12,000 and 15,000 malpractice suits were lodged in United States courts. Less than half of all malpractice claims were settled in less than eighteen months, and more than 10 per cent of such claims remain unsettled for over six years. Between 16 and 20 per cent of every dollar paid in malpractice insurance went to compensate the victim; the rest was paid to lawyers and medical experts. In such cases, doctors are vulnerable only to the charge of having acted against the medical code, of the incompetent performance of prescribed treatment, or of dereliction out of greed or laziness. The problem, however, is that most of the damage inflicted by the modern doctor does not fall into any of these categories. It occurs in the ordinary practice of well-trained men and women who have learned to bow to prevailing professional judgment and procedure, even though they know (or could and should know) what damage they do.

The United States Department of Health, Education and Welfare calculates that 7 per cent of all patients suffer compensable injuries while hospitalized, though few of them do anything about it. Moreover, the frequency of reported accidents in hospitals is higher than in all industries but mines and high-rise construction. Accidents are the major cause of death in American children. In proportion to the time spent there, these accidents seem to occur more often in hospitals than in any other kind of place. One in fifty children admitted to a hospital suffers an accident which requires specific treatment. University hospitals are relatively more pathogenic, or, in blunt language, more sickening. It has also been established that one out of every five patients admitted to a typical research hospital acquires an iatrogenic disease, sometimes trivial, usually requiring special treatment, and in one case in thirty leading to death. Half of these episodes result from complications of drug therapy; amazingly, one in ten comes from diagnostic procedures. Despite good intentions and claims to public service, a military officer with a similar record of performance would be relieved of his command, and a restaurant or amusement center would be closed by the police. No wonder that the health industry tries to shift the blame for the damage caused onto the victim, and that the dope-sheet of a multinational pharmaceutical concern tells its readers that 'iatrogenic disease is almost always of neurotic origin'.

Defenseless Patients

The undesirable side effects of approved, mistaken, callous, or contraindicated technical contacts with the medical system represent just the first level of pathogenic medicine. Such *clinical iatrogenesis* includes not only the damage that doctors inflict with the intent of curing or of exploiting the patient, but also those other torts that result from the doctor's attempt to protect himself against the possibility of a suit for malpractice. Such attempts to avoid litigation and persecution may now do more damage than any other iatrogenic stimulus.

On a second level, medical practice sponsors sickness by reinforcing a morbid society that encourages people to become consumers of curative, preventive, industrial, and environmental medicine. On the one hand defectives survive in increasing numbers and are fit only for life under institutional care, while on the other hand, medically certified symptoms exempt people from industrial work and thereby remove them from the scene of political struggle to reshape the society that has made them sick. Second-level iatrogenesis finds its expression in various symptoms of social overmedicalization that amount to what I shall call the expropriation of health. This second-level impact of medicine I designate as *social iatrogenesis*.

On the third level, the so-called health professions have an even deeper, culturally health-denying effect insofar as they destroy the potential of people to deal with their human weakness, vulnerability, and uniqueness in a personal and autonomous way. The patient in the grip of contemporary medicine is but one of mankind in the grip of its pernicious techniques. This *cultural iatrogenesis* is the ultimate backlash of hygienic progress and consists in the paralysis of healthy responses to suffering, impairment, and death. It occurs when people accept health management designed on the engineering model, when they conspire in an attempt to produce, as if it were a commodity, something called 'better health'. This inevitably results in the managed maintenance of life on high levels of sub-lethal illness. This ultimate evil of medical 'progress' must be clearly distinguished from both clinical and social iatrogenesis.

I hope to show that on each of its three levels iatrogenesis has become medically irreversible: a feature built right into the medical endeavour. The unwanted physiological social, and psychological by-products of diagnostic and therapeutic progress have become resistant to medical remedies. New devices, approaches, and organizational arrangements, which are conceived as remedies for clinical and social iatrogenesis, themselves tend to become pathogens contributing to the new epidemic. Technical and managerial measures taken on any level to avoid damaging the patient by his treatment tend to engender a self-reinforcing iatrogenic loop analogous to the escalating destruction generated by the polluting procedures used as antipollution devices.

I will designate this self-reinforcing loop of negative institutional feedback by its classical Greek equivalent and call it *medical nemesis*. The Greeks saw gods in the forces of nature. For them, nemesis represented divine vengeance visited upon mortals who infringe on those prerogatives the gods enviously guard for themselves. Nemesis was the inevitable punishment for attempts to be a hero rather than a human being. Like most abstract Greek nouns, Nemesis took the shape of a divinity. She represented nature's response to *hubris*: to the individual's presumption in seeking to acquire the attributes of a god. Our contemporary hygienic hubris has led to the new syndrome of medical nemesis.

By using the Greek term I want to emphasize that the corresponding phenomenon does not fit within the explanatory paradigm now offered by bureaucrats, therapists, and ideologues for the snowballing diseconomies and disutilities that, lacking all intuition, they have engineered and that they tend to call the 'counterintuitive behavior of large systems'. By invoking myths and ancestral gods I should make it clear that my framework for analysis of the current breakdown of medicine is foreign to the industrially determined logic and ethos. I believe that the *reversal of nemesis* can come only from within man and not from yet another managed (heteronomous) source dependent once again on presumptious expertise and subsequent mystification.

Medical nemesis is resistant to medical remedies. It can be reversed only through a recovery of the will to self-care among the laity, and through the legal, political, and institutional recognition of the right to care, which imposes limits upon the professional monopoly of physicians. I do not suggest any specific forms of health care or sick-care, and I do not advocate any new medical philosophy any more than I recommend remedies for medical technique, doctrine, or organization. However, I do propose an alternative approach to the use of medical organization and technology together with the allied bureaucracies and illusions.

Ivan Illich is a theologian and philosopher who lives and works in Cuernavaca, Mexico. He is the author of several books including *Celebration of Awareness* (1969), *Deschooling Society* (1971), *Tools for Conviviality* (1973) and *Limits to Medicine* (1976). This article originally appeared as the first chapter to the last mentioned book and was published by Marion Boyars, London. The extensive footnotes and references that accompanied the original version have been omitted here.

3.8

The Mode of State Intervention in the Health Sector

Vicente Navarro

Mechanisms of State Intervention

Let us now analyze the specific mechanisms of state intervention in capitalist societies. And let us begin by somewhat arbitrarily dividing those interventions into primarily two levels: one of negative and the other of positive selection.

A. Negative Selection Mechanisms
By negative selection, I mean that mode of intervention that systematically and continually excludes those strategies that conflict with the class nature of the capitalist society. This negative intervention takes place through (a) structural selective mechanisms, (b) ideological mechanisms, (c) decision-making mechanisms, and (d) repressive coercion mechanisms.
Structural Selective Mechanisms.
These mechanisms refer to the exclusion of alternatives that threaten the capitalist system, an exclusion that is inherent in the nature of the capitalist state. In fact, the overall priority given to property and capital accumulation explains why, when health and property conflict, the latter usually takes priority over the former. For example, the appalling lack of adequate legislation protecting the worker in most capitalist societies (including social democratic Sweden) contrasts most dramatically with the large array of laws protecting private property and its owners. The dramatic cuts in the already meager funds for federal occupational programs in the US indicate that when a conflict appears between capital accumulation and property on the one hand and health on the other, the latter is, by definition, the loser. And the present outrage voiced by the French establishment when a factory owner was jailed for negligence shows that this 'benign neglect' of workers, but strong concern for owners and property is not unique to the US.

This structural negative selective mechanism also appears in the implied assumption that all health programs and reforms have to take place within the set of class relations prevalent in capitalist societies. For example, in Britain, Bevan's Labour Party strategy of implementing the NHS (a victory for the British working class) assumed an unalterability of class relations in Britain. Indeed, the creation of the NHS was seen as taking place within the structure of capitalist Britain of 1948, respecting the class distribution of power both outside and within the health sector. Bevan relied very heavily on the consultants, who clearly were of upper class extraction and position, to break the general practitioner's resistance against the implementation of the NHS. As he proudly indicated, 'I bought them with gold.'[1] The strategy of using the nationalization of the health sector to break with the class structure outside and within the health sector, as Lenin did in the Soviet Union, was not even considered.[2]

Moreover, to reassure the medical profession in general and the consultants in particular, they were given dominant influence over the process of planning, regulation, and administration of the health sector.[3]

Ideological Mechanisms.

These mechanisms insure the exclusion from the realm of debate of ideologies that conflict with the system. In other words, it is not only programs and policies, as indicated before, that are being automatically excluded, but, more importantly, conflicting ideologies as well. This is clearly shown in the lack of attention to and the lack of research in areas that conflict with the requirements and needs of the capitalist system. Reflecting the bourgeois bias of the medical research establishment for example, much priority is given to the assumedly individual causation of disease. One instance, among others, is that most research on heart disease—one of the main killers in society—has focused on diet, exercise, and genetic inheritance. On the study of these etiologies, millions of pounds, dollars, marks, and francs have been spent. However, in a fifteen-year study of aging, cited in a most interesting report prepared by a special task force to the Secretary of Health, Education, and Welfare in the US, it was found that the most important predictor of longevity was work satisfaction. Let me quote from that report:

> ... the strongest predictor of longevity was work satisfaction. The second best predictor was over-all 'happiness' ... Other factors are undoubtedly important—diet, exercise, medical care, and genetic inheritance. But research findings suggest that these factors may account for only about 25% of the risk factors in heart disease, the major cause of death. That is, if cholesterol, blood pressure, smoking, glucose level, serum uric acid, and so forth, were perfectly controlled, only about one-fourth of coronary heart disease could be controlled. Although research on this problem has not led to conclusive answers, it appears that work role, work conditions, and other social factors may contribute heavily to this 'unexplained' 75% of risk factors.[4]

But very few studies have investigated these socio-political factors. [...] In summary, the exclusion of ideologies which question or threaten the basic assumptions of the capitalist system is a most prevalent mechanism of state intervention, i.e. the exclusion as unthinkable of any alternatives to that system.

Decision Making Mechanisms. The decision making processes are heavily weighted in favor of certain groups and classes, and thus against certain others. For example, the mechanisms of selection and appointment of members to the new regional and area health planning and administrative agencies in Britain and to the Health System Agencies in the US are conducive to the dominance over those bodies of individuals of the corporate and upper-middle classes, to the detriment of members of lower-middle and working classes.

Repressive Coercion Mechanisms.

The final form of negative selection, repressive coercion mechanisms, takes place either through the use of direct force or, more importantly, by cutting (and thus nullifying) those programs that may conflict with sources of power within the state organism.

B. Positive Selection Mechanisms

By positive selection, I mean the type of state intervention that generates, stimulates, and determines a positive response favorable to overall capital accumulation, as opposed to a negative selection which excludes anticapitalist possibilities. Offe distinguishes between two types of such intervention—allocative and productive.[5] In the former, the state regulates and coordinates the allocation of resources that have already been produced, while in the latter, the state becomes directly involved in the production of goods and services.

Allocative Intervention Policies.

These policies are based on the authority of the state in influencing, guiding and even directing the main activities of society, including the most important one—capital accumulation. The policies are put into effect primarily (although not exclusively) through laws that make certain behavior mandatory and through regulations that make certain claims legal. In the health sector, examples of the former are laws requiring doctors to register contagious disease with the state health department and for employers to install protective devices to prevent industrial accidents, while an example of the latter is regulations determining that certain categories of people receive health insurance. Both laws and regulations are determined and dictated in the world of politics. As Offe indicates, in allocative functions 'policy and politics are not differentiated'. And, as such, those policies are determined by the different degrees of dominance of the branches of the state by pressure groups and factions primarily within the dominant class.

Productive Intervention Policies.

As I have indicated, productive intervention policies are those whereby the state directly participates in the production of resources, e.g. medical education in most Western capitalist countries, production of drugs in nationalized drug industries, management of public hospitals, medical research, etc. Before analyzing these activities, let me clarify a number of points that have an important bearing on the presentation of these productive activities.

- There is not always a clear-cut distinction between allocative and productive policies. Frequently health policies include elements of both. Most allocative functions are administered by the state apparatus, mainly the civil service or the administrative branch of the executive, while productive functions take place outside the administrative bodies of the state apparatus. For example, in the production of medical knowledge (research and teaching), the allocative functions are carried out by an administrative branch of the state apparatus, while their actual production is carried out by medical schools and research institutions that, although public institutions for the most part, are not directly run by the branch of the state apparatus in charge of the allocative function, nor by any other branch for that matter.

- Both allocative and productive policies have increased dramatically in all capitalist countries since World War II and, along with that increase, a shift has taken place from allocative to productive policies. An example of the latter is the production of medical knowledge, where there has been a shift in state intervention from an allocative function (e.g. subsidies, tax benefits) to actual production (e.g. nationalization of medical schools and research institutions). Similarly, there is a trend in the health sector to move from national insurance schemes (allocative) to national health services (productive). Britain in 1948, Quebec (Canada) in 1968, and Italy in the 1970s are each examples of that trend. In all capitalist countries, there has been an impressive growth of state intervention, primarily of the productive type of intervention, as measured by either public expenditures or public employment. Moreover, this growth has taken place mainly in the social (including health) services sector. In a recent survey of expenditures carried out by OECD among its member countries, for example, it is concluded that in all of them, public expenditures have grown and will continue to grow very dramatically, both proportionally and absolutely, during the period under study (1960–80), and that the major characteristics of these changes are very substantial growth in (a) social services expenditures, including education, health and social security; (b) capital investments of an infrastructural character (e.g. roads); and (c) state aid to private industries. And in this growth of expenditures, the health sector occupies a prominent place. During the last twenty years, health expenditures in capitalist developed countries have grown faster than the GNP.[6] Similarly, in terms of employment, the social services sector (including health) has been the fastest growing. Having described that growth, let me now analyze its nature and consequences.

The Reasons for the Growth of State Intervention

The growth of the health sector in developed capitalist countries is due to the growth of social needs, which are determined by the process of capital accumulation and by the heightening of the level of class struggle. Let me expand on each.

The Growth of Social Needs as Demanded by the Process of Capital Accumulation
As indicated before, the primary role of state intervention is to facilitate the process of capital accumulation, i.e. to stimulate and strengthen the economy. Let us now discuss the main characteristics of that process of capital accumulation and analyze the sets of requirements from the different agencies of the state that are determined by that process. And a primary characteristic of that process of accumulation is, as indicated earlier, its concentration. Indeed, insurance, banking, manufacturing, and other sectors of economic life are in the hands of an increasingly small number of corporations that, for the most part, control the market in each sector. The consequences of that concentration are many but, among them, the most important is the type of technology and industrial development determined by and intended primarily to serve the needs of that concentration. And determined by that economic concentration and by that type of technological and industrial development are the following:

- *A division of labor, with a continuous demand for specialization* that fragments the process of production and ultimately the producer himself . . . In summary, and as expressed in Figure 1, increased economic concentration determines a growing concentration of political power and a greater need for state intervention to facilitate the type of industrialization demanded by that economic concentration—an industrialization that influences and determines the type of specialized medicine that is prevalent today.

    Let me clarify here that I believe the relationship among these categories to be dialectical, not linear, with a pattern of dominance that is expressed by the main direction of the arrow in Figure 1.

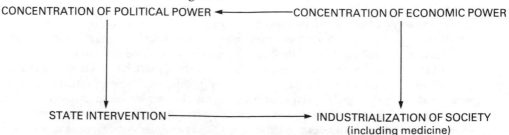

CONCENTRATION OF POLITICAL POWER ◄─────── CONCENTRATION OF ECONOMIC POWER

STATE INTERVENTION ────────────► INDUSTRIALIZATION OF SOCIETY
(including medicine)

Figure 1 The dialectical relationship between concentration of economic power and industrialization of society (including medicine)

- *An invasion of all sectors of economic life by corporate capital.* Indeed, it is a tendency of the process of capital accumulation that the search for profits invades all
  sectors of economic life, including social services such as health, education, transpor-
  tation, etc.

In summary, it is the tendency of contemporary capitalism to convert public services
into commodities to be bought and sold on the private market. Reflecting that tendency is
the push by both conservatives in the UK and conservatives and large numbers of liberals
in the US to shift the delivery of health services back to the private sector (supposedly to
enable them to be run more efficiently and more profitably) and to keep them there. And
in this scheme, the payment for services is public, while the appropriation of profit is private. In brief, the state sector is footing the bill for the profit of capital.

- *An invasion of the spheres of social life by corporate capital and its process of industrialization,* causing dislocation, diswelfare, and insecurity that state intervention,
  through social services (including medicine) is in turn supposed to mitigate. The most
  important example, of course, is the alienation that the industrialized process of production causes in the working population—an alienation that becomes reflected in
  psychosomatic conditions which medicine is supposed to care for and cure. Similarly, occupational diseases and environmental damage are, for the most part, also
  corporately caused, but, according to bourgeois ideology, individually cured
  through medical intervention. In summary, the concentration of economic activities
  and its consequent process of industrialization create a process of diswelfare that, in
  turn, determines and requires the growth of state services.
- *An invasion of corporate capital into the spheres of private life,* with the commodifi-
  cation of all processes of interpersonal relationships, from sex to the pursuit of happiness. Indeed, according to corporate ideology, happiness depends on the amount
  and type of consumption, i.e. on what the citizen has, not on what he or she does.
- *An increased proletarianization of the population,* including the medical profession.
  As a result, the health professions have shifted from being independent entrepreneurs
  to becoming employees of private medical corporations (as in the US) or employees
  of the state (as in the majority of European capitalist countries). In both cases, that
  process of proletarianization is stimulated by the state, with the assistance of the corporate segments of the capitalist class.[7]
- *An increased concentration of resources in urban areas,* and deployment of resources
  to those areas, required and needed for the realization of capital. This process of
  urbanization necessitates a growth in the allocative functions of the state (e.g. land
  use legislation and city planning) and of productive functions (e.g. roads and sanitation) so as to support, guide, and direct that process in a way that is responsive to the
  needs of capital accumulation. It is worth underlining in this context that the majority of infrastructural services are consumed by components of Capital and not by private households. For example, three-quarters of the US water supply is consumed by
  industry and agriculture (mainly corporate), while private households consume less
  than one-quarter. Water supply, however, is paid for largely from funds coming from
  the latter, not from the former.

In summary, then, the economic concentration typical of the present stage of
capitalism—usually referred to as monopoly capitalism—determines (a) an invasion
by corporate capital of all spheres of economic, social and even private life in its quest
for profits, and (b) a specific type of technological development and industrialization
that requires increased state intervention to stimulate and facilitate that concentration, as well as to rectify the dislocation of general well being created by that concentration.

Moreover, this process of economic concentration, and its concomitant industrialization determines a model of production and distribution in medicine that replicates the characteristics of the overall process of economic production and distribution, i.e. specialization, concentration, urbanization and a technical orientation of medicine. The nature of medicine, then, and its relation to the overall process of production determine in large degree its *characteristics*. And its position within that process of production explains its function, which is to take care of and solve the unsolvable—the diswelfare and dysfunctions created by that very process of production.

The Level of Class Struggle

The tendencies explained in the previous section are the result of the growing needs of capital accumulation which take place within the context of a continuous conflict between Capital and Labor—a conflict primarily between the capitalist class and the working class. Indeed, the working class aims continuously at extracting significant concessions from the state, over and above what the state considers sufficient for the needs of capital accumulation defined in the previous section. For example, it is impossible to understand the creation of the NHS in Britain without taking into account the relationship of class forces in Britain and the wartime radicalization of the working class that had called into question 'the survival of capitalism'. As Forsyth has indicated:

> Rightly or wrongly the British Government at the outbreak of war could not be sure that large sections of the working class were entirely satisfied about the reasons for fighting the war . . . For the sake of public morale the Government tried to make it clear that after the war things were going to be very different from the heartbreak conditions of the 'thirties'.[8]

The much heralded consensus on the need for a national health service that existed among Labour and Conservative politicians was the result of the radicalization of the working class on the one hand, and the concern for the survival of capitalism by the capitalist class and the state on the other. Indeed, labor movements have historically viewed social services (including health) as part of the *social wage*, to be defended and increased in the same way that *money wages* are. In fact, Wilensky has shown how the size of social wages depends, in large degree, on the level of militancy of the labor movements.[9] Thus, contrary to popular belief, the size and nature of social benefits in terms of social services is higher in France and Italy than in Scandinavia or even in Britain. And I attribute this to the greater militancy of the unions in those countries and to the existence of mass Socialist and Communist parties (whose platforms are, at least in theory, anticapitalist) that force an increase of social wages upon the state. Another indicator is the percentage of GNP spent on social security which, in 1965, was 17.5 per cent in Italy, 18.3 per cent in France, but only 7.9 per cent in the US. The practical absence of a comprehensive coverage for social benefits in the US is also undoubtedly due to the lack of an organized left party.

In summary, then, the nature and growth of the state in contemporary capitalist societies can be attributed to the increased *social needs of capital* and *social demands of labor*. And in order to understand the nature of any state policy, including health policy, we have to place our analysis within those parameters. Having said that, let me clarify two points. First, there is no single-factor explanation of social policy. Rather, it is explained by the combination of factors already mentioned. And the nature and number of those combinations will depend on the *historical* origins of each factor, the *political* form determining the facto. and its relation to others, and its *function* in that specific social formation. Second, there is no clear cut dichotomy between the social needs of capital and the social demands of labor. Any given policy can serve both. Indeed, social policies that serve the interests of the working class can be subsequently adapted to benefit the interests of the dominant class. As Miliband and others have shown so well, the 'bias of the system' has always insured that these policies can be deflected to suit the capitalist class. Indeed, history shows that concessions won by labor in the class struggle become, *in the absence of further struggle,* modified to serve the interests of the capitalist class.

In summary, I have aimed to show that if we are to understand the nature, composition, distribution and function of the medical care sector in Western developed capitalist societies, we must first understand the distribution of power in those societies and the nature, role, and instrumentality of the state. This understanding leads us to realize that (a) the assumedly transcended and diluted category of social class is a much needed category in understanding the distribution of power in our societies; and that (b) class struggle, far from being an outmoded concept of interest only to 'vulgar' Marxists, is most relevant indeed and as much needed today to understand the nature of our societies and of our health sectors as it was when Marx and Engels wrote that 'class struggle is the motor of history'.

Needless to say, this interpretation is a minority voice in our Western academic setting. It is in conflict with the prevalent explanations of the health sector, and this accounts for its exclusion from the realm of debate. Still, its veracity will be affirmed not by its 'popularity' in the corridors of power, which will be nil, but in its verification on the terrain of history. It is because of this that I dedicated this article to all those with whom I share a praxis aimed at building up a society of truly free and self-governing men and women—a society in which, as Marx indicated, the state (and I would add medicine) will be converted 'from an organ superimposed upon society into one completely subordinated to it'.[10]

References

1. See Tudor Hart, J. 'Primary care in the industrial areas of Britain: evolution and current problems', *International Journal of Health Services* 2 (3), 349–365 (1972) and 'Bevan and the Doctors', *Lancet* 2 (7839), 1196–1197 (1973).
2. For Lenin's strategy in health services, see 'Leninism and medicine'. In Navarro, V. *The Political Economy of Social Security and Medical Care in the USSR* (in press).
3. For an excellent analysis of the professional dominance in the NHS, see Robson, J. 'The NHS company inc.? the social consequence of the professional dominance in the National Health Service', *International Journal of Health Services* 3 (3), 413–426 (1973). Also Draper, P. and Smart, T. 'Social science and health policy in the United Kingdom: some contributions of the social sciences to the bureaucratization of the National Health Service', *International Journal of Health Services* 4 (3), 453–470 (1974).
4. Special Task Force to the Secretary of Health, Education and Welfare *Work in America*, M.I.T. Press, Cambridge, MA., pp. 77–79 (1973).
5. Offe, C. 'The theory of the capitalist state and the problem of policy formation'. In Lindberg, L. *et al.* (eds) *Stress and Contradiction in Modern Capitalism*, Lexington Books, London, p. 128 (1975).
6. Maxwell, R. *Health Care. The Growing Dilemma: Needs Versus Resources in Western Europe, the US and the USSR,* McKinsey and Company, New York, p. 18 (1975).
7. Editorial, 'Doctors and the State', *Wall Street Journal,* 16 January (1976).
8. Forsyth, G. *Doctors and State Medicine: A Study of the British Health Service,* Pitman and Sons, London, p. 16 (1973).
9. Wilensky, H. L. *The Welfare State and Equality,* University of California Press, Berkeley and Los Angeles (1975).
10 Marx, K. *Critique of the Gotha Program,* International Publishers, New York (1938).

Vicente Navarro is Professor of Health and Social Policy at The Johns Hopkins University, Baltimore, USA. This article is an edited extract from his book *Medicine Under Capitalism* which was published by Prodist, New York (1976).

3.9

Doctor Knows Best

Ann Oakley

> You decide when to see your doctor and let him confirm the fact of your pregnancy. From then onwards you are going to have to answer a lot of questions and be the subject of a lot of examinations. Never worry about any of these. They are necessary, they are in the interests of your baby and yourself, and none of them will ever hurt you.[1]

These admonitions, from a British Medical Association publication on pregnancy, are intended to console. Their tone is patronizing and their message clear: doctors know more about having babies than women do. (An alternative, and less charitable, construction would be that women are fundamentally stupid and doctors are inherently more intelligent.)

Obstetrics, like midwifery, in its original meaning describes a female province. The management of reproduction has been, throughout most of history and in most cultures, a female concern; what is characteristic about childbirth in the industrial world is, conversely, its control by men. The conversion of female-controlled community management to male-controlled medical management alone would suggest that the propagation of particular paradigms of women as maternity cases has been central to the whole development of medically dominated maternity care. The ideological element, as would be expected, is not part of the agenda in conventional medical histories chronicling the rise of male obstetrics—for example H. R. Spencer's *The History of British Midwifery from 1650 to 1800*.[2] Spencer terminates his discussion in a tone characteristic of the genus when he says:

> In conclusion it may be said that during the hundred and fifty years since Harvey published his 'De Generatione Animalium', a great advance had been made in the science and art of midwifery. This was due chiefly to the introduction of male practitioners, many of whom were men of learning and devoted to anatomy, the groundwork of obstetrics.

The achievements of male obstetrics over those of female midwifery are rarely argued empirically, but always *a priori*, from the double premise of male and medical superiority. More recent investigations of this argument are now revealing a different picture, in which the introduction of men into the business of reproductive management brought special dangers to mothers and babies. The easier transmission of puerperal fever in male-run lying-in hospitals is one example; the generally careless and ignorant use of technology another.[3,4] In Britain in the eighteenth and early nineteenth centuries many of the male midwives' innovations were often fatal for both mother and child. The forceps, in particular, which are frequently claimed to be the chief advantage of male medicine, were not used in more than a minority of cases attended by male midwives, and had little effect on infant mortality, except perhaps to raise it further.[4] In the 1920s in America, where female midwifery was to be most completely phased out, doctors had to contend with the fact that midwifery was obviously associated with less mortality and morbidity than the interventionist character of the new obstetrical approach.[5]

Improvements in knowledge and technique do not in retrospect justify male participation in midwifery during the eighteenth and nineteenth centuries, and if they did so at the time it was the ideological power of the claim to greater expertise that had this effect. The success of the claim seems to have had a great deal to do with the propagation of certain notions of womanhood. The nineteenth century was a crucial period both for the evolution of modern woman's position and for the consolidation of the male obstetrical takeover. Medical writing about women's diseases and reproductive capacity during this period was characterized by a curiously strong 'emotionally charged conviction' in relation to women's character.[6] Women were also seen as the 'carriers' of contagion, an intrinsic threat to the health of society. Class intersects with sexism here, for it was working-class women who were seen as 'sickening' in this sense.[7]

'It is almost a pity that a woman has a womb', exclaimed an American professor of gynaecology in the 1860s.[6] This statement neatly summarizes the low regard in which the medical profession held its female patients; through its ideological construction of the uterus as the controlling organ of womanhood, it effectively demoted reproduction as woman's unique achievement to the status of a pitiable handicap. Such a construction presented women essentially as reproductive machines, subject to a direct biological input. It enabled physicians to assert a role in the mechanical management of female disorder, thus justifying the particular techniques of drastic gynaecological surgery and obstetrical intervention, and therefore establishing the 'need' for a male medical ascendancy over the whole domain of reproductive care.

All sorts of claims were made about the womb, and its associates, the ovaries, as the site and cause of female inferiority, from physiological pathology to mental disorder, from personality characteristics to occupational qualification (or, rather, disqualification). It was not simply the process of reproduction that was perceived as disabling, but the possession of the apparatus, which evidenced its presence in a monthly flow of reminders about the incapacity of women to be anything other than slaves to their biology.[5]

Doctors contended that a woman's reproductive organs explained her femininity in a double-bind sense: women were ill because they were women, but also if they tried to avoid being women by choosing to follow masculine occupations. Medicine thus outlined the contours of woman's place—in nature, not culture, safely outside the limits of masculine society.

How and why male medicine came to assume control over the care of women in childbirth in Britain and America over the last hundred years is, of course, a complex question. But its general location is within this framework of medical concerns about the essential character of women. There are important parallels between medical and social ideologies of womanhood, yet medicine plays a particular role as social ideology. The reason for this is that the theoretical foundations of patriarchy lie in the manipulation of women's biology to constitute their social inferiority. Medicine, as the definer of biology, holds the key to its 'scientific' interpretation, and thus its cultural consequences. The power of medical ideology stems from the incorporation of social assumptions into the very language of physiological theories. The sent and received message hence has a holistic appearance.[8] To deduce the ideological component is a difficult exercise.

Ehrenreich and English[9] demonstrate how the exclusion of women from obstetrics followed a long process of staged decline in the female community health care function. They argue that male medical hostility to women is based on a fear of female procreative power—hence the corroding impact of male obstetrics on female midwifery, whether to its virtual extermination, as in North America, or to its definition as a secondary status health profession, as in Britain. Barker-Benfield's thesis is that the assault on midwives, the rise of eugenic interest in women as breeders, and the coterminous development of destructive gynaecological surgery, can only be understood as aspects of 'a persistent, defensive attempt to control and shape women's procreative power'. Among the many pungent anecdotes included in Barker-Benfield's book is his account of how J. Marion Sims 'discovered' the speculum. Sims said 'Introducing the bent handle of a spoon into a woman's vagina I saw everything as no man had ever seen before . . . I felt like an explorer . . . who first views a new and important territory.' And a contemporary commentator caught up the colonial metaphor: 'Sims' speculum has been to diseases of the womb . . . what the compass is to the mariner'. Sims saw himself as a Columbus; his New World, and that of his male gynaecological successors, was the vagina.

The tools used by traditional female midwives lack documentation, but it seems likely that they also used an instrument such as the bent handle of a spoon to examine the vagina and cervix. But the routinization of the speculum-assisted vaginal examination by doctors facilitated an opposition between male medical knowledge of women's bodies and women's own knowledge. Throughout obstetricians' long fight to establish themselves as experts, in possession of *all* the resources necessary to the care and control of women in childbirth, this clash has remained the most vulnerable link in the chain of medical command.

The conflict between reproducer as expert and doctor as expert may have five outcomes: the reproducer may accept the doctor's definition of the situation; the doctor may accept the reproducer's; the reproducer may challenge the doctor's view; the doctor may challenge the reproducer's; or the conflict between them may be manifested in a certain pattern of communication between doctor and patient that indicates the presence of unresolved questions to do with what has been termed 'intrauterine neocolonialism'.[10] In a large series of doctor–patient encounters observed for the Transition to Motherhood study, this latter outcome was much more common than direct confrontation. The woman's status as an expert may be accorded joking recognition:

DOCTOR: *First baby?*
PATIENT: *Second.*
DOCTOR: [laughing]: *So you're an expert?*

Or:

DOCTOR: *You're looking rather serious.*
PATIENT: *Well, I am rather worried about it all. It feels like a small baby—I feel much smaller with this one than I did with my first, and she weighed under six pounds. Ultrasound last week said the baby was very small, as well.*
DOCTOR: *Weighed it, did they?*
SECOND DOCTOR [entering cubicle]: *They go round the flower shows and weigh cakes, you know.*
FIRST DOCTOR: *Yes, it's a piece of cake, really.*

But frequently, patients concur in the doctor's presentation of himself (most obstetricians are male) as the possessor of privileged information:

MALE DOCTOR: *Will you keep a note in your diary of when you first feel the baby move?*
PATIENT: *Do you know—well, of course you would know—what it feels like?*
DOCTOR: *It feels like wind pains—something moving in your tummy.*

At the same time, a common feature of communication between doctor and patient is a discrepancy between their labelling of significant symptoms. The medical dilemma is that of discerning the 'presenting' symptoms of clinically significant disorders; the patient's concern is with the normalization of her subjective experience of discomfort. Of 677 statements made by patients, 12 per cent concerned symptoms of pain or discomfort, which were medically treated either by being ignored, or with a non-serious response, or through a brief and selective account of relevant physiological/anatomical data.

DOCTOR: *Feeling well?*
PATIENT: *Yes, but very tired—I can't sleep at all at night.*
DOCTOR: *Why is that?*
PATIENT: *Well, I'm very uncomfortable—I turn from one side to the other, and the baby keeps kicking. I get cramp on one side, high up in my leg. If I sleep on my back I choke myself, so I'm tossing and turning about all night long, which isn't very good.*
DOCTOR: *We need to put you in a hammock, don't we?* [Reads case notes] *Tell me, the urine specimen which you brought in today—when did you do it?*

PATIENT: *I've got a pain in my shoulder.*
DOCTOR: *Well, that's your shopping bag hand, isn't it?*

PATIENT: *I get pains in my groin, down here, why is that?*
DOCTOR: *Well, it's some time since your last pregnancy, and also your centre of gravity is changing.*
PATIENT: *I see.*
DOCTOR: *That's okay.* [Pats on back]

Such abbreviated 'commonsense' explanations are one mode in which doctors talk to patients. The contrasting mode is to 'technicalize'—to use technical language as a means of keeping the patient in her place. In maternity consultations this interactive pattern particularly characterizes those encounters in which a patient contends equality with the doctor:

DOCTOR: *I think what we have to do is assess you— see how near you are to having it.* [Does internal examination] *Right—you'll go like a bomb, and I've given you a good stirring up. So what I think you should do, is I think you should come in.*
PATIENT: *Is it possible to wait another week, and see what happens?*
DOCTOR: *You've been reading the* Sunday Times.
PATIENT: *No, I haven't. I'm married to a doctor.*
DOCTOR: *Well, you've ripened up since last week and I've given the membranes a good sweep over.*
PATIENT: *What does that mean?*
DOCTOR: *I've swept them—not with a brush, with my finger.* [Writes in notes 'give date for induction']
PATIENT: *I'd still rather wait a bit.*
DOCTOR: *Well, we know the baby's mature now, and there's no sense in waiting. The perinatal morbidity and mortality increase rapidly after forty-two weeks. They didn't say that in the* Sunday Times, *did they?*

A second classic area of dispute between reproducers and doctors is the dating of pregnancy. Six per cent of the questions asked and 5 per cent of statements made by mothers in the antenatal clinic concerned dates, mothers usually trying to negotiate the 'correct' date of expected delivery with the doctor, who did not see this as a subject for negotiation—as a legitimate area of maternal expertise. The underlying imputation is one of feminine unreliability.

DOCTOR: *Are you absolutely sure of your dates?*
PATIENT: *Yes, and I can even tell you the date of conception.*
[Doctor laughs]
PATIENT: *No, I'm serious. This is an artificial insemination baby.*

DOCTOR: *How many weeks are you now?*
PATIENT: *Twenty-six-and-a-half.*
DOCTOR [looking at notes]: *Twenty weeks now.*
PATIENT: *No, twenty-six-and-a-half.*
DOCTOR: *You can't be.*
PATIENT: *Yes I am, look at the ultrasound report.*
DOCTOR: *When was it done?*
PATIENT: *Today.*
DOCTOR: *It was done today?*
PATIENT: *Yes.*
DOCTOR [reads report]: *Oh yes, twenty-six-and-a-half weeks, that's right.*
[Patient smiles triumphantly at researcher]

Perhaps it is significant that increasingly the routine use of serial ultrasound cephalometry is providing an alternative medical technique for the assessment of gestation length. A medical rationale for the inflation of medical over maternal expertise is thus provided. It is important to note that although the efficacy, safety and technical superiority of ultrasound is widely assumed within the medical frame of reference, this does not rest on a 'scientific' basis. No randomized controlled trials have, for example, been conducted that evaluate the usefulness of routine ultrasound versus more traditional methods of clinical examination and maternal report in assessing gestation length and foetal well-being. Laboratory investigations of the physiological effects of ultrasound on developing embryonic and foetal cells are limited and contradictory. Longitudinal follow-up of children subjected to ultrasound while in the womb is sparse and restricted to a six-year period, the kind of time span known to be inadequate in showing up the long-term effects of other procedures inflicted on foetuses, such as X-rays and the administration of hormones. In animal experiments, intrauterine ultrasound has been shown to have a long-term effect on immune responses in the young.[11]

Similar kinds of scientific caveats can be levelled at other medical techniques generally used in the treatment of women as maternity cases today.[12] Unbridled medical enthusiasm for new techniques is a general feature of modern medicine and it may be not so much that obstetrics is a special case but that medical attitudes see female reproductive patienthood as a particularly passive and appropriate site for their introduction.

References

1. 'You and your baby, Part 1: From pregnancy to birth', *Family Doctor Publications*, BMA, p. 8 (1977).
2. Spencer, H. R. *The History of British Midwifery from 1650 to 1800*, John Bale, Sons and Danielsson Ltd., London (1927).

3. Oakley, A. 'Wise woman and medicine man: changes in the management of childbirth'. In Mitchell, J. and Oakley, A. (eds) *The Rights and Wrongs of Women,* Penguin, Harmondsworth (1976).
4. Versluyen, M. 'Men–midwives, professionalising strategies and the first maternity hospitals—a sociological interpretation'. Unpublished paper (n.d.).
5. Barker-Benfield, G. J. *The Horrors of the Half-known Life,* Harper and Row, New York (1976).
6. Wood, A. D. ' "The fashionable diseases": women's complaints and their treatment in nineteenth century America'. In Hartman, M. and Banner, L. W. (eds) *Clio's Consciousness Raised: New Perspectives in the History of Women,* Harper and Row, New York (1974).
7. Duffin, L. 'The conspicuous consumptive: woman as an invalid'. In Delamont, S. and Duffin, L. (eds) *The Nineteenth Century Woman: Her Cultural and Physical World,* Croom Helm, London (1978).
8. Jordanova, L. 'Medicine, personal morality and public order: an historical case study'. Paper given at British Sociological Association Medical Sociology Conference, York, 22–24 September (1978).
9. Ehrenreich, B. and English, D. *Witches, Midwives and Nurses,* Glass Mountain Pamphlets, The Feminist Press, New York (1975).
10. Swinscow, T. D. V. 'Personal view', *British Medical Journal,* 28 September (1974).
11. Rosser, J. 'Ultrasound and pregnant women'. In Association of Radical Midwives Newsletter, June (1978).
12. Chalmers, I. and Richards, M. 'Intervention and causal inference in obstetric practice'. In Chard, T. and Richards, M. (eds) *Benefits and Hazards of the New Obstetrics,* Heinemann Medical, London (1977).

Ann Oakley is a sociologist currently working with the National Perinatal Epidemiology Unit, Oxford. This article is an extract from her book *Women Confined* which was published by Martin Robertson, Oxford (1980).

3.10

The Village Health Worker: Lackey or Liberator?

David Werner

Throughout Latin America, the programmed use of health auxiliaries has, in recent years, become an important part of the new international push of 'community oriented' health care. But in Latin America village health workers are far from new. Various religious groups and non-government agencies have been training *promotores de salud* or health promoters for decades. And to a large (but diminishing) extent, villagers still rely, as they always have, on their local *curanderos*, herb doctors, bone setters, traditional midwives and spiritual healers. More recently, the *médico practicante* or empirical doctor has assumed in the villages the same role of self-made practitioner and prescriber of drugs that the neighbourhood pharmacist has assumed in larger towns and cities.

Until recently, however, the respective Health Departments of Latin America have either ignored or tried to stamp out this motley work force of non-professional healers. Yet the Health Departments have had trouble coming up with viable alternatives. Their Western-style, city-bred and city-trained MDs not only proved uneconomical in terms of cost effectiveness; they flatly refused to serve in the rural area. The first official attempt at a solution was, of course, to produce more doctors. In Mexico the National University began to recruit 5,000 new medical students per year (and still does so). The result was a surplus of poorly trained doctors who stayed in the cities.

The next attempt was through compulsory social service. Graduating medical students were required (unless they bought their way off) to spend a year in a rural health center before receiving their licenses. The young doctors were unprepared either by training or disposition to cope with the health needs in the rural area. With discouraging frequency they became resentful, irresponsible or blatantly corrupt. Next came the era of the mobile clinics. They, too, failed miserably. They created dependency and expectation without providing continuity of service. The net result was to undermine the people's capacity for self care. It was becoming increasingly clear that provision of health care in the rural area could never be accomplished by professionals alone. But the medical establishment was—and still is—reluctant to crack its legal monopoly.

At long last, and with considerable financial cajoling from foreign and international health and development agencies, the various health departments have begun to train and utilize auxiliaries. Today, in countries where they have been given half a chance, auxiliaries play an important role in the health care of rural and periurban communities.

And if given a whole chance, their impact could be far greater. But, to a large extent, politics and the medical establishment still stand in the way.

Rural health projects

My own experience in rural health care has mostly been in a remote mountainous sector of Western Mexico, where, for the past twelve years I have been involved in training local village health workers, and in helping foster a primary health care network, run by the villagers themselves. As the villagers have taken over full responsibility for the management and planning of their program, I have been phasing out my own participation to the point where I am now only an intermittent advisor. This has given me time to look more closely at what is happening in rural health care in other parts of Latin America.

Last year a group of my co-workers and I visited nearly forty rural health projects, both government and non-government, in nine Latin American countries (Mexico, Guatemala, Honduras, El Salvador, Nicaragua, Costa Rica, Venezuela, Colombia and Ecuador.) Our objective has been to encourage a dialogue among the various groups, as well as to try to draw together many respective approaches, methods, insights and problems into a sort of field guide for health planners and educators, so we can all learn from each other's experience. We specifically chose to visit projects or programs which were making significant use of local, modestly trained health workers or which were reportedly trying to involve people more effectively in their own health care.

We were inspired by some of the things we saw, and profoundly disturbed by others. While in some of the projects we visited, people were in fact regarded as a resource to control disease, in others we had the sickening impression that disease was being used as a resource to control people. We began to look at different programs, and functions, in terms of where they lay along a continuum between two poles: community supportive and community oppressive.

Community supportive programs or Community oppressive programs?

Community supportive programs, or functions, are those which favorably influence the long-range welfare of the community, that help it stand on its own feet, that genuinely encourage responsibility, initiative, decision making and self-reliance at the community level, that build upon human dignity.

Community oppressive programs, or functions, are those which, while invariably giving lip service to the above aspects of community input, are fundamentally authoritarian, paternalistic or are structured and carried out in such a way that they effectively encourage greater dependency, servility and unquestioning acceptance of outside regulations and decisions; those which in the long run are crippling to the dynamics of the community.

It is disturbing to note that, with certain exceptions, the programs which we found to be more community supportive were small non-government efforts, usually operating on a shoestring and with a more or less sub-rosa status. As for the large regional or national programs—for all their international funding, top-ranking foreign consultants and glossy bilingual brochures portraying community participation—we found that when it came down to the nitty-gritty of what was going on in the field, there was usually a minimum of effective community involvement and a maximum of dependency-creating handouts, paternalism and superimposed, initiative destroying norms.

Primary health workers

In our visits to the many rural health programs in Latin America, we found that primary workers come in a confusing array of types and titles. Generally speaking, however, they fall into two groups:

Auxiliary nurses or health technicians	Health promoters or village health workers
At least primary education plus 1–2 years training	Average of 3rd grade education plus 1–6 months training
Usually from outside the community	Usually from the community and selected by it.
Usually employed full time	
Salary usually paid by the program (not by the community)	Often a part time health worker supported in part by farm labor or with help from the community
	May be someone who has already been a traditional healer

In addition to the health workers just described, many Latin American countries have programs to provide minimal training and supervision of traditional midwives. Unfortunately, Health Departments tend to refer to these programs as 'Control de Parteras Empíricas' ('Control of Empirical Midwives')—a terminology which too often reflects an attitude. Thus to Mosquito Control and Leprosy Control has been added Midwife Control. (Small wonder so many midwives are reticent to participate!) Once again, we found the most promising work with village midwives took place in small non-government programs. In one such program the midwives had formed their own club and organized trips to hospital maternity wards to increase their knowledge.

Key questions

What skills can the village health worker perform? How well does he perform them? What are the limiting factors that determine what he can do? These were some of our key questions when we visited different rural health programs.

We found that the skills which village health workers actually performed varied enormously from program to program. In some, local health workers with minimal formal education were able to perform with remarkable competence a wide variety of skills embracing both curative and preventive medicine as well as agricultural extension, village cooperatives and other aspects of community education and mobilization. In other programs—often those sponsored by Health Departments—village workers were permitted to do discouragingly little. Safeguarding the medical profession's monopoly on curative medicine by using the standard argument that prevention is more important than cure (which it may be to us but clearly is not to a mother when her child is sick), instructors often taught these health workers fewer medical skills than many villagers had already mastered for themselves. This sometimes so reduced the people's respect for their health worker that he (or usually she) became less effective, even in preventive measures.

In the majority of cases, we found that external factors, far more than intrinsic factors, proved to be the determinants of what the primary health worker could do. We concluded that *the great variation in range and type of skills performed by village health workers in different programs has less to do with the personal potentials, local conditions or available funding than it has to do with the preconceived attitudes and biases of health program planners, consultants and instructors.* In spite of the often repeated eulogies about 'primary decision making by the communities themselves', seldom do the villagers have much, if any, say in what their health worker is taught and told to do.

The Political Context

The limitations and potentials of the village health worker—what he is permitted to do and, conversely, what he could do if permitted—can best be understood if we look at his role in its social and political context. In Latin America, as in many other parts of the world, poor nutrition, poor hygiene, low literacy and high fertility help account for the high morbidity and mortality of the impoverished masses. But as we all know, the underlying cause—or more exactly, the primary disease—is inequity: inequity of wealth, of land, of educational opportunity, of political representation and of basic human rights. Such inequities undermine the capacity of the peasantry for self care. As a result, the political/economic powers-that-be assume an increasingly paternalistic stand, under which the rural poor become the politically voiceless recipients of both aid and exploitation. In spite of national, foreign and international gestures at aid and development, in Latin America the rich continue to grow richer and the poor poorer. As anyone who has broken bread with villagers or slum dwellers knows only too well: *health of the people is far more influenced by politics and power groups, by distribution of land and wealth, than it is by treatment or prevention of disease.*

Political factors unquestionably comprise one of the major obstacles to a community supportive program. This can be as true for village politics as for national politics. However, the politico-economic structure of the country must necessarily influence the extent to which its rural health program is community supportive or not.

Let us consider the implications in the training and function of a primary health worker. If the village health worker is taught a respectable range of skills, if he is encouraged to think, to take initiative and to keep learning on his own, if his judgement is respected, if his limits are determined by what he knows and can do, if his supervision is supportive and educational, chances are he will work with energy and dedication, will make a major contribution to his community and will win his people's confidence and love. His example will serve as a role model to his neighbors, that they too can learn new skills and assume new responsibilities, that self-improvement is possible. Thus the village health worker becomes an internal agent-of-change, not only for health care, but for the awakening of his people to their human potential . . . and ultimately to their human rights.

However, in countries where social and land reforms are sorely needed, where oppression of the poor and gross disparity of wealth is taken for granted, and where the medical and political establishments jealously covet their power, it is possible that the health worker I have just described knows and does and thinks too much. Such men are dangerous! They are the germ of social change.

So we find, in certain programs, a different breed of village health worker is being molded . . . one who is taught a pathetically limited range of skills, who is trained not to think, but to follow a list of very specific instructions or 'norms', who has a neat uniform, a handsome diploma and who works in a standardized cement block health post, whose supervision is restrictive and whose limitations are rigidly predefined. Such a health worker has a limited impact on the health and even less on the growth of the community. He—or more usually she—spends much of her time filling out forms.

In a conference I attended in Washington in 1980 on Appropriate Technology in Health in Developing Countries, it was suggested that *'Technology can only be considered appropriate if it helps lead to a change in the distribution of wealth and power.'* If our goal is truly to get at the root of human ills, must we not also recognize that, likewise, health projects and health workers are appropriate only if they help bring about a healthier distribution of wealth and power?

Prevention

We say prevention is more important than cure. But how far are we willing to go? Consider diarrhea: each year millions of peasant children die of diarrhea. We tend to agree that most of these deaths could be prevented. Yet diarrhea remains the number one killer of infants in Latin America and much of the developing world. Does this mean our so-called 'preventive' measures are merely palliative? At what point in the chain of causes which makes death from diarrhea a global problem are we coming to grips with the real underlying cause? Do we do it . . .

. . . by preventing some deaths through treatment of diarrhea?

. . . by trying to interrupt the infectious cycle through construction of latrines and water systems?

. . . by reducing high risk from diarrhea through better nutrition?

. . . or by curbing land tenure inequities through land reform?

Land reform comes closest to the real problem. But the peasantry is oppressed by far more inequities than those of land tenure. Both causing and perpetuating these crushing inequities looms the existing power structure: local, national, foreign and multinational. It includes political, commercial and religious power groups as well as the legal profession and the medical establishment. In short it includes . . . ourselves. As the ultimate link in the causal chain which leads from the hungry child with diarrhea to the legalized inequities of those in power, we come face to face with the tragic flaw in our otherwise human nature, namely *greed*.

Where, then, should prevention begin? Beyond doubt, anything we can do to minimize the inequities perpetuated by the existing power structure will do far more to reduce high infant mortality than all our conventional preventive measures put together. We should, perhaps, carry on with our latrine-building rituals, nutrition centers and agricultural extension projects. But let's stop calling it prevention. We are still only treating symptoms. And unless we are very careful, we may even be making the underlying problem worse . . . through increasing dependency on outside aid, technology and control.

But this need not be the case. *If* the building of latrines brings people together and helps them look ahead, *if* a nutrition center is built and run by the community and fosters self-reliance, and *if* agricultural extension, rather than imposing outside technology encourages internal growth of the people toward more effective understanding and use of their land, their potentials and their rights . . . then, and only then, do latrines, nutrition centers and so-called extension work begin to deal with the real causes of preventable sickness and death.

The Village Health Worker

This is where the village health worker comes in. It doesn't matter much if he spends more time treating diarrhea than building latrines. Both are merely palliative in view of the larger problem. What matters is that he gets his people working together.

Yes, the most important role of the village health worker *is* preventive. But preventive in the fullest sense, in the sense that he helps put an end to oppressive inequities, in the sense that he helps his people, as individuals and as a community, liberate themselves not only from outside exploitation and oppression, but from their own short-sightedness, futility and greed.

The chief role of the village health worker, at his best, is that of liberator. This does not mean he is a revolutionary (although he may be pushed into that position). His interest is the welfare of his people. And, as Latin America's blood-streaked history bears witness, revolution without evolution too often means trading one oppressive power group for another. Clearly, any viable answer to the abuses of man by man can only come through evolution, in all of us, toward human relations which are no longer founded on short-sighted self-interest, but rather on tolerance, sharing and compassion.

I know it sounds like I am dreaming. But the exciting thing in Latin America is that there already exist a few programs that are actually working toward making these things happen—where health care for and by the people is important, but where the main role of the primary health worker is to assist in the humanization or, to use Paulo Freire's term, *conscientización* of his people.

Misconceptions

I shall try to clear up some common misconceptions. Many persons still tend to think of the primary health worker as a temporary second-best substitute for the doctor . . . that, if it were financially feasible, the peasantry would be better off with more doctors and fewer primary health workers. I disagree. After twelve years working and learning from village health workers—and dealing with doctors—I have come to realize that the role of the village health workers is not only very distinct from that of the doctor, but, in terms of health and well-being of a given community, is far more important.

You may notice I have shied away from calling the primary health worker an 'aux-iliary'. Rather I think of him as the primary member of the health team. Not only is he willing to work on the front line of health care, where the needs are greatest, but his job is more difficult than that of the average doctor. And his skills are more varied. Whereas the doctor can limit himself to diagnosis and treatment of individual 'cases', the health worker's concern is not only for individuals—as people—but with the whole community. He must not only answer to his people's needs but he must also help them look ahead, and work together to overcome oppression and to stop sickness before it starts. His responsibility is to share rather than hoard his knowledge, not only because informed self-care is more health conducing than ignorance and dependence, but because the principle of sharing is basic to the well-being of man.

Perhaps the most important difference between the village health worker and the doctor is that the health worker's background and training, as well as his membership in and selection by the community, help reinforce his will to serve rather than bleed his people. This is not to say that the village health worker cannot become money-hungry and corrupt. After all, he is as human as the rest of us. It is simply to say that for the village health worker the privilege to grow fat off the illness and misfortune of his fellow man has still not become socially acceptable.

The day must come when we look at the primary health worker as the key member of the health team, and at the doctor as the auxiliary. The doctor, as a specialist in advanced curative technology, would be on call as needed by the primary health worker for referrals and advice. He would attend those 2–3 per cent of illnesses which lie beyond the capacity of an informed people and their health worker, and he even might, under supportive supervision, help out in the training of the primary health worker in that narrow area of health care called 'Medicine'.

Health care will only become equitable when the skills pyramid has been tipped on its side, so that the primary health worker takes the lead, and so that the doctor is on *tap* and not on *top* (Figure 1).

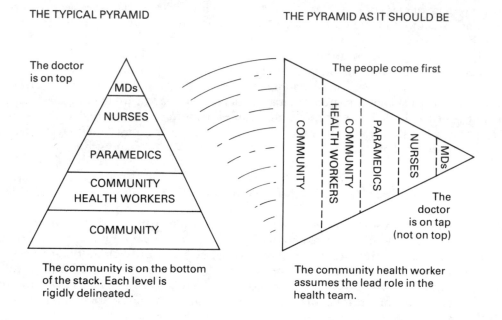

Figure 1 Tipping the health manpower pyramid on its side.

David Werner is an American biologist and Director of the Hesperian Foundation in California, who has spent many years living and working in Mexico. This article previously appeared in *Health Auxiliaries and the Health Team*, edited by Muriel Skeet and Katherine Elliott and published by Croom Helm (1978).

Part 4

Health-care systems

Introduction

As the collection of articles in this part shows, health-care means different things in different places. In the UK and the USA, complex systems have evolved with time. These reveal many divergences that have their roots in the social structure of the two countries in the last century. Health-care as practised in the East is based upon traditional concepts on which have been superimposed Western ideas, legacies of colonial rule. Changes in economic, social and political structures within a country initiate a cascade of events. For health-care, these may be beneficial or retrograde depending on the direction of change and the priorities of the new rulers. For example, in Nicaragua the popular revolution of the late 1970s transformed health-care from that catering for the wealthy to a more equitable system that encompassed the population as a whole. Even so, a country which is attempting to gain greater control of its own economy has to set up an order of priorities, which means that the development of different aspects of health care must proceed at different rates.

Although individual countries have initiated national systems of health-care, there has also been a trend in the past forty years towards the establishment of international organisations to tackle those issues in health with a common, indeed global, relevance. The most important of these is the World Health Organisation (WHO), with its programmes to contain infectious diseases and to improve basic living standards via the provision of food and uncontaminated water. The eradication of smallpox is often held up as a shining example of the effectiveness of international collaboration in the provision of health-care. There are, however, still some problems, such as drug-dependency, which prove elusive to the formulation of a successful and practical international policy. The reasons for this failure lie within the perceived causes of drug-dependency, which differ between countries east and west, north and south.

The first four articles deal with national systems of health-care—how these have evolved with time and to what extent they are developing still. Rosemary Stevens and Gwyn Bevan reveal the nature of health-care in two Western industrialised societies that have a history of cross-fertilisation—the UK and its former colony, the USA. The feature that distinguishes between the two systems is the persistence in the UK of the general practitioner, the majority of whose earnings derive from the state. In the UK modern medical practice has its roots in the trade guilds of earlier centuries. The Royal Colleges of Physicians and of Surgeons catered largely for the upper levels of society, though they also practised in hospitals for the poor which were set up by charitable (often religious) organisations. It is here that the modern hospital specialities originated. By contrast, general practitioners had more humble beginnings in the traditional apothecary. However, the position of the general practitioner was secured when, in the early part of the century, the National Insurance Act provided for basic health-care by GPs with referral to specialists—at least for men. However, in the USA at this time the GP had all but disappeared. Medical practitioners in the United States had specialised early on (the system was based on competition) and probably from this arose the scientific emphasis on medicine. As Stevens points out, the health-care individuals receive under the American system is based on what they can afford to pay for, whereas in the UK a system of primary health-care has not only remained, but is provided along with the other components of the National Health Service through general taxation, and is open to all.

While the health system in one former British colony has evolved *de novo*, that in another (India) has accommodated colonial influence and yet maintained its traditional base. In their study of indigenous medical practice in Madras, Professor Ramesh and Dr Hyma point to the prevalence and obvious success of this form of health-care which is, so they claim, integrated with the needs of society, requiring little in the way of resources, and which extracts fees from patients on the basis of what they can afford. Fifty per cent of India's population is served by indigenous practitioners. In contrast to Western medical practice, there is little specialisation but, in common with it, indigenous medicine is still evolving.

Thomas Bossert's account of the rapid changes in health-care in Nicaragua after the revolution indicates how dramatically policy can be shifted, but it also shows that a government has to decide what price it is prepared to pay. Under the Somoza regime, the policy was to have hospital care rather than preventive medicine. This denied essential medical services to the mass of the population, as hospitals were concentrated in the large cities and responsibility for the medical programme lay with Somoza's relatives and friends. While this gained urban political support for Somoza, the Sandinista movement was dependent on the rural people, who were the majority, for its success. Health policy became a key political issue, and the revolutionary government has attempted to transform the former, largely curative, policy into a more preventive and equitable one. Bossert illustrates how such a change in policy is dependent upon both good administration and the necessary resources. In a country that is rebuilding its social and economic structure, it is possible to make such a dramatic change (as happened to a lesser extent in the UK in the late 1940s), but there are many other enormous demands on resources, not the least of which is the maintenance of a defence force to protect the country against outside influences with vested interests. The key to the new health policy in Nicaragua is participation within the local community and the basic provision of vaccination, sanitation and child care.

The remaining articles in the section illustrate attempts to formulate and then implement health policy at an international level. Although, as Marc Strassburg describes, smallpox had been eradicated from Europe and North America by the 1970s, a number of reservoirs of the virus still existed. By 1980 the WHO declared the world to be free of smallpox, a feat that had been achieved by the application of two key principles in any health-care programme—organisation and resources. If smallpox can be eradicated, will a future world be free of disease? Will such a programme work for everything, given the input of enough resources? The answer is probably no. Smallpox was a prime candidate because much was known of the process and progress of the disease, and a vaccine was available. A similar programme to eliminate malaria has not been successful, largely because of the existence of a reservoir of the malaria parasite in mosquitoes.

Though the smallpox eradication programme was planned and organised centrally it became clear very early on that the programme would need to be modified to suit differing local conditions. The mass vaccination programmes were subordinated to existing local practices of isolation of patients and confinement. Tailoring a programme to suit local conditions is the clear message in the three articles concerned with drug-dependency. The approach in the United States, described by Jerome Jaffe, has been to make possession of narcotics a criminal offence, thus making criminals of those who take drugs and so driving the whole issue firmly into the realm of the law. Those dependent upon heroin are offered treatment (drug substitution) only in special clinics which cost the country millions of dollars each year to run. While this model was at first used in Egypt, as revealed by Gamel Mady Abu El Azayem, it was soon replaced by a programme that did not alienate patients and that was a good deal cheaper. Compulsory treatment was replaced by a voluntary system and the number of people involved in the programme increased sizeably. This aspect of community care is epitomised in the article by Vichai Poshyachinda. In Thailand, the responsibility for drug addicts is taken on by the main religious order. Though the treatment is basic, and appears harsh, it is cheap and voluntary, and has a success rate (in terms of abstinence) equivalent to that of the specialised clinics in the West.

These articles show the variety of approaches to providing health-care. The construction of any health-care system must, of necessity, not only take into account the local needs but also be available to those most in need. What price is put on the provision of such a system—i.e. where health ranks on the scale of a nation's spending—is a political question.

4.1

The Evolution of the Health-Care Systems in the United States and the United Kingdom: Similarities and Differences

Rosemary Stevens

I should like to present some ideas about the nature of the health-care systems of the two countries. For in the two systems there are some fundamental differences which long antedate the National Health Service in Britain or more recent Government initiatives here. Basic professional and social assumptions as they have evolved over the centuries, suggest that medical care itself means different things in different places. We are not always using common assumptions, rationalizations, or even definitions.

Specialization: Common Developments

For 100 years we have been under the spell of a movement toward increased technical specialization in medicine. Now this movement is virtually completed. Specialized departments in hospitals sprang up on both sides of the Atlantic only in the 1870s and 1880s, marking organizational acceptance that specialization was here to stay. St Thomas's Hospital in London set up outpatient departments for ophthalmology in 1871, for otolaryngology in 1882, for dermatology in 1884.[1] Over here, the Massachusetts General Hospital was setting up its own departments of dermatology (1870), neurology (1872), laryngology (1872), ophthalmology (1873), and aural surgery (1886) during the same period.[2] While specialization was accepted reluctantly by leaders of the medical professions in both countries—the first neurologist appointed to the Massachusetts General Hospital was barely dignified by the title of 'electrician'—the movement toward specialization had become inevitable.

By the early 1900s it appeared in America that general practice was moribund, if not dead. While the role of the family doctor as adviser and counselor was idealized as the ultimate in the doctor-patient relationship after 1890, a certain aura of myth and nostalgia surrounded this idealization—as it has, indeed, to the present. The family physician, that 'chum of the old people, the intimate of confiding girlhood, the uncle and oracle of the kids',[3] had largely disappeared by 1915. Outpatient departments of city hospitals provided general services for the indigent masses. The American middle class was already going directly to specialists.

Even in England, where the general practitioner was more readily defined and firmly established, outpatient departments of general hospitals and the rise of special hospitals in the last quarter of the nineteenth century threatened the generalist's position. It has been estimated that, before the National Health Insurance Act of 1911, only 10 to 20 per cent of the British population had family practitioners.[4] Hospitals had become 'temples of research, and the avenues leading to additional medical knowledge'.[5]

By World War I the specialization movement was in full swing. New professions added vertical specialization to the horizontal specialization developing in medicine. Besides the great rise of the nursing profession, there were social workers, optometrists, X-ray technicians, laboratory workers, physical therapists, and (in the American Midwest) nurse-anesthetists. Medicine was no longer a single matter of a conference between two individuals: one patient and one practitioner.

Specialization demanded some response to the questionable relationship between the new specialists and general practitioners—if, indeed, the generalists were to survive. Generalist–specialist relations, transmitted later to questions of primary versus secondary (and tertiary) care, became one set of issues for discussion in the modern health-care system. A related set of issues concerned the emerging role of the hospital, that center of specialized knowledge and techniques. Was it to be the center of all medical care, the temple of service as well as scientific excellence? Such questions were engaging writers on both sides of the Atlantic well before World War I and became intense in the 1920s and 30s.

Other themes with which we still contend have been apparent over many decades. Problems of cost increases and cost containment in medical care have been discussed, particularly on this side of the Atlantic, for at least six decades. The distribution of medical services—questions of urban–rural distributions and the concentration of specialists in major cities—was already of concern in the 1920s. The medical profession, a rag-bag of individuals with varying training and from varying backgrounds on both sides of the Atlantic in the late nineteenth century, became homogenized, standardized, and middle class in the years between the two World Wars. As the status of the profession rose with its advancing techniques so, from World War I, did the social background of its students.

Yet, while some of the dilemmas of modern medicine are clear—the relationship between generalists and specialists, the role of the hospital, the nature of the 'physician', and the role of medical education—the specific responses to medical specialization in Britain and America have been, and may continue to be, quite different, because of the way each health system has developed.

Professional Distinction and Social Differences

Most of the basic characteristics of British and American medicine existed in embryonic form in the 1870s and were clearly evident by 1914. Differences existed in the relative development of professional patterns of medical practice in the two countries, in professional regulation and medical education, in general social attitudes toward the provision of medical care, and even in the behavior of patients.

A quite conservative student of the hospital scene, Henry Burdett,[6] noted with some criticism: 'Free relief has now become so general that the majority of the population in England consider it not only not a disgrace, but the most natural thing in the world, when they fall ill, to demand and receive free medical treatment without question or delay.'

In contrast, he commented, 'America, owing no doubt to the fact of its being a relatively new country, possessing few endowed charities, and an energetic population consisting largely of those who resort to it in the hope of earning an independence may be regarded as the home of the pay system.'

Most patients in American hospitals occupied pay beds or paying wards, in contrast to the largely charitable English hospital system. Moreover, patients were already characterized as being, in England, relatively passive recipients of medical care, while Americans were both more adventurous and more litigious.

Trying to explain the difference a generation earlier, a leading Californian physician had remarked: 'Patients in old countries are more timid: they are not anxious to be the subjects of experiments. In new countries, they bite at all new medicines.'[7]

But while this adventurousness might appeal to the desires of American physicians to show initiative, it resulted equally in 'serious annoyance' from malpractice claims. Modern Californians may be reassured to learn that malpractice claims similar to those of today were being made 100 years ago: 'A certain class of patients make it a business to extort money in this way, by the aid of a certain class of lawyers who go halves in the speculation'.[7]

There would inevitably have been differences in the type of medical organization developing for the small, densely populated, and relatively homogeneous population of Britain and the diverse population of America, scattered over a vast continent. But coupled with these topographical distinctions and with the more general distinctions between the rough and tumble of life in a rapidly growing country and one with centuries of social stability, there were already marked distinctions in patterns of professional organization in medicine.

Medicine in England grew from centralized professional guilds and from a professional system clearly stratified by social status. Before 1858, there were technically three recognized medical professions in England. The Royal College of Physicians, established in 1518, was the traditional domain of the educated elite. The Royal College of Surgeons, founded in 1800, represented the growing prestige of surgeons—well before the technological revolution in surgery made such a distinction functionally inevitable. Apothecaries formed a third strain. Systematic training of apothecaries for medical practice was achieved through an act of 1815, and the resulting apothecaries' license rapidly became the most popular way to become a licensed practitioner. In fact, the most common way of becoming licensed by the mid-nineteenth century was to become both an apothecary and a surgeon.[8]

The early existence of the guilds of physicians, surgeons, and apothecaries has left an enduring imprint on medical care in England. Physicians, as the elite of the medical profession, were a relatively small—if powerful—body, whose clientele during the nineteenth century was divided into two extraordinarily diverse groups. As private practitioners, members of the Royal College of Physicians catered largely to the upper segments of society, although they might function as general consultants to apothecaries when called upon to do so. Yet at the same time, because physicians had been instrumental in founding the great charitable hospitals of England in the eighteenth century, physicians were also the honorary medical staffs of the most prestigious hospitals—which, in turn, catered largely to the poverty-stricken.

Surgeon-apothecaries, on the other hand, found themselves a growing role during the nineteenth century as practitioners to the middle class in the expanding industrial cities. When the three branches of practice were combined into one medical register under the Medical Acts of 1858 and 1886, the earlier distinctions did not evaporate. There was now one medical profession, with a training supposedly designed for general practice, but distinctions remained at the graduate level. The elite of the profession (members of the Royal College of Physicians and fellows of the Royal College of Surgeons) continued to control major hospital positions. Indeed, the struggle for an honorary appointment could become the dominant motive of a doctor's career. In 1900, when American hospital building was in full swing and hospital appointments tended to be open to most recognized physicians, the British voluntary hospital was controlled by a small number of leading practitioners. Each was usually responsible for an identifiable group of beds in a particular ward and thus for the patients who occupied those beds. Surgeon-apothecaries, meanwhile, were general practitioners who worked almost entirely outside the voluntary hospital system.

National health insurance provided the final endorsement of this system in 1911 by creating a central role for the general practitioner. Members of the working population below a specified income level were now insured for the services of general practitioners, but not for hospital or specialist care.

General or family practice became, and has remained, central to the organization of the British system. It has been bolstered, it is true, by further government action: the National Health Service Act of 1946, which incorporated general practice as the basis of the health-care system, and changes in reimbursement following the profession's 'Doctor's Charter' of 1965, equalizing generalist and specialist incomes. But such actions would have been unthinkable had the earlier traditions not existed.

Modern medical care in Britain relies, in short, on the system of checks and balances which emerged from the prespecialization era. General practitioners control access to the health-care system; salaried hospital staff, the consultants (who are now, of course, all specialists), control access to hospital care. When each round of specialist treatment is completed, the patient returns to his family practitioner. The old social division between the branches of practice have been continued in the separate *functions* of primary and secondary care, and there continue to be far more general practitioners than specialists.

In the United States there were no guilds, no national focus for an elite such as London provided to British practitioners, and until the 1870s there were relatively few hospitals. American medicine was a profession without institutions. If the professional development of British medicine can be characterized as the history of guilds which eventually came together, establishing mutually acceptable positions, the development of American medicine for most of its history has been a search for *itself*, for identity and professional unity. Out of this movement was to come a medical profession commited to university-centered education and technological advancement, organizationally based on an array of specialists.

Defining the Practice of Medicine

From time to time efforts were made to establish guilds on this side of the Atlantic. John Morgan was one of several Scottish-trained physicians returning to the Colonies who tried before Independence to establish the educated 'physician' as a separate rank of practitioner along British lines. But such efforts were doomed to failure in the competitive and social climate of the day. One continuing theme of American medicine was already evident. Even in the Revolutionary era there were relatively large *numbers* of doctors in America. Clearly medicine was felt to be a desirable occupation.

One estimate for New York in 1750 gives a ratio of one doctor to every 350 members of the population; in Williamsburg in 1730 there was one doctor to every 135 members of the population, relatively a far greater density of doctors than today. It was just not practicable for the American doctor (unless he had considerable private income) to say he would do no surgery and dispense no drugs, but merely be an educated physician. Almost from the beginning, the American doctor has been an individual in a competitive market situation, dependent on his success—not on family connections or institutional affiliations (as is clearly the case of physicians in England), but on the exercise of his own initiative.

Even in the eighteenth century, any suggestion of a guild also suggested the imposition of a potentially dangerous monopoly. Social elitism in medical practice as in other fields has consistently been regarded as un-American. Early licensing laws were repealed in the 1830s and 1840s, leaving the field of medicine open to all comers. (Modern licensing laws date from the 1870s.) The rise of proprietary or profitmaking medical schools during the century added another component for untrammelled competition.

Instead of creating distinctions within the profession, medical societies arose in America to protect all 'regular' practitioners from the common threat of 'irregulars' or quacks.[10] The American College of Surgeons and the American College of Physicians, which followed in 1915, came much too late to direct basic patterns of the medical profession.

Probably the most important early impact of the College of Surgeons was its accreditation and upgrading of the standards of hospitals, which had sprung up like mushrooms from the 1880s in the American doctor's enthusiastic desire to do surgery. The British response to the technological possibilities or relatively 'safe' surgery in the post-asepsis, post-anesthetics era had been to exclude any remaining general practitioners from the staffs of hospitals, restricting operations to the small staff of consulting surgeons. But no such constraints existed in America, and there was a ready market for hospital construction in the expanding cities. Surgery, indeed, was so instantly popular that it was to become a lasting characteristic of American medicine: about a fourth of all American physicians have been surgeons in recent decades, a much larger proportion than in England. While England was consolidating the general practitioner, America was hailing the virtuosity of the surgeon and sometimes criticizing his excesses and deploring his greed.

But in all fields, compared with the individualism, exuberance, and ingenuity of American medical practice at the beginning of this century, medicine in England seemed tame and settled. Abraham Flexner, reporting on England in 1912, found educational standards there low and medical education regarded among clinicians as merely a 'professional incident', with any interest in research mostly missing. The guild system was, he remarked, 'admirably calculated to protect honor and dignity, to conserve ceremony, and to transmit tradition'.[11]

While there were relatively large numbers of doctors in Britain in the first decade of the century, social and ethical structures in Britain precluded out-and-out competition. The British doctor, accustomed to working for the Poor Law and for public health authorities, might welcome National Health Insurance as a means of upgrading his financial status. In America, while there was also discussion of health insurance through the state, the mood was different. Fee-splitting was rife, there were kickbacks, usually from surgeons to referring practitioners. It was acknowledged that fees and services were related: the higher the fee, the better the care. The California state medical journal put forward as its primary objection to contract practice in 1913 *not* the argument that the rates paid were too low, but that patients for whom only 10 cents were paid would get only 10 cents worth of treatment.[12] Cost and quality were inextricably combined, as indeed they have remained to this day.

Since there was no entrenched social structure for general practice, there was no ethical or other barrier against specialization or direct competition for patients by American physicians. There were both money and social advancement in specialism through private office practice—in contrast to the British system of social advancement through hospital positions. Virginia doctors, even in the 1870s, advertised in such areas as 'Speciality Surgery', 'Diseases of Females', 'Diseases of Urinary Organs', 'Diseases of the Ear and Eye'. A formal social class system for medical education had failed in America; there was now an emergence of a self-proclaimed technological elite, competing directly with generalists for patients.

The standardization movement in American medical practice was well underway at the turn of the century. There was a gradual 'leveling up of the masses of the profession'.[14] The reorganization of the Harvard curriculum in 1870 had been followed by upgrading of standards in other schools, and the foundation of the Johns Hopkins school in 1893 provided a paradigm for the future development of scientific, laboratory-oriented medical schools based on universities.

The American Medical Association, unifying its scattered organization over the same period, rose on the banner of standardization. There was to be one American doctor, produced by medical schools of equivalent quality. While the profession in Britain was grappling with the problems of introducing general practitioner services under National Health Insurance in 1911, American medical education was set on the road to an increasingly scientific emphasis for medicine. The movement was rapid. By 1920, America had replaced Germany as the world leader of scientific medicine. Medical education was based on universities, with a strong research emphasis. It was not surprising that the graduates of these schools would turn increasingly to the specialities. Nor, indeed, was there any social structure such as National Health Insurance to encourage the continuation of general practice as a means of making a reasonable living; nor any ethical arrangement such as the referral system, which existed in England, to establish primary care as a central function of the emerging health system. In America generalists continued to compete with specialists, and one specialist with another.

References

1. McInnes, E. M. *St Thomas's Hospital,* Allen and Unwin, London (1963).
2. Washburn, F. A. *The Massachusetts General Hospital: Its Development, 1900–1935,* Houghton Mifflin Co., Boston (1939).
3. Jacobi, A., quoted by Michael M. Davis 'Organization of medical service', *American Labor Legislation Review,* 6 16–20 (1916).
4. Titmuss, R. M. 'Trends of social policy'. In *Law and Opinion in England in the Twentieth Century,* Ginsberg, M. (ed) Greenwood, London (1959).
5. Kershaw, R. *Special Hospitals: Their Origin, Development, and Relationship to Medical Education,* Pulman, London (1909).
6. Burdett, H. C. *Hospitals and Asylums of the World,* Vol. III, J. and A. Churchill, London (1893).
7. Gibbons, H. Annual Address to the California State Medical Society. *Transactions of the Medical Society of California,* privately printed (1872).
8. Newman, C. *The Evolution of Medical Education in the Nineteenth Century,* Oxford University Press, London (1957).
9. Shryock, R. H. *Medicine and Society in America 1660–1860,* New York University Press, New York (1962).
10. Kett, J. *The Formation of the American Medical Profession: The Role of Institutions 1760–1860,* Yale University Press, New Haven (1968).
11. Flexner, A. *Medical Education in Europe,* Carnegie Foundation, New York (1912).

12. *California State Journal of Medicine*, Editorial, **11**, 41 (1913).
13. Blanton, W. B. *Medicine in Virginia in the Nineteenth Century*, Garrett and Massie, Richmond (1933).
14. Mumford, J. G. *A Narrative of Medicine in America*, Lippincott, Philadelphia (1903).

Rosemary Stevens is in the Department of History and Sociology of Science, University of Pennsylvania, though at the time of writing the article she was at Tulane University in Louisiana. The article has been edited from a longer version that appeared in 1976 in *Priorities in the Use of Resources in Medicine*, Number 40 in the Fogarty International Center Proceedings, published by the US Department of Health, Education and Welfare.

4.2

The Structure of the National Health Service

Gwyn Bevan

The NHS is a highly complex organisation in a state of flux. The first consultative document to propose reorganising the NHS was issued by the Ministry of Health in 1968, twenty years after the original structure was created. During the subsequent fifteen years those working in the NHS have been either discussing or implementing radical changes (and in 1984 still implementing one whilst discussing its successor). It is, therefore, essential to situate any description of the structure of the NHS in the context of its past and proposals for the future. It is also important to understand the characteristics of the NHS, which have meant that some of these facts have endured whilst others have been changed. This article therefore begins with a description of the characteristics of the NHS which the various organisational changes have tried to incorporate or modify, before going on to describe the structure of the NHS, how its performance is monitored and evaluated; the different kinds of occupational and professional groups who work in the NHS; and how decisions on resources are made.

The article is mainly concerned with how the NHS is (and has been) organised in England. However, each country of the UK has distinctive organisational characteristics. One worth mentioning here is that the Department of Health and Social Security (DHSS) relates to a Regional tier in England (Regional Health Authorities) whereas Scotland, Wales and Northern Ireland each have government departments which also fulfil some regional responsibilities. The different government departments are the Scottish Home and Health Department; the Welsh Office; and the Department of Health and Social Services (Northern Ireland).

Throughout these descriptions references are made, when necessary, to changes proposed in the Report of the Management Inquiry of 1983 chaired by Mr Roy Griffiths, the Managing Director of Sainsburys (The Griffiths Report). At the time of writing (1984) these proposals have been accepted by the Government, and are being implemented. What does seem clear is that the Inquiry report marks an important phase in the debate over how the NHS should be organised.

Key issues in managing health services

(i) Clinical autonomy

When the NHS was created, doctors secured organisational arrangements which gave them *clinical autonomy*: each doctor is responsible for treating his or her patients and is given autonomy to decide what is appropriate. Fundamental tasks in the NHS are the responsibility of autonomous clinicians. The style of running the NHS has, so far, been to give them administrative support to enable them to discharge their responsibilities to patients, rather than to attempt to manage clinicians and encroach on the delicate (and ill-defined) area of clinical autonomy.

(ii) Hospitals

Many of the initiatives for changes in the management of the NHS originate from the tensions that hospitals necessarily create. On the one hand, there is the sense that health services ought to prevent, as far as possible, the need for hospital services, and it is therefore misplaced to have a health service which is focused on running hospitals. On the other hand, acute hospitals (short-stay) are complex, expensive and require sophisticated management techniques to operate smoothly. The 1948 structure for England and Wales was criticised for its focus on hospitals; it was alleged that what had been created was not a National Health Service but a National Hospitals Service. The 1974 reorganisation sought to alter this but was in turn criticised for providing hospitals (in particular) with a poor management structure. The restructuring of 1982 and the proposals in the Griffiths Report in 1983 both include changes intended to improve management of hospitals (and community services).

(iii) The tripartite structure

The original structure of the NHS was also criticised for fragmenting three services which ought to be coordinated: hospital services, community services and family practitioner services. Community health services were the responsibility of local authorities; they included the work of the medical officer of health (MOH), environmental health officers, school health services and health visitors. The 1974 reorganisation was intended to integrate health services. The post of MOH was abolished. The new health authorities employed many of these workers as community physicians, as well as taking over the school health services and employing health visitors. There is, however, need for coordination with social services which are still (except in Northern Ireland) the responsibility of local authorities. Family Practitioner Services had (and still have) an administrative structure which is largely independent of the Health Authorities. General practitioners were (and still are) independent contractors and not salaried employees of the NHS (unlike hospital doctors).

(iv) Infinite demand, finite resources

Between the publication of the Beveridge Report in 1942 and the launching of the NHS in 1948, the assumption of that report that spending on an NHS would be stable for twenty years (then probably decline) was not challenged even by the Treasury (which is invariably concerned about innovations in expenditure and is particularly on its guard for innovations that have an inbuilt tendency to increase expenditure). The report assumed that as a result of free access to health services, people would become healthier and there would be less need for those services. The Treasury did not question that assumption and the Ministry of Health was able to guarantee clinical autonomy to the doctors without alarming the Treasury.

The failure to question the naive assumptions of the Beveridge Report eased the launching of the NHS. But the failure to achieve financial control of the NHS was not understood during the first decade of its existence. It is only in recent years that the problems posed by seeking to reconcile that control with clinical autonomy are being seriously considered.

The 1974 reorganisation was based on (what appears in retrospect to be) an equally naive assumption: that the problems of resource management had ceased to be serious because of economic growth. The oil that fuelled that growth was, unfortunately, at the time that reorganisation was being accomplished, being so increased in price that even the limited economic growth of the UK stopped.

The assumptions behind subsequent changes to the NHS are that these will lead to improvements in the management of the service and the efficiency with which services are delivered. In future, the NHS is expected to generate much of the extra resources that are needed by its own efforts.

History of NHS and Management

Figure 1 gives the three different structures of the NHS in England: from 1948 to 1974; from 1974 to 1982; and since 1982. There has always been: a regional structure for hospital services, initially Regional Hospital Boards (RHBs) and, from 1974, Regional Health Authorities (RHAs); and a separate administration for Family Practitioner Services, initially through Executive Councils, and, from 1974, through Family Practitioner Committees. Fundamental changes have taken place within the regional structure in 1974: undergraduate teaching hospitals were integrated with other hospitals (i.e. abolition of their autonomous Board of Governors); Hospital Management Committees were abolished; Area Health Authorities (AHAs) and Districts were created. In 1982: AHAs were abolished and District Health Authorities (DHAs) created; DHAs were to strengthen management at unit level by creating Unit Management Groups (UMGs). This section attempts to explain why the changes took place and what the functions of the different administrative bodies are.

The 1948 organisation of the NHS encouraged a bias towards institutions and particularly acute hospitals: RHBs saw planning in terms of new acute hospitals; their constituent Hospital Management Committees and the independent Boards of Governors were concerned with running hospitals. The priorities appeared to be: first, teaching hospitals; second, other acute hospitals; third, long-stay care; and finally, within long-stay care, services for the mentally handicapped.

The 1974 reorganisation, which created RHAs, AHAs and Districts, introduced four main features specifically directed at mobilising the biases of these organisations away from institutions and acute services. The first was the establishment of management teams at District level which include a general practitioner and a community physician. This also applies to the DHAs created in 1982 (see below).

A second feature was a new planning system (launched in 1976) which emphasised services rather than buildings and enabled multidisciplinary teams (including, for example, general practitioners and social workers) to consider developments for 'priority' care groups (such as the elderly, the mentally ill and the mentally handicapped). This planning system continues to develop.

The third feature was the creation of AHAs in England and Wales (and Health Boards in Scotland) which were normally coterminous with the boundaries of the local authorities responsible for social services, and with the administration of Family Practitioner Services. In Northern Ireland, the Health Boards were made jointly responsible for health and social services, the latter being transferred from local authorities. The creation of AHAs (and Health Boards) can be seen as the cornerstone of the objectives of the 1974 reorganisation in terms of facilitating coordination of the different services.

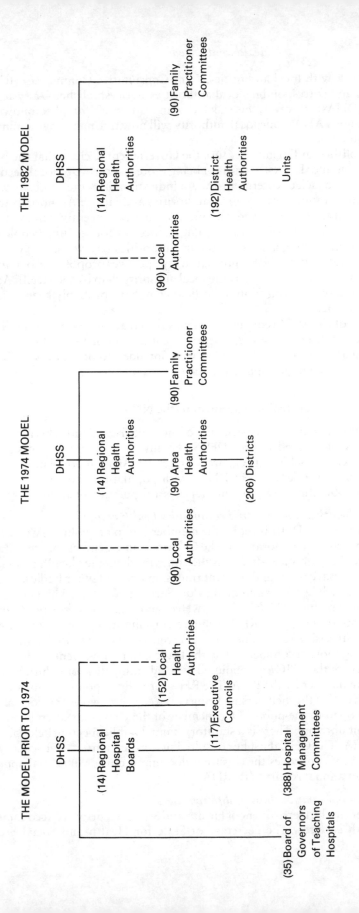

THE MODEL PRIOR TO 1974

DHSS

(14) Regional Hospital Boards

(152) Local Health Authorities

(117) Executive Councils

(388) Hospital Management Committees

(35) Board of Governors of Teaching Hospitals

THE 1974 MODEL

DHSS

(14) Regional Health Authorities

(90) Local Authorities

(90) Area Health Authorities

(90) Family Practitioner Committees

(206) Districts

THE 1982 MODEL

DHSS

(14) Regional Health Authorities

(90) Local Authorities

(90) Family Practitioner Committees

(192) District Health Authorities

Units

―――― Indicates direct managerial authority

– – – Indicates consultative/coordinating relationships

Figure 1 The changing management structure of the NHS in England since 1948

To facilitate work with local authorities, Joint Consultative Committees (JCCs) of officers from AHAs and corresponding local authorities were established—a system that has continued with DHAs. However, this task has been made more complex following the abolition of coterminous AHAs: one local authority will now normally have a number of DHAs with which to work.

AHAs were abolished in England because the Government decided that the benefits of the creation of the smaller DHAs, in terms of being more responsive to local needs, outweighed the losses from a lack of coterminosity. An indication that coterminosity was not sufficient to foster cooperation between local authorities and Health Authorities was the introduction in 1977, and the continued use since, of financial incentives in the form of joint finance to encourage such cooperation. Joint finance is about getting people out of hospital, or stopping them being admitted. Health Authorities receive monies which can only be spent by local authorities; the Health Authority approves proposals providing that the money can be more effectively spent by the local authority than by the Health Authority. However, the total sums involved in 'joint financing' have probably been much too small to have much impact.

A fourth feature of the 1974 reorganisation was the creation of Community Health Councils (CHCs) for each District to represent the consumers of the NHS. They were encouraged to pay particular attention to what were intended to be services for priority groups, such as the mentally handicapped and the elderly.

Current management of the NHS

Figure 2 shows the current management structure of the NHS in England. This includes the various organisations mentioned above: DHSS; Family Practitioner Services; RHAs, DHAs, and Units; JCCs and CHCs. There are fourteen RHAs with populations ranging from two to six million people and 192 DHAs with populations ranging from under 100,000 to about 860,000 (the average size of a DHA is a population of around 200,000).

(i) Membership of health authorities and community health councils
The policy of each RHA and DHA is set by the members, who are voluntary apart from the Chairman, who receives an honorarium. The Chairman and members of each RHA are appointed by the Secretary of State after consultation with the major health professions, main local authorities, universities and relevant trades unions and other bodies.

The Chairman of each DHA is appointed by the Secretary of State, whereas the other members are appointed by the RHA (normally twelve) and by local authorities (normally four). The members appointed by the RHA include a consultant; a general practitioner; a nurse, midwife or health visitor; a nominee of the university medical school in the region; a member from among those recommended by the trade union movement.

Half the members of the CHC are appointed by local authorities, one-third by voluntary bodies and the remainder by the RHA. The RHA formally appoints the members for four-year terms, with half of the membership being renewed every two years. Formal meetings of the CHC are open to the public. One member of the CHC may attend and speak at DHA meetings, but not vote. There is a statutory annual public meeting held jointly by the CHC and the DHA. The CHC must be consulted on certain matters, particularly hospital closures: if the CHC approves the closure it does not require Ministerial approval. Each CHC submits an annual report to its RHA.

(ii) Responsibilities and relationships of different tiers
Government Ministers in the Department of Health and Social Security are accountable to Parliament for health services. The Secretary of State for Health and Social Security

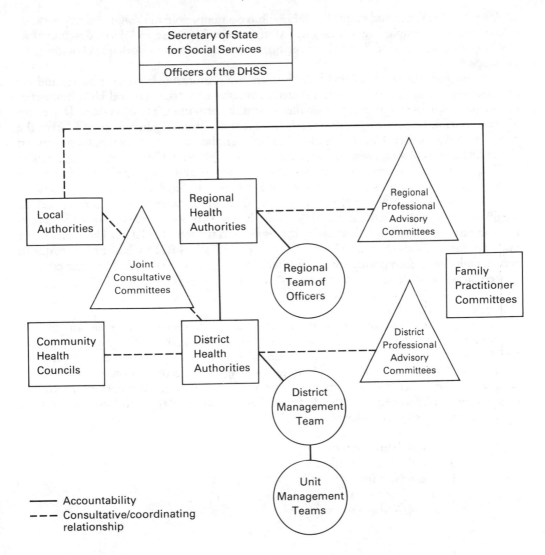

Figure 2 The management structure of the NHS in England from 1982

negotiates in Cabinet for resources for the NHS (as well as for Social Security and Social Services). The DHSS decides allocations of capital and revenue to the RHAs. Ministers are responsible for broad, national direction on policies. These include decisions on priorities and changes in the provision of services. DHSS officials advise Ministers and have had to tread a delicate path between formulating policy and leaving management to those in the NHS. This practice, as might be expected, has not been wholly successful and the Griffiths Report called for the creation of two national boards: the Government has established one (the Supervisory Board) and the other (the Management Board) will (at the time of writing) be established as soon as its chairman has been appointed.

The Regional Health Authorities are mainly policy-making bodies (their policies being subject to approval by the DHSS). They produce strategies for the development of services and are accountable to the DHSS for the delivery of services by DHAs. They decide allocations of revenue and capital to DHAs; have a major role in design and approval of major hospitals; employ senior medical staff (except for those in DHAs designated as teaching authorities); and decide how regional services (such as radiotherapy) ought to be developed.

In contrast, the District Health Authorities are responsible both for policies and for the running of health services. Each District contains a District General Hospital, either one large hospital or a number of smaller hospitals, providing acute services. DHAs are also responsible for services for the elderly, the mentally ill and the handicapped. Given the nature of RHAs and DHAs, the relationship between them is more complex than between subordinate tiers of a commercial organisation. The operational principle still appears to be that of the 1974 reorganisation: maximising accountability upwards and delegation downwards. There is no simple line relationship between officers in one tier and officers in its superior in the hierarchy. Exceptionally, there are differences over policy, such as Regional Chairmen criticising the DHSS, and Health Authorities refusing to make reductions in finance or staffing called for by the DHSS and the relevant RHA. The Secretary of State appoints Chairmen of RHAs and DHAs. In 1982 all 14 RHA Chairmen were due to retire; eight were re-appointed for a further term, six were replaced. The replacements caused 'acrimonious public recriminations' (*The Health Services,* 9 July 1982).

(iii) Management teams

There are two vital issues in managing the NHS: the need to secure 'consensus' and the role of clinicians. The importance of securing consensus was seen to be so important in the 1974 reorganisation that it became institutionalised for each administrative tier. At each level of the NHS a 'team' is specified in terms of its membership; 'consensus' has been defined as all members of the team agreeing on a decision, or no members disagreeing so strongly that *they* would veto the decision. Teams exist at Regional, District and Unit levels and are constituted as follows:

Regional: Regional Administrator
              Regional Medical Officer
              Regional Nursing Officer
              Regional Treasurer
              Regional Works Officer

District: District Administrator
              District Medical Officer
              District Nursing Officer
              District Treasurer
              A consultant representative
              A general practitioner representative

Unit: Unit Administrator
              Unit Nursing Officer
              A medical representative

The Griffiths Report recommended the appointment of General Managers at each level. The Government, in June 1984, asked health authorities in England to identify individual general managers (drawn from inside and outside the NHS), for these to be introduced at health authority level as soon as possible and at unit level by the end of 1985. This means that an individual rather than a team is identified with the responsibility of general management at each level. Although this means the end of 'consensus management' it does not mean the end of management by consensus: the style through which consensus is achieved will be changed.

There are important distinctions between the posts of executive officers, such as the administrators, medical officers, nursing officers and treasurers, and the representatives of consultants and general practitioners. The administrator, nurse and treasurer are the senior persons at the top of the hierarchy of that function. The consultants and general practitioners have no hierarchy and elect their representatives. The medical officer is a community physician whose prime function as an officer of the Authority is to provide a broad community-based view of health needs.

(iv) Monitoring and evaluation by central government

Monitoring takes place both within the NHS and by external bodies. Within the NHS each level is expected to monitor and evaluate the performance of its subordinate tier: the DHSS of RHAs, RHAs of DHAs and DHAs of Units. The planning system is intended to enable the different levels to agree on objectives and future policies and to provide a basis for monitoring subsequent action. Since 1981, a system of Annual Performance Reviews has given a formal procedure through which monitoring and review are conducted. The monitoring and evaluation of performance would seem to be a natural, routine activity for any organisation and may therefore appear to merit no discussion. What is remarkable is the piecemeal, *ad hoc*, nature of the developments of such processes in the NHS. This was seized on by the Griffiths Report which hopes, through its proposed recommendations, to ensure routine and systematic monitoring and evaluation of the performance of the NHS. These hopes depend, however, on finding an acceptable way of measuring the performance of an organisation as complex as the NHS.

Some monitoring of some parts of the NHS is carried out by national bodies set up and controlled by the DHSS, such as the Health Advisory Service (HAS). This was set up first as the Hospital Advisory Service, following the Ely Hospital scandal when the administration of services for the mentally handicapped in a Cardiff hospital was severely criticised in an official report. The Hospital Advisory Service concentrated on inspecting conditions in long-stay hospitals. The Health Advisory Service has a broader remit and now covers health and personal social services. Other central government monitoring is carried out by the Health Service Commissioner (or so-called health ombudsman).

The final level of monitoring occurs in Parliament where Ministers are accountable for the NHS and have to answer a variety of questions. Two committees have specific concern: the Gladstonian Public Accounts Committee (PAC) and the recently established (1979) Select Committee on Health and Social Services. The PAC has long been influential in its examination of waste and inefficiency (it is seen as an embodiment of the spirit of Parliamentary scrutiny of the management of public money). The PAC routinely considers reports by the Comptroller and Auditor General on total expenditure and examines subjects which he draws to the Committee's attention. In Parliament, the DHSS is monitored by a Select Committee which has produced a number of influential reports. This Committee routinely reports on the annual White Paper on public expenditure on the Government's plans for the NHS.

Occupations in the NHS

The data on staff employed in the NHS show that nurses are by far the most numerous, followed by ancillary workers, with administrative and clerical staff being ranked third

(Table 1). The number of doctors is relatively small. In the NHS, the importance of employing doctors, nurses and midwives is naturally unchallenged. Other jobs of a professional and technical nature (such as laboratory technicians) are also seen to be essential for a modern health service. The value of the jobs of ancillary workers (such as porters, cleaners, laundry and catering workers) can also be readily understood.

Table 1 Staff directly employed by the NHS in England in 1980

Type of Staff	Number (whole time equivalent)
Medical and dental	38,200
Nursing and midwifery	370,100
Professional and technical	61,900
Works professional	5,900
Maintenance	20,600
Administrative and clerical	105,430
Ambulance officers, etc.	3,200
Ambulance men/women, etc.	14,560
Ancillary	172,000
Total	791,900

The question of who might be dispensable tends to be focused on administrators. Does the NHS need all those administrators? Could not the money be better spent on patient care? Although it is conventional to question the value of administrators in public services, it is worth challenging this convention. Administrators provide the management and the information essential for the functioning, monitoring and evaluation of the NHS. Consider the various administrative tasks involved in admitting someone to hospital: first, it is necessary to make sure that a bed is available in the appropriate ward. Second, caring for the person in hospital requires: administration of supplies (e.g. bed linen, food, drugs, dressing, equipment); arrangements of diagnostic tests; coordination of the tasks involved in an operation. The myriad administrative functions that go on in hospitals (which, of course, are only part of administration; other tasks include running community services, budgeting and planning) indicate the essential nature of administration. This does not mean that current practice is perfect, nor that the number currently employed in administration is just right. But questions about improving performance or about the numbers employed can, of course, also be asked about everyone employed in the NHS.

Professional organisations and unions

The influence of the medical profession on the policy of the NHS goes back to 1948; that of nursing is more recent, having been formally introduced in 1974. The 1974 reorganisation also introduced a plethora of advisory groups for the various professions of the NHS: doctors, dentists, nurses and midwives, pharmacists, ophthalmic and dispensing opticians. The medical and nursing professions are represented on management teams at District and Regional levels and on DHAs and RHAs.

Groups which lack professional status do have a voice on policy, albeit limited, through the trade union representation on authorities. Unionisation has grown apace in the NHS, the two principal unions being the Confederation of Health Services Employees (COHSE) and the National Union of Public Employees (NUPE). Workers in the NHS also belong to other unions, such as the National and Local Government Officers Association (NALGO) and the Association of Scientific, Technical and Managerial Staffs (ASTMS). There is some overlap and competition between unions and professional organisations, particularly for nurses among NUPE, COHSE and the Royal College of Nursing (RCN). However, NUPE mainly recruits ancillary workers, porters, ward orderlies and cooks; COHSE mainly recruits those with the least prestigious qualifications, such as the less-skilled nurses working in long-stay hospitals. There are no clear lines of demarcation, and the unions have increasingly challenged the RCN's capacity to act as both trade union and professional organisation.

The General Medical Council (GMC) is a statutory national body which is responsible for recognition of the right to be a medical practitioner (whether in hospital, community services or general practice). The GMC vets hospitals which provide clinical training for medical students as house officers after they have passed their university exams, and is responsible for striking off a doctor's name from the medical register for misconduct.

The Royal Colleges are run by the doctors to regulate their own specialities. They are also sources of advice on national policy for the different specialities. Some Royal Colleges are ancient (those of Physicians and Surgeons); others are more recent (such as that of General Practitioners). Individuals appointed to consultant posts are usually members of the appropriate Royal College, which means that they have received a postgraduate training recognised as suitable by that College and have passed the membership exams. The Royal College of General Practitioners is developing a similar role in general practice.

The British Medical Association (BMA) is the most famous organisation of medical practitioners but has no statutory or regulatory responsibilities (these being vested in the Royal Colleges and the GMC). The BMA claims to represent the whole of the medical profession. One of its important functions is that of being the main doctors' 'trade union', although it has carefully eschewed this description (even to the extent that its application, in December 1971, for registration as a trade union under the Industrial Relations Act was accompanied by an official statement that 'we shall not, by registering, become a Trade Union').

Financial Management of the NHS

Finally, it is necessary to consider briefly one of the most crucial aspects of managing the NHS—that of finance. Governments of all developed countries have major problems in financing health care. When we say the NHS is 'free', this means that few charges are levied for the services provided; it does not mean that often painful choices and decisions about spending on the NHS can be avoided. The NHS is financed mainly from general taxation (and not from National Insurance contributions). Because the NHS does not have its own ear-marked source of funding, decisions on its total expenditure have to be made by setting its claim against those for less taxation and for increase in expenditure on social security, defence, education, etc. These necessarily political judgements are made by the Cabinet in the annual Public Expenditure Survey. Arguments have been made about altering this process, in particular to some kind of earmarked finance on the assumption that people would be prepared to pay more for health services under such an arrangement. However, the Report of Royal Commission on the NHS (published in 1979) reviewed these arguments and concluded that they would have little impact on the total sums available for the NHS (and would increase administrative costs).

The outcome of the Public Expenditure Survey is a plan in cash for three forward years, published in annual White Papers on public expenditure. The first year provides the cash budget for the NHS for the coming financial year; this is one of the Estimates presented to the House of Commons before the start of the financial year to gain the Commons' approval for the supply of money.

In 1976 the Resource Allocation Working Party (RAWP), which had been set up by the DHSS, produced a report that recommended methods to distribute revenue and capital in England between different regions. These methods calculate for Health Authorities future *targets* that are intended to indicate each authority's resource entitlement from a given total. The intention is to move each authority's allocation toward its target. The DHSS has used the RAWP methods for making allocations of revenue to RHAs (the methods for capital are less sound, were used after some delay, and are under review). Resource allocation working parties of the other government departments of health and of most RHAs followed the RAWP methods in calculating revenue targets for their district authorities and boards.

The processes of resource allocation decide how much money each authority and board has available. How the money is spent on different services is decided through budgeting. Since 1974 budgeting has been organised in terms of different functions, such as nursing, catering and laundry. It is important to note that clinicians, unless responsible for a function (such as pathology), are not budget holders; they make demands for treating patients (either implicitly or explicitly) on budgets managed by others. This is one of the main issues which the Griffiths Report attempted to tackle. The report called for greater involvement by clinicians in budgeting. This was seen as one way of creating greater accountability in the NHS, which in turn, it was hoped, would lead to better management. Whether or not such changes take place is uncertain at the time of writing. The effect that such changes might have is even less clear.

Gwyn Bevan is a health economist working in the Department of Community Medicine, St Thomas' Hospital Medical School, London. This article which has not previously been published, was written while Gwyn Bevan was working at the University of Warwick.

4.3

Traditional Indian Medicine in Practice in an Indian Metropolitan City

A. Ramesh and B. Hyma

Indigenous medical beliefs and practices have always been an integral part of many human cultures. A recent WHO [World Health Organization] Meeting on the Promotion and Development of Traditional Medicine observed that even though many health professionals and institutions often viewed traditional medicine 'as a practice on the decline and of no importance' it is still important and has vitality. Traditional systems of medicine continued to meet the health needs of most rural populations of the developing world and find patronage in urban areas as well.

There are many reasons cited for the promotion and development of traditional medicine: its approach is unique and holistic. It is culturally, socially and environmentally close to people, i.e. it is the people's own health care system and is accepted and utilized by them. It has a potential for wider application at low cost. It uses local resources (herbs, metals, minerals, etc.), local technology and local labor. It is not dependent on alien technology, materials, expertise and knowledge. It is found particularly effective in dealing with many chronic ailments, allergic conditions, culturally linked psychosomatic diseases and illnesses. It is also recognized that the services of traditional healers and practitioners could be utilized with advantage at various levels of preventive and curative techniques in the health care programs. It has the potential to contribute to scientific and universal medicine.

Practitioners of traditional medicine represent a vast human resource outside the official health services. It is well known that many of the traditional medical practitioners of various categories (such as healers, herbalists, spiritualists, birth attendants or midwives) 'have already undergone elaborate training in ancient systems of medicine that had evolved reliable methods of treatment and pattern of medications long before modern medicine came along. Other healers have had their skill handed down through generations—the distillation of a surprising degree of practical knowledge, skills and wisdom about the physical, mental and psychological ills of mankind'.

To assess the effectiveness of traditional medicine in practice, this paper concentrates its investigation in a metropolitan city of India where the traditional Indian medical systems continue to flourish. This study was restricted itself to examining the size, distribution and the current social, economic and political status and practice characteristics of traditional practitioners in the city of Madras, India.

A Note on the Traditional Medicine in India

In the history of medical systems in India, traditional medicine has not been static, but has continually evolved and progressed even in urban settings. In India there are two parallel systems of medicine, the modern system commonly referred to as allopathy and homoeopathy, and the Ayurvedic, Siddha and Unani system of medicine, commonly known as indigenous system. Naturopathy and Yoga also attract followers for their therapeutic values. Of the three indigenous systems of medicine, Ayurveda is used all over the country.[1] Siddha is extensively used in the southern state of Tamil Nadu and in the neighboring states.[2] The Unani system is used predominantly in areas of Muslim culture.[3]

On the basis of National Health Policy formulated in 1948, after the Independence of India, the Government is committed to promote and develop the indigenous system of medicine along with the modern medicine. The indigenous system of medicine is practiced by a large number of hereditary medical practitioners and by persons trained in teaching institutions run by the State Governments and other approved bodies. India now has a large number of qualified practitioners of integrated medicine and an estimated total of 7,000–8,000 professionally qualified practitioners of Ayurveda, Siddha, Unani and homoeopathy are entering the profession every year.

Carl E. Taylor has estimated that 'in India organized health services provide only 10% of the medical care. Another 10% is provided by qualified physicians in towns and cities. The balance is split between home medical care and indigenous practitioners.'

Though modern scientific medicine forms the basis for the development of the National Health Services in the country, ultimate objectives are to facilitate the integration and emergence of one system of medicine with its various sub-systems. Modern health care systems continue to expand and command people's respect, yet traditional systems are by no means on the decrease. However, it is still not very clear how the two approaches to medicine can be integrated or to what extent they can cooperate and interact. In the search for effective ways either to integrate or develop these two systems it becomes necessary to examine their competence and capacity, to serve and satisfy the basic health needs of the populations concerned and to be integrated into public health systems in primary health care.

The Research Setting and Methods

Madras is the fourth largest city in India with a population of nearly 3 million (1977 estimate), in which approximately 30 per cent live in 1,200 slums and squatter settlements where the basic needs of these people are not fully satisfied. Madras is also one of the major centers of modern medicine in India, with its established medical schools, numerous hospitals (both private and public), nursing homes, clinics, dispensaries and medical practitioners (general and specialists, etc.). It is also one of the centers of traditional medicine where numerous Ayurveda, Siddha, Unani and homoeopathy practitioners, clinical and pharmacological research centers and other clinics and dispensaries (both private and public) are found scattered at various parts of the city.

These centers of traditional medicine, large and small, serve a significant majority of the city's population, and also draw a large number of patients seeking treatment from the immediate metropolitan region as well as from other parts of the State and out of the State. Very little is known about the way the two divergent approaches (modern medicine vs indigenous medicine) to healing operate side by side in the same metropolitan setting. We seem to know even less about the reasons for the persistence of indigenous medical practices in the most expanding urban cultures, or about the structural accommodation which must be made in the urban environment with the advent of modern medical establishments and practices, and the people's health needs and behavioral responses to such rapid changes in the health care systems. Even though overall trends may appear to be moving towards adoption of modern scientific therapy in urban areas, general observations indicate that Indian systems of herbal medicine and practitioners are in no way diminishing in size in serving some of the basic health needs of the people in the city.

Spatial distribution of IMPs in Madras city—a general observation
A heavy concentration (more than 50 per cent of the total IMPs [Indigenous Medical Practitioners]) has occurred in the old residential highly populated areas of the city followed by significant numbers clustered in the old commercial and manufacturing sectors in the northern parts of the city. In the newly developed residential neighborhoods their numbers are very low, below 0.1 per cent, indicating a distinct spatial pattern of concentration in the diffusion of IMPs in Madras City.

With regard to the three indigenous systems of medicine (viz. Siddha, Ayurveda and Unani), it is observed that Siddha practitioners, numbering 635 out of a total of 956 IMPS, dominate the spatial pattern in Madras City. This is again reflected in the very high concentration of Siddha IMPs in old residential areas. The Ayurveda practitioners (200) do not exhibit any definite pattern with regard to their spatial distribution. However, small concentrations are found in some old parts of the city. The Unani practitioners are concentrated in the same area as Siddha vaidyas.

An Analysis of the Questionnaire Survey

In order to analyse in detail the spatial phenomena with regard to the IMPs in Madras, the sample practitioners (private and registered), 95 in all were interviewed by a detailed questionnaire. A total of 35 questions relating to the following 10 major socio-economic and practice characteristics were asked: (1) System of practice; (2) Practitioner's personal dimensions; (3) Training background; (4) Practice; (5) Characteristic features of the patients seen; (6) Diagnostic methods; (7) Prescription of medicine; (8) Procurement of medicine; (9) Specialization; and (10) Attitude and opinion.

System of practice
Though there are three major types, Ayurveda, Siddha and Unani, still a number of practitioners practiced integrated medicine. The survey showed that 36.4 per cent of the IMPs belong to Siddha System, followed by Ayurveda (36.4 per cent), Unani (10.4 per cent) and Integrated (20 per cent) which clearly indicates the importance of Siddha and Ayurveda systems in meeting the basic health care needs.

Practitioner's personal dimensions
The bulk of them were male members. Only a handful of them were females in all the three

systems. These few female practitioners are found to practice mainly integrated medicine specializing in gynecology and obstetrics. It is interesting to note that practitioners of ancient Ayurveda and Siddha were traditionally males. It is reported however, that a few females are now being trained in Ayurveda, Siddha and Unani Colleges. Unani medicine seems to be the domain of males.

Two-thirds of the practitioners interviewed were found in the age group between 40 and 60. It is interesting to note they were equally divided into the 40–50 and 50–60 age groups. The low figure in the age group between 20–40 clearly indicated that fewer practitioners have entered the profession in recent years in the city.

Though most of the IMPs belonged to the Hindu religious community, a small proportion of them were Muslims. There were only two Christians who practiced Indian medicine in our sample. Further, it can be pointed out that a fifth of the Muslims practiced Siddha and Ayurveda systems rather than Unani which is favoured by Muslim culture.

About a third of the practitioners had college education. Thirty persons indicated that they had diplomas/certificates and practiced Siddha or Ayurvedic medicine but received no formal education. The rest of the practitioners had 8–11 years of school education.

More than 50 per cent of the IMPs were born and brought up in Madras City itself, but of these the bulk of them practice Siddha medicine. About 16 per cent of the practitioners had rural background and another 10 per cent who came from outside the State of Tamil Nadu. It is interesting to note that most of the practitioners who came from outside the state are engaged in Ayurvedic practice, indicating that a strong base for Ayurveda exists outside the State of Tamil Nadu.

Nearly half of the practitioners interviewed entered the profession because of its tradition within the family. It was also observed that a small proportion (15 per cent) of the practitioners have indicated that some of their relatives also practice Indian indigenous medicine.

Practice

A small percentage (10 per cent) of practitioners worked in more than two clinics in the city. It is also observed that most of the practitioners had not changed their location of practice since their registration, indicating either the stability of their practice or lack of other alternatives!

The location choice seems to be either older populated residential areas or economically viable areas. However, a quarter of the practitioners had their clinics in areas where they acquired them through hereditary practices. In general, the location choice exhibited a definite pattern. The high class and upper middle class neighbourhoods did not seem to attract the IMPs. Further, the middle income group were concentrated mainly in the residential areas in the old congested parts of the city. This is, however, not to say that the elites had no access to this health care system. Their ease of mobility made it possible for them to select practitioners, clinics and dispensaries offering indigenous medicine.

The general procedure (in contrast with modern medical practices) is to spend 10–20 minutes (25 per cent of the practitioners) or 20–40 minutes (35 per cent) per patient per day. In other words, this norm confirmed previous findings that 'the more traditional an indigenous medical practitioner was in his approach to diagnosis and treatment, the more likely he was to spend more than 10 minutes with a given patient'.

Characteristics of patients

With regard to age or sex, there seems to be no definite pattern. Data from interviews with patients of practitioners showed that 50 per cent of those interviewed were in the age group 20–50. A large number of housewives, and men in government services were met. A sizeable group of middle class people also attended the dispensaries run by these practitioners. At least 20 per cent of the patients said they had college education and 50 per cent of them have had no formal schooling. Most of the patients were drawn from within the city and from the immediate neighborhood of the practitioner's place of practice.

Most of the practitioners settled their fees with the patients at the time of each visit. A few of the patients received treatment on credit. Though most of the practitioners said that they do not collect money from the economically poorer sections of the community, the minimum charge for consultation ranged between Rs. 2 to Rs. 5 per patient. Thirty per cent of the patients interviewed said that it cost them less than Rs. 2 per visit. This indicated that the practitioners charge for their service on the ability of their clients to pay rather than conforming to fixed consultation fees. Most of the patients appeared satisfied with their practitioners and said they are warm and friendly and placed their confidence in them.

Diagnostic methods

Few of the IMPs exhibited modern medical instruments such as stethoscopes, thermometers, blood pressure apparatus, syringes and needles. These were used mainly by those who practiced integrated medicine. These practitioners also occasionally sent their patients for laboratory tests for blood, stools, urine and X-rays. About 30 per cent said they performed minor surgery like stitching, incising or dressing wounds, etc. A quarter would not treat any cases relating to minor surgery.

Most of the IMPs use physical examination such as viewing the patient's body (darsanam in Sanskrit), touching (sparsanam) and eliciting information by questioning (prasanam). It appeared that nearly 50 per cent of the practitioners use pulse rates, 32 per cent diagnose by eye examination and 25 per cent by examination of hair and ears. However, pathological methods of diagnosis seem to still play a less important role in their method of practice.

Prescription of medicine

Less than 15 per cent of the practitioners said they prescribe Indian medicine as well as allopathy medicine. Nearly two-thirds of them said they prescribe only indigenous medicine. There were no responses from the rest. The prescription of medicine seems to be influenced to some extent by the hereditary formulae for preparing local herbs, powders, minerals, etc. and by local cultural knowledge and concepts related to the prevalent diseases in the area. Many methods and techniques employed are closely guarded secrets.

Specialization

There were some clear indications of the kinds of cases which the practitioners preferred to treat. However, 25 per cent of them would not treat any cases relating to the surgical side. Most of the practitioners were of the view that all types of diseases could be treated by indigenous medicine.

In the most commonly treated diseases noted in our survey, ailments like coughs, diarrhoea, dysentery, fever, indigestion, etc. have been given primary importance (by 80 per cent of the practitioners) followed by skin disorders (45 per cent of the IMPs treated these), ulcer (50 per cent), nervous disorders (42 per cent), rheumatism (24 per cent) and lung and bronchial ailments (24 per cent). About 5–6 per cent of the practitioners claimed that they can treat specific cases like anemia, arthritis, colics, cellulitis, dermatitis, diabetes, jaundice, obesity, rheumatism, sexual disorders, menstrual disorders, mental diseases, children's diseases, infertility, impotence, etc.

There appears to be little formal specialization, in contrast with modern medicine. A handful of practitioners, however, claimed that they have developed special formulae in treating specific ailments like rheumatism, arthritis, children's diseases, skin diseases, etc. About 5 per cent claimed that they practiced witchcraft and black magic. However, there are no clear records of potent medicines and their effects on patients. No written records nor files were maintained by the practitioners. Those few who did maintain some records were reluctant to produce them. So valuable information on types of diseases treated and the associated medicaments used is often lacking or unavailable to assess the efficacy of treatment.

The Concluding Discussion

This survey was carried out with an aim of ascertaining some of the strengths and weaknesses of traditional medical practices in an urban setting.

The indigenous medical systems still remain a significant contributor to medical care of the people not only in rural areas but also in the cities. They seem to have survived in their present independent form, with each system retaining its own special features. From our survey it is not possible to identify definitely or clearly whether a particular branch (Ayurveda, Siddha or Unani) of this system is able more effectively to meet the health needs of the population. All three seem to provide fairly satisfactory solutions for common local ailments. However, observations indicate that in Madras city, Ayurvedic institutions and clinics in general continue to enjoy more public support than Siddha and Unani. The proportion of the total urban population receiving Ayurvedic care has steadily increased as evidenced by an increase in the sale of its popular products as well as expansion of some of its dispensaries.

Lack of standardized training and qualification of the practitioners is still evident, even though a large number are entering the profession every year. All grades and levels of training, with different knowledge, skills and sophistication of practice exist in the city. Most of the practitioners operate in isolation and their bargaining power is weak. This may be partly due to their inability or failure to form effective associations or societies or to belong to those few in existence so as to improve the quality of their services as well as to protect their interests.

Adoption of modern scientific and technical methods of practice is very incomplete. Even the lack of precision in diagnostic methods was observed. Techniques for preparation and preserving medical remedies are not standardized nor inspected closely. Absence of toxicological and pharmacodynamic analysis is noted except for those conducted on a small scale in a handful of government and private research clinics and laboratories.

In the informal sector of the city, many of the IMPs seem much more secure and confident and continue to offer a useful public service in the city. Though not all IMPs may be suited for integration into modern health care organizations, certainly a sizeable number may be eligible for incorporation. Even where there is competition from modern practitioners in the same community, these IMPs are able to maintain stable practices and enjoy social prestige if not great economic prosperity.

A number of favorable factors support them: they charge less for their services; they are located in centers where effective demand for their services still exists; they provide many dietary prescriptions which are expected by people of Indian culture when they are ill.

All indications are that indigenous medical systems will probably continue to provide services as long as the central and state governments continue to sponsor the indigenous systems officially, and promote medical relief, education and training, and clinical and pharmacological research. At present indigenous medical services freely cut across all socio-economic groups as well as rural and urban areas. However, they still continue to occupy an insignificant position under the programmes for health planning in the states.

The possibility of bringing Indian medical practitioners into the national/regional/ local health care programmes needs to be continually evaluated especially in view of the shortages of trained health personnel to provide services for the development of rural as well as urban health care systems.

Strong governmental commitment, support and planning for this system are still lacking. State aid to institutions, dispensaries and private practitioners still remains a minor part of total health expenditures. The status of many of the private practitioners remains economically backward compared to allopathic doctors. Male domination to some extent may limit direct female access to health care in this system.

The practical and survival value of Indian medical practitioners is certainly high. Thus given proper understanding, publicity and financial support, traditional systems of medicine can play a vital role in a country's health care delivery programmes, i.e. the capacity of health care can be considerably increased by the use of doctors trained in indigenous medicine. Understanding the complementarity of functions between the modern and the traditional medicine also awaits further exploration and research in the Indian urban setting.

This brings us to a final question as to whether one should advance the development of a dual health care system from which patients can select modern or traditional health services or an integrated system, where it is certain that traditional systems would occupy a subordinate role and lose their individual cultural heritage characteristics. This policy-implementation decision continues to pose a dilemma to many governments of developing nations.[4]

Notes and References

1. Ayurveda is the traditional Hindu system of medicine based on Vedic scriptures; it utilizes herbs, minerals and diet restrictions in treatment of illnesses. Literature available on Ayurveda was found to be compiled sometime during the fifth century BC.
2. Siddha system of medicine in Tamil Nadu, an explanatory note: This system is considered as an independent entity. Its antiquity is well recognized. The exact period of its origin is not known (some claim that it existed before Vedic period). The therapeutics of Siddha medicine consist mainly of the use of metals and minerals, whereas in the earlier Ayurvedic texts there is no mention of metals. It has, however, many similarities with Ayurvedic medicine. It uses also products of vegetable and animal origins. There were 18 Siddhars who were basically responsible for many branches of knowledge and their works were written in Tamil. There are at least 500 works written and 3,000 formulae. Initially they were recorded on palm leaves. Many examples of palm leaf literature are still being transcribed and printed in Tamil. The exact figure of Siddha Vaidyas (practitioners) is not known. However, they are known to exist in thousands in the state of Tamil Nadu.
3. The Unani system, also known as the Greek/Arab system of medicine, brought into India by the Muslim conquerors, has also been in use for several hundred years. It uses herbs, minerals and metallic salts.
4. Birchman, W. 'Primary health care and traditional medicine—considering the background of changing health care concepts in Africa', *Soc. Sci. Med.* **13B**, 175 (1979). Dunlop, D. W. 'Alternatives to "Modern" health delivery systems in Africa: public policy issues of traditional health systems', *Soc. Sci. Med.* **9**, 581 (1975).

Professor A. Ramesh is Chairman of the Department of Geography in the University of Madras and B. Hyma is in the Department of Geography in the University of Waterloo, Canada. The article has been edited from a longer version that appeared in *Social Science and Medicine* (Vol. 15D, pp. 69–81) which was published by Pergamon Press, Oxford, UK (1981).

4.4

Health Policy Making in a Revolutionary Context: Nicaragua, 1979–81

Thomas John Bossert

Passing signs proclaiming 'The Revolution is Health', I wandered into a health center in one of the major towns in the Central Highlands. I was genially welcomed by the energetic and busy nurse, who easily incorporated my interruption into her more pressing activities—giving me a detailed description of the local health programs while at the same time assisting the rest of the health center staff and village volunteers in search of vaccines, food supplements for infants, and materials for latrine construction. Her programs included finishing the third phase of the national polio vaccination campaign, sponsoring tetanus vaccinations in the local elementary school (which she reported had already reached 75 per cent of its largest population), promoting a sanitation campaign that had installed 300 latrines in six months, and initiating a local census of the children under five, mothers and pregnant women—the population most 'at risk' medically. She and other members of the health center staff also delivered weekly 'health talks' informing the community members about how best to care for their own health through nutrition, sanitation and pre-natal care.

I had been in health posts in Nicaragua before the revolution and what impressed me most was the amount of new activity and the excitement and enthusiasm of all those involved. This health center was now engaged in activities it had not done before. It was not only distributing more vaccines and food supplements than it had under Somoza but it was integrating these activities into the newly formed community organizations: the *Sandinista* Defense Committees (CDS), the local Council of Reconstruction and the new Nicaraguan Women's Association (AMNLAE). For the first time on a large scale, the government was encouraging communities to participate in activities to improve their health conditions and was supplying many of the needed materials—milk, vaccinations, latrine construction materials.

The sign over the small health center—'Revolution is Health'—posed a difficult question: what kind of health care is revolutionary. On the face of it, the answer appears deceptively simple. The public health system of the Somoza regime was so extremely inequitable, and so clearly emphasised curative hospital care rather than sorely needed preventive

programs, that a new approach which brought more equal distribution of services and
began to emphasise preventive programs would be revolutionary for Nicaragua. However, in comparison with other countries, it is difficult to specify a particular health policy
as revolutionary, both because existing revolutionary regimes have quite different
approaches and because even the least reform-minded regimes, such as that of Guatemala,
have begun to adopt new policies that represent a more equitable distribution of health services. Indeed, there is now a general commitment by both revolutionary and non-
revolutionary regimes to the achievement of several goals embodied in the internationally
approved 'primary care approach'.[1] These goals may be summarized as: (1) the achievement of greater equality of access to health services—by both increasing services to lower
classes and, most importantly, by improving access in the rural areas where large populations still have no access at all; (2) a decisive commitment to improved preventive measures
such as provision of clean water, sanitation, nutrition, immunizations, maternal and child
health—activities which are more likely to improve health than are physician-oriented
curative services; (3) considerable participation of communities in both establishing local
health priorities and in implementing local health programs. A fourth, less explicit goal is
to achieve the goals of equity, prevention and participation within a relatively restricted
national health budget. This last goal in part recognizes the limited contribution of health
services to improved health levels of a population.[2] It is likely that expanded production
and more equitable distribution of wealth have a greater impact on health than do health
services themselves.

While all national governments are officially committed to these goals one could
expect a greater commitment from revolutionary regimes to at least the first three goals of
greater equity, prevention and participation. If we consider revolutionary regimes to be
those ideologically committed to achieving economic equity, popular participation, and
rationally planned allocation of goods and services, these health goals fit the general com-
mitments. There is no doubt empirically that revolutionary regimes such as those of China,
Cuba and Tanzania have made remarkable progress toward the achievement of these
health goals—far greater progress than most non-revolutionary regimes.[3]

A central issue, however, is raised by the fourth goal: a restricted health budget.
Revolutionary commitment may be measured in terms of a willingness to devote national
resources to a social service such as health. Provision of more health services could be seen
as a means of redistribution of wealth and as a response to popular demand. As such it
moves toward achieving economic equity while also gaining popular legitimacy. Following this logic the Cuban revolution appears to have chosen to devote considerable
resources to the provision of high levels of health care. However, few regimes are capable
of making this choice which, even for revolutionary regimes, means a sacrifice of other
sectors. Furthermore, it seems unwise to devote massive resources to the health sector
in the absence of clear evidence that health service expenditures are the most cost-effective
means of improving health. Also, to assume that provision of health services contributes to a regime's legitimacy is problematical. Health services are a costly means of
distributing wealth and of responding to popular demand, and they will become more
costly if regimes are to respond to accelerating demand for higher quality care. Effective
policies to increase economic production are likely to be a more useful means of gaining
legitimacy.

The Nicaraguan revolutionaries were faced with the problem of restructuring
the Nicaraguan health system in such a way as to achieve equity, prevention, and participation within a relatively restricted budget. Their task was difficult under any circumstances. It was complicated by the severe problems of the health system they inherited from
Somoza.

Health and Health Services under Somoza

There is little doubt that the health conditions of Nicaraguans during the Somoza dictator-ship were extremely poor, although they were not notably worse in Nicaragua than in other comparable Central American countries like Guatemala and Honduras. Life expec-tancy was 53 years, and infant mortality, often taken as an indicator of general health status of the whole population, was estimated at the extremely high rate of between 120 and 146 per 1,000 live births. Guatemala and Honduras had similar high rates, while by contrast the wealthier and progressive Costa Rica had a life expectancy of 70 years and infant mortality of 29 per 1,000. As in Guatemala and Honduras, preventable diseases were the principal causes of death: diarrhea and infectious diseases accounted for 31.4 per cent of all deaths and over 50 per cent of infant mortality. Nutrition levels were also extremely low, contributing to mortality from other causes. Sixty-six per cent of children under five years of age were estimated to have some degree of malnutrition.

Nicaragua had an extremely inequitable health system. Like most public health sys-tems, the Nicaraguan system did not serve the upper class—those who could easily afford private medical care and who could go to the United States for specialized treatment. While the public hospital system was officially responsible for both urban and rural areas, it overwhelmingly favored the former, a phenomenon not unusual in Central America but perhaps more extreme in Nicaragua. In 1973 over half of the hospitals beds in the country were in the three major cities and only five health facilities with beds were in rural areas. Even the most simple facilities—the health centers without beds—were much more preva-lent in urban than in rural areas. Only 35 of the 119 health centers were in rural areas and most were staffed with untrained auxiliary nurses. While Managua had only 25 per cent of the population, 50 per cent of the physicians and 70 per cent of the professional nurses worked there. Urban areas had averages of more than 11 physicians per 10,000 popula-tion, while the countryside had 2.5 or fewer. Provision of potable water was also skewed toward urban areas, where most habitations had direct water connections, while only 14 per cent in the rural areas had any access at all to potable water.

A general problem of public health systems in Latin America is that usually two major institutions are responsible for health facilities—the Ministry of Health and the Social Sec-urity Institute. This dual system often leads to duplication of services and tremendous inefficiencies. The Nicaraguan system was unusual in that it not only had this dual charac-ter but was actually even more fragmented. This fragmentation added to the confusion in a sector which also had the Social Security Institute, an autonomous water and sewer agency and military hospitals. Furthermore, even the Ministry of Health was fragmented internally with several vertically-run programs that functioned with relative autonomy. Like most other institutions in Nicaragua, the fragmented health system was dominated by personal associates of Somoza. His wife, Doña Hope, headed the hospital sector, and his last Minister of Health was one of his personal physicians.

What really set Somoza's Nicaragua apart from other Central American countries was that there was no major attempt to improve the system and redress the inequalities. In the early 1970s Guatemala, Honduras and Costa Rica began significant new programs that emphasized primary care and preventive activities for their extremely underserved rural areas. These programs actually did shift the expenditure patterns of the governments, demonstrating a major commitment to public health programs for rural areas which was not apparent in Somoza's Nicaragua, where only a few small primary care programs were initiated in the late 1970s.

Insurrection and the Destruction of The Somoza Health System

The period of insurrection beginning after the assassination of Pedro Joaquin Chamorro had several implications for the future health system. It marked a period of brutal destruction of hospitals, raised the need for curative and rehabilitative services for those wounded in the war, weakened the capacity of the Somoza government to maintain even the inadequate services that existed and inhibited small reform initiatives. On the positive side, it also marked a period of construction within the insurrectionary forces of a cadre of physicians and a model of volunteer community services.

The war also produced a tremendous number of casualties that required curative and rehabilitative services. After the *Sandinista* victory three new centers for rehabilitation were created, but the need was much greater than these centers could supply. Some war victims were sent to Cuba, Spain, Costa Rica and East Germany for special treatments and teams of plastic surgeons visited from the United States.

The period of insurrection was also one in which part of the medical profession played a visible public role in opposition to Somoza. Although the traditional association of physicians, the *Colegio de Médicos*, was strongly *Somocista* (its president was one of Somoza's personal physicians), a second physician organization, more closely associated with the medical school of the National University, was openly opposed to the Somoza regime. This organization, the *Federación de Sociedades Medicales de Nicaragua*, however, was extremely weak and apparently did not play the radicalizing role that its counterpart in Cuba did.[3] The more important opposition came from the health workers' union, FETSALUD, which was dominated by non-physician hospital staff. FETSALUD organized several long strikes in hospitals during the last years of the Somoza regime. While these strikes did not fully disrupt services, they did rally popular support in opposition to Somoza.

During the insurrectionary period, the *Sandinista* army, as well as other popular organizations, did attract and incorporate in its ranks many medically trained people. Physicians abandoned their practices to join the guerilla fronts and care for the wounded. Medical students joined the organizing efforts and engaged in training of paraprofessionals. These activities not only involved care for the insurrectional military forces but also marked the beginnings of a popularly oriented volunteer health system which would be expanded and institutionalized after the victory.

First Steps toward building a New Health System

Even before the new Nicaraguan leadership left Costa Rica, it declared its commitment to improving the health of Nicaraguans. One of the first acts of the Government was to unite the fragmented health organizations of the Somoza period into a single system under the authority of the Ministry of Health.

Following the Government's theme that emphasized reconstruction, the most immediate and pressing needs appeared to be for the physicians and hospital care. During the first months the Ministry assessed the damage done to hospitals and almost immediately began reconstruction of the worst damaged. They were aided in these tasks by donations from West Germany, Sweden and Switzerland. Also, in response to an international commitment of solidarity, the Ministry assumed responsibility for international brigades of more than 500 physicians who arrived from many countries.

There was a clear popular demand for these services. In sharp contrast to the under-utilization of the Somoza health facilities, the Government now found itself flooded with people in the hospitals and clinics around the country. People claimed that these services were now 'theirs' and not Somoza's. The Ministry estimated that while the Somoza health system covered only 30 per cent of the population, in the first few months of the revolution they were covering around 70 per cent. Furthermore, the people were not simply waiting for the government to supply services. Many communities were using local resources— often the confiscated homes and goods of Somoza supporters who had left the country—to provide hospital beds, medicines, office equipment, refrigerators, and even buildings for clinics and warehouses.

The Ministry, however, did not devote itself entirely to curative activities. In the early months, the regime initiated three major programs in preventive medicine. It began a wide-spread vaccination campaign against polio, measles and other infectious diseases, which reached an estimated 85 per cent of the target population. In the first six months a sanitation campaign distributed 4,200 latrines—twice the number the Somoza regime distributed in all of 1978. Using materials supplied by UNICEF, the Ministry established 250 centers for oral rehydration for the treatment of diarrhea. These centers, located in health facilities all over the country, provided an easily administered solution of salts and sugar that is perhaps the most effective and inexpensive means of reducing mortality from diarrhea.

The Ministry also took charge of the training of all health personnel. One of the early decisions was to encourage the medical school to increase the number of graduates from 50 per year to around 500. This decision may have been ill advised, since physicians only increase the demand for curative care; however, plans were made to increase the preventive medicine component of medical education and to discourage the pursuit of esoteric specialities. Efforts were also begun to improve the training and expand the number of non-physician health workers, especially nurses and lab technicians.

Perhaps the most significant feature of the new health system was the open commitment to the participation of the community in health programs. Through popular organizations the Ministry implemented its immunization campaigns, promoted the installation of latrines, distributed food supplements and completed a census of children at risk. These organizations began their own initiatives in providing materials, labor and equipment for construction of health posts and for preventive programs. They also took responsibility for assuring that price controls for some food items were respected.

A final area of concern for the new regime was the improvement of planning and administration, which proved to be a major task. In the absence of specific data, health planning was practically impossible and efforts in this area were postponed. Shortage of administrative skills was also a problem. While many people in the Somoza ministry stayed on to contribute to the revolution, the most important decision-making positions at all levels tended to be taken over by a new group of officials with little administrative experience and almost no training in public health.

The lack of administrative and public health experience was partially compensated by an enthusiastic collective decision-making process that particularly marked the early months of the regime. It was clear that no firm hierarchy of administrative decisions had yet been established and that the national level was not rigidly imposing a predetermined policy on the regional offices. The effort emphasized the collective nature of the enterprise of problem-solving and decision-making. This process was later viewed as having a considerable cost in terms of time and efficiency, but it did contribute to knowledge sharing in the initial period when few could claim expertise or authority for decision-making.

The new health policy was first initiated without clear budget guidelines. By February 1980, however, the Ministry was beginning to draw up a budget for that fiscal year. The basis for the budget was the 1979 Somoza budget projections. It was clear that the budget allocation for the health sector would not be significantly higher than that allocated by the Somoza Government. The revolutionary health policy would have to achieve its goals within these rather restrictive budgetary constraints.

Revolutionary Health Policy

The new regime had clearly made progress toward achieving the goals of equity, prevention, and participation within a reasonable budget restraint. They made major advances over the previous regime's extremely inadequate system. More Nicaraguans, especially those in lower classes, were being served in the hospitals and clinics. Immunization campaigns and other preventive programs were more widespread than they had been under Somoza. An extensive system of popular participation in health activities had begun. Furthermore, all this activity was apparently accomplished within a national budget not significantly greater than that of the Somoza regime. There remained, however, some critical problems which suggested that the initial policy was not as clearly oriented toward equity and prevention as it might have been. Although some activities were targeted for rural areas, by far the major emphasis was on providing care in the urban areas, leaving the urban-rural imbalance observed under Somoza virtually intact. In addition, while the revolution had begun preventive primary care programs (such as those of our energetic nurse cited above), such programs were still severely restricted in relation to the expenditures on curative care, especially for urban hospitals.

The central question for this analysis is why, when they had a chance early in the regime, did the Nicaraguan revolutionaries not choose to give greater emphasis to equity and prevention. One reason has to do with the apparent general policy commitment of the regime to restore basic services to their pre-war status. Most government programs in other areas, not only health, emphasized 'reconstruction' in 1980. The National Plan of Reconstruction clearly reflected this orientation. It included few original new programs but rather was based largely on programs that were planned during the last two years of the Somoza regime. This general policy appeared to respond to the immediate demands from the crucial urban and semi-urban areas where the revolution drew its initial and most important political support.

A second reason for this policy is in part the result of the administrative disarray during the initial period. The lack of administrative control implicit in this period made it necessary not to overextend the limited administrative capacity of the Ministry.

During the initial period of administrative confusion, a second condition shaped health policy. The new team of policy makers was made up almost entirely of physicians whose training was primarily curatively oriented.

What was the potential for a change in health policy toward a greater commitment to equity and prevention? A shift in policy would have been difficult. Already in February 1980 there were growing pressures to increase, not decrease, the emphasis on hospital care in urban areas.

There were, however, some reasons to expect that the initial policy could change significantly in the future. Growing awareness of the budgetary constraint and the need to limit costs in the hospital sector in order to achieve goals of prevention and equity, as well as growing administrative capacity to manage new programs, were likely to have an impact on policy-making.

Perhaps a more potent source of change could come from a more active participation in health policy by the *Sandinistas*, the FSLN, who would have the political capacity to restrict responsiveness to popular demands in urban areas and to resist physician reference for curative policies.

During the first months of the new regime, the health sector was not a priority sector for the FSLN. Few FSLN members were assigned to the Ministry. Gradually the FSLN increased its presence in the Ministry, until by mid-1980 the neurosurgeon who had been Minister was replaced by Lea Guido, a *Sandinista* leader who was not a physician. Also, in the *Junta de Gobierno,* Daniel Ortega of the FSLN assumed greater responsibility for health activities.

The FSLN, more than the physicians in the Ministry, had an interest in imposing its national austerity program and enforcing trade-off choices in the health sector. With pressing needs for national resources in productive sectors and concern for restrictions on foreign exchange, the FSLN could reorient Ministry priorities away from high-cost, low-effectiveness curative services and toward more equitable and more preventive programs. Also, using its greater influence in mass organizations, the FSLN could place emphasis on channeling popular participation toward preventive activities and away from the creation of new clinics.

The Nicaraguan revolution teaches us the difficulty of achieving revolutionary goals in health policy. It had achieved great advances over the Somoza regime's health policies, but it still faced difficult choices if it was to achieve greater emphasis on preventive programs and equal distribution of services.

References

1. There is a growing literature on international health and primary care. See, for example, World Health Organization and United Nations Children's Fund, *Primary Health Care,* World Health Organization, Geneva (1978); World Bank, *Health Sector Policy Paper,* World Bank, Washington, DC (1980).
2. See McKeown. T. *The Role of Medicine: Dream, Mirage or Nemesis?,* Blackwell, Oxford (1979); also, Gwatkin, Davidson, R., Wilcox, Janet R. and Wray, Joe D. *Can Health and Nutrition Interventions Make a Difference?,* Overseas Development Council, Washington, DC (1980).
3. On Cuba see: Danielson, R. *Cuban Medicine,* Transaction Books, New Brunswick, NJ (1979) and Navarro, V. 'Health, health services and health planning in Cuba'. *Int. J. Hlth. Serv.* 2, 3397 (1972). On China see: Sidel, Victor W. and Sidel, R. *Serve the People: Observations on Medicine in the People's Republic of China,* Josiah Macy, Jr Foundation, New York (1973) and Chen, P. *Population and Health Policy in the People's Republic of China,* Smithsonian Institution, Washington, DC (1976). On Tanzania see Gish, O. *Planning the Health Sector: The Tanzanian Experience,* Croom Helm, London (1975).

Thomas Bossert is now a member of the Faculty of Political Science, Sarah Lawrence College, Bronxville, New York. At the time of writing the article he was associated with Dartmouth Medical School and the Harvard School of Public Health in the United States. The article has been edited from a longer version that appeared in *Social Science and Medicine* (Vol. 15C, pp. 225–231) which was published by Pergamon Press, Oxford, UK (1981).

4.5

The Global Eradication of Smallpox

Marc A. Strassburg

On 8 May 1980, the 33rd World Health Authority Assembly declared the world free of smallpox. This followed approximately 2½ years after the last documented naturally occurring case of smallpox was diagnosed in a hospital worker in Merca, Somalia. A major breakthrough for the eventual control of this disease was the discovery of an effective vaccine by Edward Jenner in 1796. In 1966 the World Health Assembly voted a special budget to eliminate smallpox from the world. At that time, smallpox was endemic in more than 30 countries. Mass vaccination programs were successful in many Western countries; however, a different approach was taken in developing countries. This approach was known as surveillance and containment. Surveillance was aided by extensive house-to-house searches and rewards offered for persons reporting smallpox cases. Containment measures included ring vaccination and isolation of cases and contacts. Hospitals played a major role in transmission in a number of smallpox outbreaks. The World Health Organization (WHO) is currently supporting several control programs and has not singled out another disease for eradication. The lessons learned from the smallpox campaign can be readily applied to other public health programs.

The last documented case of naturally occurring smallpox in the world was diagnosed on 31 October 1977 in a 23-year-old male hospital cook living in Merca, Somalia. This was five days after rash had appeared and after exposure of friends, neighbors and other hospital staff members.[1] No additional cases of smallpox resulted, which was fortunate, since hospitals had commonly been the site of secondary spread to physicians, nurses, patients, and hospital visitors.[2,3]

To certify a country as smallpox-free, two years had to have elapsed without a case of smallpox being detected by an active and sensitive surveillance system. Almost two years to the day (26 October 1979) after this last case in Somalia, the (WHO) Global Commission for the Certification of Smallpox Eradication confirmed that smallpox also had been eradicated in Ethiopia, Somalia, and Kenya. Eradication efforts had been successful in this last endemic area, despite the ongoing war between Ethiopia and Somalia in the rugged and inaccessible Ogaden desert.

Also during 1979, 76 other countries were certified as smallpox-free, and, on 8 May 1980, the 33rd World Health Assembly declared the world free of smallpox.[4]

History

The origin of smallpox probably predates written history. Epidemics of smallpox-like illnesses have been described in ancient Chinese and Sanskrit texts. Historical accounts beginning in the sixth century describe pandemics both in Europe and Asia. In the Americas, the disease was probably introduced during the 1500s by slave ships from Africa. Reported fatality rates for smallpox have varied between less than 1 per cent and 50 per cent. Differences in fatality rates were probably related to both the virulence of a particular strain (variola major and variola minor as well as intermediate strains have been described) and the nutritional status of the affected population.

Prior to the eighteenth century, few effective measures for the control of smallpox were known. Although quarantine proved useful for a number of diseases, the procedure had limited success in smallpox control, since the disease was communicable during the prodromal period before the onset of rash. Prior to Jenner's discovery of vaccination, a procedure known as variolation was used to confer immunity.[5] Variolation was accomplished by obtaining material from the pustules of a smallpox patient and scratching the material onto the skin of a susceptible person. Many persons so variolated had symptoms of reduced severity, although they were capable of transmitting fully virulent cases of smallpox to others. Of special concern was that many of the variolated persons did not require bed rest, and thus they promoted a rapid spread of the disease. This practice, which originally had been described by the Chinese in 1000 BC, was still found in a number of countries in the twentieth century.[6]

The Vaccine

A major breakthrough in providing an effective measure for the control of smallpox occurred in 1796 when Edward Jenner[7] observed that persons who contracted cowpox, a relatively mild disease, developed immunity to smallpox. Jenner prepared a vaccine consisting of material from cowpox lesions. He fully understood the implication of the discovery of his new vaccine when he predicted that 'the annihilation of smallpox must be the final result of this practice.'

In America, Benjamin Waterhouse published an account of Jenner's work in an article entitled, 'A Prospect of Exterminating the Smallpox: Being the History of the Variolae Vaccine, or Kine-pox, Commonly Called the Cowpox; As It Appeared in England: With an Account of a Series of Inoculations Performed for the Kinepox, in Massachusetts.' Although much controversy surrounded Waterhouse's distribution of the vaccine, he is noted for conducting one of the first controlled clinical trials with the smallpox vaccine and for promoting its acceptance in the Americas.[8]

Despite the discovery of such an effective vaccine, it took nearly 200 years to bring about the eradication of smallpox. Several explanations for this delay may be offered. First, it was not until the 1950s that a heat-stable, freeze-dried vaccine was available. This important advance prolonged the viability of the vaccine in parts of the world where strict maintenance of the cold chain was difficult. Second, it was not until the 1960s that the bifurcated needle was developed. The bifurcated needle (used in the multiple-puncture vaccination technique) was easier to use, required less vaccine, and resulted in higher 'take' rates than other methods. Third, even with an improved vaccine and vaccination technique, not all countries were capable of carrying out a successful mass vaccination campaign. Although mass vaccination campaigns had been effective in eliminating smallpox in many Western countries, the limited resources and the organizational problems common to many health service systems in the developing world made complete vaccination coverage nearly impossible.

The World Health Organization's Program for Eradication

In 1966 the World Health Assembly, which is the controlling body for WHO, voted a special budget ($2.5 million) to begin the global program aimed at eliminating smallpox from the world. Although it would seem that all involved in such a program would be highly motivated, many participants, both at national and local levels, were skeptical that smallpox or any other disease could be eradicated. One possible explanation for this lack of enthusiasm was that the WHO eradication program for another disease—malaria—was not succeeding.

In 1967, when the smallpox campaign began, more than 30 countries were considered endemic, with importations being reported in another 12 countries. At that time four major reservoirs existed: Brazil; Africa south of the Sahara; Asia, including Bangladesh, Nepal, India and Pakistan; and the Indonesian Archipelago. Although only 130,000 cases were reported in 1967, it was estimated that there were closer to 10 million cases.[6]

Of paramount importance to the success of the smallpox eradication program was administrative and logistical support. Under the able leadership of Donald A. Henderson of WHO, precise objectives and goals for each country were established. WHO trained both international and national epidemiologists and was responsible for securing additional supporting funds for the eradication program.

New Approach to Eradication

A new strategy for smallpox eradication, one which did not rely on mass vaccination, was eventually adopted. This new strategy was called surveillance and containment and was developed by smallpox workers in West Africa.[9] The development of this strategy was greatly influenced by a thorough knowledge of the following important elements in the natural history of smallpox.[10] (1) The spread of smallpox was relatively slow, and a case usually infected only from two to five other persons. (2) Smallpox tended to cluster within villages or in a single area. (3) Man was the only reservoir of infection, and no carrier state was known. (4) Immunity was of long duration after either infection or vaccination.

Surveillance consisted of case-finding through systematic searches, improved reporting systems, and active source tracing. Many countries offered cash rewards to persons providing information leading to the discovery of a smallpox case. Containment efforts included isolation of patients and vaccination of all known or suspected contacts. The principal objective of this approach was to seal off outbreaks within specific geographical areas, thereby reducing transmission into unaffected areas. Although large-scale vaccination programs were still conducted, mass vaccination was no longer solely relied upon for control of the disease.

The Hospital's Role in Transmission

Important to the success of this new strategy was the development of effective isolation and quarantine measures. Historically, special huts, 'pest-houses', or isolation hospitals were principally used to remove affected persons from the community. The most unusual of these was probably the floating smallpox hospital employed at Long Reach, Dartford, England, about 1900. Later, as countries with improved medical services developed specialized departments for infectious disease patients, an increasing number of acutely ill patients, including smallpox patients, were admitted. In England, this seems to have first appeared in Chester in 1784.[11] It is probable that many of these early hospitals played major roles in smallpox transmission. This was well documented during the 1950s and 1960s when numerous hospitals were implicated as the principal source of spread in outbreaks.[3, 12–14]

After analyzing 30 epidemics of smallpox in Western countries between 1946 and 1964, Thomas Mack of the Centers for Disease Control reported that, of 516 cases of smallpox, 280 had been hospital-acquired. Among the hospital-acquired cases were included 130 patients, 35 nurses, 25 physicians, 50 other hospital staff and mortuary personnel, and 40 visitors and outpatients.[15] The last major outbreak of smallpox in the United States, which occurred in January 1947, began after an immigrant with smallpox (from Mexico) was hospitalized at Willard Parker, the communicable diseases hospital in Manhattan. The first secondary cases included another patient and a hospital staff member. A total of 12 secondary cases resulted, and within 1 month's time over 6 million persons were vaccinated in New York City.[16] Common to many hospital-centered outbreaks was (1) misdiagnosis or late diagnosis of the smallpox case, (2) inadequate isolation of the patient, (3) spread among unvaccinated hospital staff, and (4) spread to the surrounding community.

In the Federal Republic of Germany (Meschede 1970 and in Monschau 1961) two unusual nosocomial smallpox outbreaks resulted from a hospitalized smallpox patient when transmission occurred without face-to-face contact. The study of these two hospital-centered outbreaks revealed that virus particles were disseminated by air over considerable distance within a facility. This unusual airborne transmission most likely occurred because (1) the source cases had extensive rash and cough; (2) the humidity in the hospitals was relatively low at the time; and (3) air currents were present that caused rapid spread of the virus.[17]

With the new emphasis on surveillance and containment, the necessity for effective isolation was even more critical to success. During 1975, I worked as a consultant in the Bangladesh Eradication Program in the crowded capital of Dacca City. At the Infectious Diseases Hospital there, it was necessary to post vaccinator guards around the clock to vaccinate routinely all persons going into the facility who did not have proof of a recent vaccination. In many countries the practice of hospitalizing smallpox patients was openly discouraged, and the patients remained at home accompanied by a vaccinator until the patient fully recovered.

Between 1967 and 1977 the eradication campaign moved steadily forward, with smallpox successively eliminated in Western and Central Africa, Brazil, Indonesia, Southern Africa, Asia, and finally in East Africa.

Still Cause for Concern?

Although four years have passed without a reported case of naturally occurring smallpox, there are some who believe that smallpox may emerge from some hidden focus of infection, an unknown animal reservoir, or from some old smallpox crusts that are lying dormant somewhere in the world. This concern has been heightened by the recent discovery of a disease called monkeypox, which was first identified in a captive cynomolgus monkey in 1958 in Denmark. Monkeypox can be transmitted to man, although this is thought to be infrequent. Humans who have monkeypox present a picture clinically similar to humans with smallpox. Fifty cases have been reported for West and Central Africa between 1970 and 1980; however, in only five instances has secondary transmission possibly occurred. Both the low frequency of disease and the low transmission rate appear to indicate that monkeypox is not a public health problem of any significance. The source of human monkeypox is unknown but it is thought to be a zoonotic disease of rodents.[18]

There may be some who believe that smallpox eradication will not be complete until those strains maintained in laboratory freezers are destroyed. Concern over the maintenance of such a virus was heightened recently by events in Birmingham, England. There, in August 1978, a photographer who worked above a laboratory housing the smallpox virus contracted the disease. Only one secondary case was reported—the photographer's mother.[19]

In 1976, 76 laboratories were known to stock smallpox virus; as of December 1981 there were four reporting that they still maintained the virus. Currently, one of the laboratories designated for WHO poxvirus research is the Centers for Disease Control, Atlanta.[20] Some scientists point to the present need to maintain the virus in the laboratory in order to help to investigate the ecology of monkeypox and other poxviruses,[21] and it is conceivable that some military personnel may want to keep this virus in their biological arsenals.

What's Next?

Now that smallpox appears conquered, many public health workers are looking for another candidate for eradication. Although not everyone agrees on a single definition of the word 'eradication', for smallpox it implied an absence of clinical cases of the disease on a continent, with little or zero likelihood of the disease reoccurring. In the selection of a new candidate for eradication, a number of factors need consideration: (1) the degree of understanding of the natural history of the disease; (2) types of appropriate control measures available; (3) mortality produced by the disease; (4) morbidity, including suffering and disability; (5) availability of adequate funding; (6) the cost-benefit of such an eradication effort; and (7) the probability of success within a given time period.

Many of these factors are interdependent. For example, malaria, which is considered by many as the leading cause of mortality in the world today, may require in excess of one billion dollars for the first years of an eradication program.[22] Similar expenses would accompany attempts to eradicate other diseases transmitted by arthropod vectors (e.g. yellow fever, trypanosomiasis, and onchocerciasis).

Zoonotic diseases are also difficult to eradicate because animal populations serve as principal reservoirs and are difficult to control. Possibly from the group of diseases that, like smallpox, is transmitted chiefly from person to person and for which man is either the principal or only reservoir of infection, a candidate can be found. From this group, measles clearly stands out as a potential candidate for eradication. Although the effect of measles on world mortality and morbidity may not be as great as was that of smallpox, the natural history of measles is well understood, there is a good vaccine (though not as heat-stable as the smallpox vaccine), and man is the only reservoir of infection. Thus measles would require a similar strategy and organization to carry out a successful eradication effort.

References

1. Deria, A., Jezek, Z., Markvart, K., Carrasco, P. and Weisfeld, J. 'The world's last endemic case of smallpox: surveillance and containment measures', *Bull. WHO* 58, 279–283 (1980).
2. WHO Scientific Group on Smallpox Eradication, World Health Organisation Tech. Rep. Ser. No. 393 (1978).
3. Millar, J. D. 'Smallpox: a continuing threat', *Hospitals* 39, 57–58 (1965).
4. (Anonymous) 'Global eradication of smallpox', *Bull. WHO* 58, 161–163 (1980).
5. Langer, W. L. 'Immunization against smallpox before Jenner', *Sci. Am.* 235 (4), 112–117 (1976).
6. WHO Expert Committee on Smallpox Eradication, World Health Organization Tech. Rep. Ser. No.493 (1972).
7. Jenner, E. *An inquiry into the causes and effects of the variolae vaccine, a disease discovered in some of the western counties of England, particularly Gloucestershire, and known by the name of the cow pox,* Sampson Low, London (1798).
8. Hopkins, D. R. 'Benjamin Waterhouse (1754–1846), the "Jenner of America" ', *Am. J. Trop. Med. Hyg.* 26, 1060–1063 (1977).
9. Foege, W. H., Miller, J. D. and Lane, J. M. 'Selective epidemiologic control in smallpox eradication', *Am. J. Epidemiol.* 94, 311–315 (1971).
10. Rao, A. R., Jacob, E. S., Kamalakshi, S., Appaswamy, S. and Bradbury, B. D. 'Epidemiological studies in smallpox: a study of intrafamilial transmission in a series of 254 infected families', *Indian J. Med. Res.* 56, 1826–1854 (1968).
11. Dixon, C. W. *Smallpox,* J. & A. Churchill Ltd., London (1962).
12. Arita, I., Shafa, E. and Kader, M. A. 'Role of hospital in smallpox outbreak in Kuwait', *Am. J. Public Health* 60, 1960–1966 (1970).
13. Zetterberg, B., Ringertz, O., Svedmyr, A., Wallmark, G. and Alin, K. 'Epidemiology of smallpox in Stockholm 1963'. In Strom, J. and Zetterberg, B. (eds) 'Smallpox outbreak and vaccination problems in Stockholm, Sweden, 1963', *Acta. Med. Scand. Suppl.* 464, 8–35 (1963).
14. Morris, L., de Lemos, A. L. and de Silva, O. J. 'Investigations of hospital-associated smallpox— Vitoria, Espirito Santo', *Am. J. Public Health* 37, 2331–2334 (1970).
15. Mack, T. 'Six hospitals study best means of assuring smallpox immunity among personnel', *Hospitals* 39, 59–61 (1965).
16. Weinstein, I. 'An outbreak of smallpox in New York City', *Am. J. Public Health* 37, 1376–1384 (1947).
17. Wehrle, P. F., Posch, J., Richter, K. H., Henderson, D. A. 'An airborne outbreak of smallpox in a German hospital and its significance with respect to other recent outbreaks in Europe', *Bull. WHO* 43, 669–679 (1970).
18. Breman, J. G. Kalisa-Ruti, Steniowski, M. V., Zanotto, E., Gromyko, A. I. and Arita, I. 'Human monkeypox, 1970–79', *Bull. WHO* 58, 165–182 (1980).
19. Hawkes, N. 'Smallpox death in Britain challenges presumption of laboratory safety: peer review failed dismally', *Science* 203, 855–856 (1979).
20. Global eradication of smallpox. *WHO Weekly Epidemiol. Rec.* 56, 393–400 (1981).
21. Foege, W. H. 'Should the smallpox virus be allowed to survive?' *N. Engl. J. Med.* 300, 670–671 (1979).
22. Wood, C. (ed) *Tropical Medicine: From romance to reality,* Academic Press, Inc., London, Chap. 5 (1978).
23. Henderson, D. A. 'Smallpox shows the way', *World health,* pp. 22–27 (February 1977).

Marc Strassburg is an epidemiologist and currently head of programme evaluation in the Department of Health Services, County of Los Angeles, California. The article is reprinted in its entirety from the *American Journal of Infection Control* (19, 53–59, 1982), which is published by C. V. Mosby, St Louis, Missouri, USA.

4.6

Drug Problems in the Sociocultural Context

'Thailand: Treatment at the Tam Kraborg Temple' by Vichai Poshyachinda

Since Thailand became a united free country over 700 years ago, Buddhism has been the national religion. The culture and tradition of the people are closely woven with the philosophical concepts of their religion. The temple and the priest stand as dominating influences in society.

It has been a natural evolution for the Buddhist temple to assume the role of treatment centre in response to the growth of drug dependence. There are no less than five of these centres in the country. Each temple offers its own model of help, conceived from traditional experience and belief. The temples can be regarded as providing the genuine indigenous treatment of drug dependence in Thailand.

The Tam Kraborg temple

The Tam Kraborg provides simple treatment facilities. A few wooden benches and tables placed on an open verandah serve as the intake registration unit. A small plain open hall is used as the shrine for the administration of the vow. The living quarters for the clients are a single spacious hall not unlike a military barracks. During the first five days after admission the clients stay on one side of the hall; they then move across to the other side.

When full, the temple holds 300–400 resident clients and about 100 priests. About 40 of the priests are former clients who were ordained after treatment.

Treatment is carried out by a priest. The giving of the vow to the Buddha is a rite at which either the abbot or a priest from a small chosen group always presides. Although the turnover rate indicates a substantial work-load, the temple never has to resort to hired staff.

Like any other Buddhist temple in Thailand, this temple is largely supported by voluntary contributions from the public, and at times subsidized by various government bodies. While the treatment is free, the charge for subsistence for each case is about US$1.00 per day.

The treatment model

There is only one treatment model offered at the Tam Kraborg. The goal is complete drug abstinence for life. To enter the programme, the client must make a clear statement of determination to seek treatment. The four principal rules of conduct are explained to the client on admission. These rules are: complete abstinence from drugs causing dependence; obedience to the priest; no disruptive behaviour; and, to remain within the temple compound throughout the treatment period without any excuses.

Then the client makes his vow to the Buddha. The new admission group for the day performs the ceremony in a small shrine under the guidance of a priest. The vow is in essence a pledge of abstinence for life from opium, morphine, heroin, *ganja* and other drugs that cause dependence. Clients who belong to religions other than Buddhism can pledge their vow according to their own belief.

The daily treatment schedule for the first five days comprises two principal sessions. A dose of herbal medicine is given in the morning, which induces immediate vomiting for about 10–15 minutes. In the afternoon session the clients take a herbal steam bath for 10– 15 minutes. This cycle of sessions is explained to the client as the means to purge drugs from the body. In the morning session, clients who have already participated in the first five days join actively in the treatment. Some assist by nursing others through the vomiting session, while others cheer their fellows with spirited native tunes and jokes. The atmosphere is not unlike that of a lively competitive game at a temple festival.

Occasionally, in the evening after dinner, the priest gives a discourse on Buddhist doctrine or on a client's problem which he has submitted as a subject for the discourse. This religious session is informal and attendance is left to the motivation of the individual but all clients are encouraged to join in it.

For the remaining five days, there is no prescribed schedule. The client is left to recover from his physical exhaustion. The priest usually encourages those who feel physically strong enough and are so inclined to help in the daily chores or assist in the treatment session for newcomers.

On the tenth and last day of admission, the clients are assembled again in the shrine and reminded of their pledge; they are then free to leave the temple.

The clients

The admission records of the temple from 1963 to the end of 1977 show that slightly more than 40,000 cases have been treated. Almost all were men; fewer then 1 per cent were women. About 40 per cent came from Bangkok, and the rest from the 72 provincial cities in the country. The principal drugs misused were opium and heroin.

An epidemiological study was carried out by the Institute of Health Research on a cohort of 1,054 males admitted from October 1976 to February 1977. It revealed a clear picture of an epidemic spread of heroin starting around 1969. Although the use of cannabis and opium by this cohort reflected the same epidemic trend, data also show that the use of these two substances was prevalent much earlier in an endemic pattern. The cohort can be divided into two main groups: the heroin users from Bangkok and the provincial cities, and the opium users of the rural areas.

The heroin users were, in general, young adults aged between 15 and 25 years and socioeconomically unstable as shown, for example, by a high unemployment rate of about 35 per cent. About one-third admitted to illegal activities to support their habit. The average expenditure on heroin was around US$2.70 per day. Two-thirds of the users took the drug intravenously.

The opium users presented a totally different picture. Approximately 80 per cent were above 30 years of age and they were economically stable. Almost all were fully employed in various rural occupations. Self-reported illegal activity was negligible. The money spent on opium smoking averaged US$0.75 per day. They seemed to be comparatively well adjusted in their society.

Treatment outcome

The abstinence rate six months after discharge for the heroin users from Bangkok was about 20 per cent, and for those from the provincial cities, about 30 per cent. Most of the recidivists had resumed heroin use within three months. However, they were spending less money on the drug: the Bangkok recidivists were spending on an average about 30 per cent, and those from the provincial cities about 40 per cent, of the amount spent during the thirty days before admission. The employment status of about 60 per cent of the heroin users who reported drug abstinence was unchanged, and improvement was reported by about 30 per cent. One-third of the recidivists showed further deterioration in employment status, half remained the same, and about 10 per cent reported improvement.

The opium smokers, who mostly came from the provincial cities, had an abstinence rate of about 50 per cent at six months. Their employment status remained unchanged, but it should be noted that this group was fairly stable economically to begin with.

Conclusion

The treatment model of these temples finds its support in the strong popular belief in religion and in herbal medicine. The service rendered by these temples probably covers a significant part of the drug-dependent population in the country. Active participation of the community in the treatment programme is very notable.

What is undoubted is that the Buddhist temples have developed a treatment approach which is eminently worth further close research, a model highly congruent with the indigenous culture, and a treatment programme which is remarkably practical in terms of its staffing and cost.

'Egypt: A Community-Based Outpatient Clinic' by G. M. Abu El Azayem

At the beginning of the present political regime in Egypt, in 1952, severe penalties were inflicted on those who trafficked in drugs or consumed them, and in 1960, capital punishment was introduced for recidivism. At the same time, drug dependents were considered patients and the law permitted them to have treatment, including hospital care. In 1961, dependents who accepted medical treatment were exempted from punishment. They were sent for compulsory treatment to mental hospitals. However, it was noticed that they were reluctant to carry on with treatment in hospital. Those who were admitted asked to be discharged before the prescribed treatment was completed. Also, they were very troublesome in hospital and the rate of relapse was very high. As a result of these problems, staff as well as the general public asked for more suitable facilities and a change in therapeutic policy. It should be noted that treatment was available only for those who were arrested as a result of breaking the law that prohibited drug-taking.

In 1969, the first outpatient clinic for the treatment of alcohol and drug dependence was opened by the Central Association for the Treatment of Alcohol and Drug Dependents, a community based-organization. The Board of this organization includes doctors, lawyers, police officers, social workers, a clergyman and representatives of the Socialist Arab Union.

Aspects of the new therapeutic policy

The Board was unanimous that the new treatment should have the following aspects:

(a) it should be on a voluntary basis and dependents should be encouraged to ask for treatment of their own free will;
(b) it should be available for every dependent;
(c) it should overcome the disadvantages associated with previous therapies;
(d) it should be reasonably cheap; the previous approach with methadone was too expensive for the middle and poorer classes: besides, drug dependence took the form of

methadone dependence;

(e) it should accord in other ways too with the needs of patients of different socioeconomic strata, and;

(f) it should succeed in overcoming the inherent reluctance of many of these patients to seek treatment.

Application of the new therapeutic programme

To start applying the new therapeutic policy, a clinic was chosen in the most crowded quarter of Cairo. Thus the clinic was within reach of dependents and was soon noticed by almost all the inhabitants of the district. Patients are generally adults over 25 years; 68 per cent are between 40 and 60 years old. They come from the poorer sector, with a median monthly income of less than US$50.00. Almost all are employed. About 40 per cent are totally illiterate. Almost all (95 per cent) are married with a large number of children. Treatment is on a voluntary basis, and privacy is closely protected. Patients are examined physically and mentally to treat any accompanying physical or mental disorder. The social worker investigates and helps with family and other social problems. The clergyman discusses their problems with them and strengthens their will by spiritual approaches.

Social therapy aims at guiding patients in dealing with their own problems whether in the family or at work. An effort is also made to correct family misbeliefs about addiction; most patients think that drugs give more energy for work and increase sexual ability. Patients are then helped to find work.

It was noticed that 95 per cent of those coming for treatment were opium addicts. They weighed about 50 kg and most of them were suffering from loss of appetite. We therefore used insulin treatment to treat the loss of weight and the accompanying loss of appetite. Opium addicts get through the withdrawal state rapidly and painlessly with the help of insulin treatment. We believe that insulin helps to reduce the craving for opium. As it is given by injection, it is regarded by the patients as a potent therapy.

Patients with accompanying depression were treated with antidepressant drugs, and those suffering from insomnia were given appropriate drug treatment.

Group psychotherapy is used to change attitudes and behaviour, and to motivate the dependents to solve their personal, family and social problems. Group therapy is carried out by the psychiatrist, the social worker and clergymen, in the form of free dialogue. A club has been opened in the clinic where patients gather before and after treatment. It helps to reinforce the group therapy.

Merits of the new therapeutic policy

The cost of this outpatient treatment programme is very low, and thus accords with the economic realities of many patients' lives. Being painless and offering quick benefits, it has stimulated the addicts to persuade their friends to come for treatment. The voluntary nature of the programme has stimulated the addicts to develop their own willpower and to share actively in the treatment, in marked contrast with compulsory treatment. Dependents were permitted to come in the afternoon so that they could carry on with their regular work in the morning—an important advantage over compulsory treatment, for which patients are shut off from gainful employment. Before the introduction of voluntary treatment only 950 dependents were treated over ten years; with voluntary treatment 1,500 cases enrolled during the first year alone. Very fundamentally, the community treatment respects the personality of the dependent and does not humiliate him as was the case with the compulsory method.

All these advantages help to overcome inherent resistance and to foster a feeling of trust and willingness for a speedy recovery. Analysis of the statistics reveals that 70 per cent of the dependents who consult the clinic come voluntarily six times per week in the afternoon, for about two months. This regular attendance shows their increasing confidence in the treatment. Follow-up of 100 opium addicts showed that 65 per cent had improved and had had no relapses up to one year after the end of treatment.

This approach has dealt with many difficult practical questions in the field of drug dependence, and has piloted the way for a new, readily available, cheap and reliable therapy that suits the sociocultural characteristics of our opium addicts.

'United States of America: Methadone—an Alien Technology?' by J. H. Jaffe

The use of oral methadone as a form of treatment for addiction to heroin was introduced in the USA in 1964. This approach to the problem of heroin use was a sharp departure from previous practice. The use of an opioid generated controversy, but the behaviour of patients was so consistently better than it had been previously that methadone treatment spread rapidly. It was not long, however, before questions were raised about the suitability of methadone maintenance as treatment in less developed countries.

Early reports about methadone maintenance
Investigators began to use oral methadone in the treatment of heroin addicts, and the early reports were almost unanimous in finding that those who remained on treatment showed a sharp drop in their use of heroin, a marked decrease in criminal activity and an increase in the amount of legitimate employment.

Oral methadone has several advantages that made it particularly useful at the time of its introduction. The most important is its long duration of action. This property has several implications. First, since a key issue in the USA was to assure the public that the opioids provided to addicts would not be sold to others, it was important to use a drug that could be given once a day (so that addicts could ingest their entire dose at the clinic). Second, it was also important to have a drug that would produce a stable level of tolerance so that progressive escalation of dosage would be unnecessary. Methadone given orally exhibits this characteristic: people can remain on the same dose for years. Third, the long duration of action produces a rather stable level of drug effect over the course of the day [and so] permits a more normal pattern of behaviour. To a very large degree, individuals tolerant to oral methadone seem quite normal even to trained clinical observers.

Critics of the methadone maintenance approach pointed out that patients were still taking a 'narcotic drug', that they were obliged to remain on treatment indefinitely, that methadone did not change the basic personality of the addict and that many patients were beginning to use alcohol to excess. Despite these criticisms a substantial number of heroin addicts who had not shown much interest in detoxification programmes or therapeutic communities sought treatment in methadone programmes.

In part because of attitudes toward opiates and opiate addiction, the early methadone programmes were highly structured organizations; as well as providing methadone, they gave counselling, medical care and legal aid. Careful records were kept and patients who showed progress were permitted to take medication from the clinic. Linking this privilege to behavioural adjustment was designed to motivate patients to change their behaviour as well as to minimize the diversion of drugs from the clinics. Such structured clinics were expensive: in 1972, total costs ranged from US$1,200 to $2,500 per patient per year; the cost of the medication itself was trivial. Although this was expensive, other treatment approaches, especially inpatient detoxification, were even more so. Furthermore, heroin addicts who were unwilling to enter other types of treatment were eager to try methadone maintenance.

By 1973, there were doubts about the efficacy of methadone maintenance treatment. When programmes were no longer selecting their patients or refusing to admit patients with alcohol problems, it was becoming clear that the remarkable results obtained in the early years could not always be reproduced. Some programmes were unable to demonstrate decreases in crime rates (except drug-possession crimes) or significant increases in employment rates; and alcoholism among patients was proving troublesome. Some critics pronounced the programmes failures.

Subsequent studies comparing the outcomes of a variety of treatments concluded that for the older addict with a longer history of drug use, methadone led to a better than expected level of social adjustment and a decrease in criminal activity while the individual was on treatment.

While on treatment most patients also showed sharp decreases in the use of illicit heroin and modest increases in productive legitimate activity. Thus, despite certain criticisms, it is clear that many addicts who might have done poorly in other programmes are helped by methadone programmes.

The early methadone programmes were viewed as providing comprehensive care and not merely as a means of distributing opioids legitimately. While inexpensive when weighed against the possibility that the untreated addict would commit a great deal of crime, the actual cost of treatment was substantial. In 1972, the least expensive clinics in the USA, those that treated only outpatients and at least 100 patients at one place, cost approximately US$1,200 per patient per year. This figure included the costs of the facility itself (usually rented), nurses to dispense methadone, doctors to see the patients, counsellors to help them change their life-style, administrative costs and urine testing. Obviously, it would have been much cheaper simply to dispense methadone, but public opinion in the USA against mere dispensing of an opiate was so strong that the government regulations made counselling and medical supervision mandatory.

No one knows to what degree clinics which merely provided an oral opioid would have produced the same behavioural changes or what kinds of problems might have arisen in the absence of government regulations. The major disadvantages of methadone for developing countries would appear to be economic because a structured system would be expensive, and psychological because in many cultures it would replace an indigenous behaviour that had been a comprehensible part of the common experience by an alien one.

Vichai Posyachinda is at the Institute of Health Research, Chulalongkem University, Bangkok; Gamal Mady Abu El Azayem is Director of the General Abbossia Mental Hospital, Cairo; Jerome Jaffe is at the Department of Psychiatry, College of Physicians and Surgeons of Columbia University, New York. All three articles are edited from longer versions that appeared in *Drug Problems in the Sociocultural Context*, edited by Griffith Edwards and Awni Arif and published by the World Health Organisation on Public Health Paper, Number 73 (1980).

Part 5

Organisations and occupations

Introduction

Most of the material in this part is devoted to the perception and performance of the roles of different health service staff. Social roles are the patterns of behaviour expected of those occupying any social position. Social positions may be occupationally specified, such as those of doctors, nurses and kitchen maids. They may be defined with reference to illness and the work that this creates, as is the case with patients. People also fill positions such as those of a parent, spouse and family member. The performance of roles, therefore, involves a social relationship, or interaction, between people who hold similar or different social positions, such as a doctor with another doctor or with a patient.

Because of differences in rank and in the distribution of economic resources and other powers, these positions are often accorded different social status. Those participating in social relations are often of unequal status and therefore interacting within some form of hierarchy. Their relative status shapes these relationships, as well as the value and significance they attach to themselves. It is not merely that hospital consultants have posts that are officially superior to junior doctors but that some specialities are accorded more esteem. Patients are essential to the health service as its 'raw material', but they tend to be ranked low or outside the pattern of working relationships. This part is therefore concerned with the ways in which patients and health service staff give meaning to their roles and their interaction with one another in the organisation.

In his article on the containment of mental illness in the community, Erving Goffman, an American sociologist, describes how fundamentally different is the situation from that of physical illness. Given what is normally expected of people at work or in families, mental illness can be a social offence which involves behaviour that could otherwise be considered wilfully disruptive. Within a hospital, other people, such as staff and relations, can control the contacts that patients make, but outside, in the family and local community, bizarre behaviour can be contained only by breaking the normal pattern of family life. The patient's closest relations are expected to collude with outsiders and, as the patient seeks support for his or her perception of the situation, so members of families may abdicate their supportive roles and become divided against themselves.

Social roles and occupational activities are not, of course, fixed. They can be perceived very differently, both by different people and at different times. As described in the Report of the Committee on Nursing that was chaired by Professor Asa Briggs, nursing has inherited a popular image that is shared both by many nurses and by some of those, like doctors, who work closely with nurses. The hierarchical code of discipline and the setting of work in some types of hospital perpetuates both a Victorian legacy and elements of romantic fiction. The problems created by the destruction of initiative and unstimulating exhaustion remain, and lead to frustration, dissatisfaction and often the abandonment of nursing by those most interested in patient care.

The work of hospital kitchen maids would appear to have little direct association with patient care, although the 'hotel-side' of hospital life is of great importance to the well-being of patients. Elizabeth Paterson, a British sociologist, describes how the low status of kitchen maids is reflected in their dirty and sometimes hazardous work and how their world of work is dominated by the characteristics of the actual food they have to prepare. Despite being at the bottom of the staff hierarchy, they have developed ways of distancing themselves from this demeaning status and even ways of structuring their time and other activities to escape from it. Nevertheless, their subordinate position is reflected in the relative importance that the maids attach to food preparation for staff and private patients, both categories of consumer who command power in the organisation and expect value for money.

The different statuses associated with different working roles in an organisation, and the particular position of patients classified as mentally ill, are not aberrations. They are part of the complex pattern of relationships and perception of tasks and roles within the field of health and disease. This is very clearly demonstrated in Roger Jeffrey's sociological analysis of casualty departments. This sort of hospital work is among the least specialised; it also involves working closely with members of the public, many of whom fail to honour the more acceptable requirements of the sick role. Casualty work tends to be done by overworked junior doctors in poor conditions. Some patients have suffered through no fault of their own, and treating them may involve some special skill or unusual degree of responsibility. These are viewed as the 'good patients'. But the rest are seen as 'rubbish'—trivial callers, drunks, overdosers, tramps and nutcases—because they are considered to have created their own condition and, far from being disabled by it, may be seeking to use it for purposes other than recovery. As such, they seem to serve no useful purpose to the staff and reinforce the low status of their work.

Hospitals are hierarchical organisations and this hierarchy is reflected not only within and between professions but also in the status of the different types of patient each occupation attracts. What these articles show is that the work of all occupations, from kitchen maids to doctors, contains elements of good or attractive work and dirty work. The doctors' loathing of tramps and overdoses is mirrored in the kitchen maids' feelings towards dealing with the slop-bins. Similarly, both occupations enjoy occasional perks— for doctors it's the 'real' patient displaying classical signs of a rare disease, for the kitchen maids it's the 'nicest tomatoes'.

5.1

The Insanity of Place

Erving Goffman

In the last twenty years we have learned that the management of mental illness under medical auspices has been an uncertain blessing. The best treatment that money has been able to buy, prolonged individual psychotherapy, has not proven very efficacious. The treatment most patients have received—hospitalization—has proven to be questionable indeed. Patients recover more often than not, at least temporarily, but this seems in spite of the mental hospital, not because of it. Upon examination, many of these establishments have proven to be hopeless storage dumps trimmed in psychiatric paper.

Given the life still enforced in most mental hospitals and the stigma still placed on mental illness, the philosophy of community containment seems the only desirable one. Nonetheless, it is worth looking at some implications of this approach for the patient's various 'others', that is, persons he identifies as playing a significant role in his life. To do this we must examine the meaning of the patient's symptoms for his others. If we do this we will learn not only what containment implies, we will learn about mental disorder.

The interesting thing about medical symptoms is how utterly nice, how utterly plucky the patient can be in managing them. There may be physical acts of an ordinary kind he cannot perform; there may be various parts of the body he must keep bandaged and hidden from view; he may have to stay home from work for a spell or even spend time in a hospital bed. But for each of these deviations from normal social appearance and functioning, the patient will be able to furnish a compensating mode of address. He gives accounts, belittles his discomfort, and presents an apologetic air, as if to say that in spite of appearance he is, deep in his social soul, someone to be counted on to know his place, someone who appreciates what he ought to be as a normal person and who is this person in spirit, regardless of what has happened to his flesh. He is someone who does not will to be demanding and useless. Tuberculosis patients, formerly isolated in sanitaria, sent home progress notes that were fumigated but cheerful. Brave little troops of colostomites and ileostomites make their brief appearances disguised as nice clean people, while stoically concealing the hours of hellish toilet work required for each appearance in public as a normal person. We even have our Beckett player buried up to his head in an iron lung, unable to blow his own nose, who yet somehow expresses by means of his eyebrows that a full-fledged person is present who knows how to behave and would certainly behave that way were he physically able.

And more than an air is involved. Howsoever demanding the sick person's illness is, almost always there will be some consideration his keepers will *not* have to give. There will be some physical cooperation that can be counted on; there will be some task he can do to help out, often one that would not fall to his lot were he well. And this helpfulness can be *absolutely* counted on, just as though he were no less a responsible participant than anyone else. In the context, these little bits of substantive helpfulness take on a large symbolic function.

Now obviously, physically sick persons do not always keep a stiff upper lip (not even to mention appreciable ethnic differences in the management of the sick role); hypochondriasis is common, and control of others through illness is not uncommon. But even in these cases I think close examination would find that the culprit tends to acknowledge proper sick-role etiquette. This may not only be a front, a gloss, a way of styling behaviour. But it says: 'Whatever my medical condition demands, the enduring me is to be dissociated from these needs, for I am someone who would make only modest reasonable claims and take a modest and standard role in the affairs of the group were I able.'

The family's treatment of the patient nicely supports this definition of the situation, as does the employer's. In effect they say that special licence can temporarily be accorded the sick person because, were he able to do anything about it, he would not make such demands. Since the patient's spirit and will and intentions are those of a loyal and seemly member, his old place should be kept waiting for him, for he will fill it well, as if nothing untoward has happened, as soon as his outer behaviour can again be dictated by, and be an expression of, the inner man. His increased demands are saved from expressing what they might because it is plain that he has 'good' reasons for making them, that is, reasons that nullify what these claims would otherwise be taken to mean. I do not say that the members of the family will be happy about their destiny. In the case of incurable disorders that are messy or severely incapacitating, the compensatory work required by the well members may cost them the life chances their peers enjoy, blunt their personal careers, paint their lives with tragedy, and turn all their feelings to bitterness. But the fact that all of this hardship can be contained shows how clearly the way has been marked for the unfortunate family, a way that obliges them to close ranks and somehow make do as long as the illness lasts.

Now turn to symptoms of mental disorder as a form of social deviation. In our society, what is the nature of the social offence to which the frame of reference 'mental illness' is likely to be applied?

The offence is often one to which formal means of social control do not apply. The offender appears to make little effort to conceal his offence or ritually neutralize it. Mental symptoms are not, by and large, *incidentally* a social infraction. By and large they are specifically and pointedly offensive. As far as the patient's others are concerned, the troublesome acts do not merely happen to coincide partly with what is socially offensive, as is true of medical symptoms; rather these troublesome acts are perceived, at least initially, to be intrinsically a matter of wilful social deviation.

It is important now to emphasize that a social deviation can hardly be reckoned apart from the relationships and organizational memberships of the offender and offended, since there is hardly a social act that in itself is not appropriate or at least excusable in some social context. The delusions of a private can be the rights of a general; the obscene invitations of a man to a strange girl can be the spicy endearments of a husband to his wife; the wariness of a paranoid is the warranted practice of thousands of undercover agents.

Mental symptoms, then, are neither something in themselves nor whatever is so labelled; mental symptoms are acts by an individual which openly proclaim to others that he must have assumptions about himself which the relevant bit of social organization can neither allow him nor do much about.

It follows that if the patient persists in his symptomatic behavior, then he must create organizational havoc in the minds of members. This havoc indicates that medical symptoms and mental symptoms are radically different in their social consequences and in their character. It is this havoc that the philosophy of containment must deal with. It is this havoc that psychiatrists have dismally failed to examine and that sociologists ignore when they treat mental illness merely as a labelling process. It is this havoc that we must explore.

Mental hospitals can manage such diffusions and distortions of identity without too much difficulty. In these establishments much of the person's usual involvement in the undertakings of others and much of his ordinary capacity to make contact with the world are cut off. There is little he can set in motion. A patient who thinks he is a potentate does not worry attendants about their being his minions. That he is in dominion over them is never given any credence. They merely watch him and laugh, as if watching impromptu theatre. Similarly, when a mental hospital patient treats his wife as if she were a suspect stranger, she can deal with this impossible situation merely by adjusting downward the frequency and length of her visits. So, too, the office therapist can withstand the splotches of love and hate that the patient brings to a session, being supported in this disinvolvement by the wonderfully convenient doctrine that direct intercession for the patient, or talk that lasts more than fifty minutes, can only undermine the therapeutic relationship. In all of these cases, distance allows a coming to terms; the patient may express impossible assumptions about himself, but the hospital, the family, or the therapist need not become involved in them.

Matters are quite different, however, when the patient is outside the walls of the hospital or office—outside, where his others commit their persons into his keeping, where his actions make authorized claims and are not symptoms or skits or something disheartening that can be walked away from. Outside the barricades, dramatically wrong self-identification is not necessary in order to produce trouble. Every form of social organization in which the patient participates has its special set of offences perceivable as mental illness that can create organizational havoc.

The maintenance of the internal and external functioning of the family is so central that when family members think of the essential character, the perduring personality of any one of their numbers, it is usually his habitual pattern of support for family-organized activity and family relationships, his style of acceptance of his place in the family, that they have in mind. Any marked change in his pattern of support will tend to be perceived as a marked change in his character. The deepest nature of an individual is only skin-deep, the deepness of his others' skin.

In the case of withdrawals—depressions and regressions—it is chiefly the internal functioning of the family that suffers. The burden of enthusiasm and domestic work must now be carried by fewer numbers. Note that by artfully curtailing its social life, the family can conceal these disorders from the public at large and sustain conventional external functioning. Quiet alcoholism can similarly be contained, provided that economic resources are not jeopardized.

It is the manic disorders and the active phases of a paranoid kind that produce the real trouble. It is these patterns that constitute the insanity of place.

The beginnings are unclear and varied. In some cases something causes the prepatient—whether husband, wife, or child—to feel that the life his others have been allowing him is not sufficient, not right, and no longer tenable. He makes conventional demands for relief and change which are not granted, perhaps not even attended. Then, instead of falling back to the *status quo ante*, he begins his manic activity. As suggested, there are no doubt other etiologies and other precipitating sequences. But all end at the same point—the manic activity the family comes to be concerned with. We shall begin with this, although it is a late point from some perspectives.

The manic begins by promoting himself in the family hierarchy. He finds he no longer has the time to do his accustomed share of family chores. He increasingly orders other members around, displays anger and impatience, makes promises he feels he can break, encroaches on the equipment and space allocated to other members, only fitfully displays affection and respect, and finds he cannot bother adhering to the family schedule for meals, for going to bed and rising. He also becomes hypercritical and derogatory of family members. He moves backward to grandiose statements of the high rank and quality of his forbears, and forward to an exalted view of what he proposes soon to accomplish. He begins to sprinkle his speech with unassimilated technical vocabularies. He talks loudly and constantly, arrogating to himself the place at the centre of things this role assumes. The great events and personages of the day uncharacteristically evoke from him a considered and definitive opinion. He seizes on magazine articles, movies, and TV shows as containing important wisdom that everyone ought to hear about in detail right now.

In addition to these disturbances of rank, there are those related to the minor obligations which symbolize membership and relatedness. He alone ceases to exercise the easy care that keeps household equipment safe and keeps members safe from it. He alone becomes capricious in performing the little courtesy-favours that all grown members offer one another if only because of the minute cost of these services to the giver compared to their appreciable value to the recipient. And he voices groundless beliefs, sometimes in response to hallucinations, which imply to his kin that he has ceased to regulate his thought by the standards that form the common ground of all those to whom they are closely related.

The constant effort of the family to argue the patient out of his foolish notions, to disprove his allegations, to make him take a reasonable view—an argumentation so despaired of by some therapists—can similarly be understood as the family's needs and the family's effort to bring the patient back into appropriate relationship to them. They cannot let him have his wrong beliefs because they cannot let him go. Further, if he reverses his behaviour and becomes more collected, they must try to get him to admit that he has been ill, else his present saneness will raise doubts about the family's warrant for the way they have been treating him, doubts about their motivation and *their* relationship to him. For these reasons, admission of insanity has to be sought. And what is sought is an extraordinary thing indeed. If ritual work is a means of retaining a constancy of image in the face of deviations in behaviour, then a self-admission that one is mentally ill is the biggest piece of ritual work of all, for this stance to one's conduct discounts the greatest deviations. A week of mayhem in a family can be set aside and readied to be forgotten the moment the offender admits he has been ill. Small wonder, then, that the patient will be put under great pressure to agree to the diagnosis, and that he may give in, even though this can mean that he must permanently lower the conception he has of his own character and must never again be adamant in presenting his views.

The issue here is not that the family finds that home life is made unpleasant by the sick person. Perhaps most home life is unpleasant. The issue is that meaningful existence is threatened.

Let me repeat: the self is the code that makes sense out of almost all the individual's activities and provides a basis for organizing them. This self is what can be read about the individual by interpreting the place he takes in an organization of social activity, as confirmed by his expressive behaviour. The individual's failure to encode through deeds and expressive cues a *workable* definition of himself, one which closely enmeshed others can accord him through the regard they show his person, is to block and trip up and threaten them in almost every movement that they make. The selves that had been the reciprocals of his are undermined. And that which should not have been able to change—the character of a loved one lived with—appears to be changing fundamentally and for the worse before their eyes. In ceasing to know the sick person, they cease to be sure of themselves. In ceasing to be sure of him and themselves, they can even cease to be sure of their way of knowing. A deep bewilderment results. [Consider] now some further aspects of the family's response.

One issue concerns the structure of attention. Put simply, the patient becomes someone who has to be watched. Each time he holds a sharp or heavy object, each time he answers the phone, each time he nears the window, each time he holds a cup of coffee above a rug, each time he is present when someone comes to the door or drops in, each time he handles the car keys, each time he begins to fill a sink or tub, each time he lights a match—on each of these occasions the family will have to be ready to jump.

Three points are to be made concerning the family's watchfulness. First, households tend to be informally organized, in the sense that each member is allowed considerable leeway in scheduling his own tasks and diverting himself in his own directions. He will have his own matters, then, to which he feels a need to attend. The necessity, instead, of his having to stand watch over the patient blocks rightful and pleasurable calls upon time and generates a surprising amount of fatigue, impatience, and hostility. Second, the watching will have to be dissimulated and disguised lest the patient suspect he is under constant surveillance, and this covering requires extra involvement and attention. Third, in order to increase their efficiency and maintain their morale, the watchers are likely to engage in collaboration, which perforce must be collusive.

The family must respond not only to what the patient is doing to its internal life, but also to the spectacle he seems to be making of himself in the community. At first the family will be greatly concerned that one of its emissaries is letting down the side. The family therefore tries to cover up and intercede so as to keep up his front and theirs. This strengthens the collusive alignment in the family against the patient.

As the dispute within the family continues and grows concerning the selves in whose terms activity ought to be organized, the family begins to turn outward, first to the patient's kinsmen, then to friends, to professionals, to employers. The family's purpose is not merely to obtain help in the secretive management of the patient, but also to get much needed affirmation of its view of events. There is a reversal of the family information rule. Acquaintances or other potential sources of aid who had once been personally distant from the family will now be drawn into the centre of things as part of a new solidarity of those who are helping to manage the patient, just as some of those who were once close may now be dropped because apparently they do not confirm the family's definition of the situation.

Finally, the family finds that in order to prevent others from giving weight to the initiatory activity of the patient, relatively distant persons must be let in on the family secret. There may even be necessity for recourse to the courts to block extravagances by conservator proceedings, to undo unsuitable marriages by annulments, and the like. The family will frankly allow indications that it can no longer handle its own problems, for the family cat must be belled. By that time the family members will have learned to live exposed. There will be less pride and less self-respect. They will be engaged in establishing that one of their members is mentally ill, and in whatever degree they succeed in this, they will be exposing themselves to the current conception that they constitute the kind of family which produces mental illness.

The family's conspiracy is benign, but this conspiracy breeds what others do. The patient finds himself in a world that has only the appearance of innocence, in which small signs can be found—and therefore sought out and wrongly imputed—showing that things are anything but what they seem. At home, when his glance suddenly shifts in a conversation, he may find naked evidence of collusive teamwork against him—teamwork unlike the kind which evaporates when a butt is let in on a good-natured joke that is being played at his expense. He rightly comes to feel that statements made to him are spoken so as to be monitored by the others present, ensuring that they will keep up with the managing of him, and that statements made to others in his presence are designed and delivered for his overhearing. He will find this communication arrangement very unsettling and come to feel that he is purposely being kept out of touch with what is happening.

In addition, the patient is likely to detect that he is being watched. He will sense that he is being treated as a child who can't be trusted around the house, but in this case one who cannot be trusted to be frankly shown that he is not trusted. If he lights a match or takes up a knife, he may find as he turns from these tasks that others present seem to have been watching him and now are trying to cover up their watchfulness.

In response to the response he is creating, the patient, too, will come to feel that life in the family has become deranged. He is likely to try to muster up some support for his own view of what his close ones are up to. And he is likely to have some success.

The result is two collusive factions, each enveloping the other in uncertainties, each drawing on a new and changing set of secret members. The household ceases to be a place where there is the easy fulfilment of a thousand mutually anticipated proper acts. It ceases to be a solid front organized by a stable set of persons against the world, entrenched and buffered by a stable set of friends and servers. The household becomes a no-man's land where changing factions are obliged to negotiate daily, their weapons being collusive communication and their armour selective inattention to the machinations of the other side—an inattention difficult to achieve, since each faction must devote itself to reading the other's furtive signs. The home, where wounds were meant to be licked, becomes precisely where they are inflicted. Boundaries are broken. The family is turned inside out.

Acknowledgement

I am much indebted to Edwin Lemert and Sheldon Messinger and to Helen and Stewart Parry for help in writing this paper.

Erving Goffman, late Professor of Sociology at the University of Pennsylvania, was author of *Asylums, Stigma* and *The Presentation of Self in Everyday Life.* This article consists of edited extracts from an article that originally appeared in *Psychiatry: Journal for the Study of Interpersonal Processes,* **XXXII**, No. 4 (November 1969).

5.2

Food-work: Maids in a Hospital Kitchen

Elizabeth Paterson

Introduction

Whilst an undergraduate I spent several vacations working as a maid in the kitchens of a fairly large teaching hospital, and became interested in the implications of performing that type of work. As a result the job developed into participant observation and an attempt to examine the setting in a manner which contrasted with many traditional organisational analyses, which often neglected the purposes and definition of the actors concerned and stressed organisational goals.[1]

What follows is an ethnographic account of how the maids did 'food-work' for all practical purposes, given a variety of organisational and architectural constraints. The paper outlines the routines in which they engaged, some of which proved to be dirty, menial and boring; the common sense assumptions they made about the tasks, the materials used to perform them and the people destined to receive the final product; the 'strain' this type of work placed on the maids' conception of self; and finally the strategies utilised to combat these undesirable effects.

Kitchen maid routine

It was from the daily institutionalised routines that passed as 'maids' work' that the meaning of 'food-work' emerged and description of these processes may lead to some understanding of the everyday assumptions that the maids, and to some extent the other kitchen staff also, made while dealing with the food.

The kitchen provided meals for around 700 patients, for the doctors', sisters' and nurses' dining rooms, the service room in the maternity hospital, the staff of the sterilisation department and for the canteen which catered primarily for technical staff.

During observation the maids' routine consisted of a variety of tasks. They emptied food containers from the heated trolleys returned from the wards and placed them in their appropriate storage areas. They prepared carrots for soup-making by processing sackfuls through 'the machine' (skinner), scraping off the remaining black sections, chopping and mincing them. Similar vegetables had to be processed in an equally tedious manner, including the washing of lettuce for salad. Maids also cleaned, battered and coated large boxes of fish. They pared, cored and sliced apples for puddings and prepared any other fruit which appeared on the menu. They removed from chickens any giblets remaining after factory processing and any excess fat, while generally up to the elbows in tepid, greasy water.

Routinely from eight a.m. onwards food was being cooked for lunch in immense vessels, stirred by wooden 'oars', dished into assorted containers and placed in heated trolleys to wait until noon. In addition each meal necessitated a succession of trolley-emptying, dish-washing and plugging-in, the process being repeated continually throughout the day, although by supper time most of the daily maids had gone off duty and had been replaced by others.

When all the food had been processed for that day, and occasionally even before, ingredients were prepared for the *next* day's dishes. Consequently besides regular accepted routines, the week's menu fleshed out the structure of the day. It indicated not only what had to be prepared or cooked immediately, but what had to be prepared that day for the next or even subsequent days.

Working assumptions

From the above description of the grinding forward of a routine day it is clear that food is very much work to those within a kitchen, just as death is work to the staff of a hospital and old people are work to the staff of an old people's home. The need to 'get through the day' has an important effect on how they conceive of what they work upon and around.

As a result the typical, common sense ways of thinking about food and its preparation within kitchen walls are different from those outside an area catering for such large numbers and where food is not the object of work. Elsewhere, food is usually considered in small quantities, carefully washed, prepared, cooked to exact times, dished when ready and consumed in small amounts by the person concerned, family or acquaintances. On the other hand, to maids dealing with it in bulk the food became like a factory product and its preparation had meaning in that sense.

As an extension of this type of thinking—food as work—it was categorised in relation to the routines of work and its easy completion. When busy—and during the period of study the maids generally were—foods were typified as 'bad' or 'good', not according to taste but by their relevance for work control.[2]

Washing lettuce for salad was a job which maids tried to avoid. It was a long, boring task and also a back-breaking one, because it necessitated bending over a low sink while holding each leaf under the tap. It had to be performed in such a tedious fashion because lettuce, above most other foods, worried both providers and receivers. Because lettuce is uncooked and tends to lie unadorned on the plate (in the hospital at least), it is patently obvious if it has brown patches, is dirty or is harbouring some wildlife. As a result a maxim about lettuce-washing existed: 'Rather get into trouble for taking a long time than get into trouble for missing slugs'. Hence 'doing lettuce' elicited sympathy from colleagues, a maid was considered brave to tackle it on her own and therefore it was a tactic which led to being classed as a 'good worker'.

On the other hand, 'good' foods were those which required little or no preparation by maids, such as macaroni and cheese, or ones which meant that few boilers or friers had to be washed afterwards. So in this additional way the menu gave meaning to the day's routine, whether it would mean hard work or not, by indicating whether 'good' or 'bad' foods had to be prepared.

'Unexpected' practices

From the description of how the food was routinely prepared, cooked and dished, and how maids typically thought about food in the kitchen, practices in that part of the hospital might seem incompatible with typical notions concerning the aims and standards of hospitals in general. One notable example of 'unexpected' practices concerned cooks rather than maids, but it very clearly illustrates the pervading attitude. Even in an area of patient catering to which one would expect careful attention to be given, special diets, the approach to food was similar.

After consultations about the health and choices of patients, dieticians made out diet sheets for specific diseases and conditions. For salt-free, high- and low-protein and sugar-free diets one would expect that the food would be carefully weighed and prepared. Despite this impression of scientific control, science seemed to be abandoned when the diet sheet left the hands of the dietician. She made frequent visits to the diet's cook, but the latter seemed more concerned with the arrangement and control of work routine than with any desire to achieve accuracy. The cook wanted to receive the diet sheet as early as possible in the morning in order to begin preparing dishes for tea. Any late adjustments meant that the cook's routine was upset; dieticians who were late were invariably labelled 'lazy'. In addition, cooks on diet duty often experienced great difficulty in obtaining from the supervisor the foods indicated on the sheet, so they often had to make do with second (or third) best. Many discovered only too late that a certain food did contain the forbidden salt or sugar.

However, such unexpected practices in doing food-work might appear less surprising when we reflect on some earlier points—that food is *work* to maids and others within the kitchen, certain expected routines had to be got through in the day with only limited staff and materials being made available. They 'do what they can' given the circumstances.

Visibility

In addition to these considerations the concept of visibility is central to any discussion of dirty and careless practices. The hospital kitchen was situated far from the visitors' entrance with few wards beyond it, with the result that there was seldom sufficient reason for outsiders to pass and glance in. Doctors and other non-domestic staff would only be interested in entering the kitchen while 'food-work' was in progress if they had a specific aim, which was unlikely given their preoccupations.

Since control is more likely to be exercised when behaviour is conspicuous and when violation of standards leaves tangible evidence, when it *was* expected that any deviation from expectations would be noticed, a conscious presentation of cleanliness was required by the supervisor. We have seen how much care was taken over lettuce-washing. In sum the kitchen and its staff were presented as clean and savoury in line with the 'front' that the rest of the hospital maintained, and any discrepant information and 'dirty work' concealed.

'Staff' and 'patients'

Up to this point the discussion appears to indicate that the 'unexpected' standards of food production were similar for all categories served by the kitchen. However this was not the case. Standards differed for doctors and sisters, who were considered of high social worth, for nurses and technical staff who were lower in the hierarchy, for private patients who were considered almost as worthy as staff, and for 'ordinary' patients, whose status was considered lowest of all. This was related to the power of the respective categories; their power to demand accounts for food that was deemed unsatisfactory; the power resting in the fact that all groups except 'ordinary' patients could be said to pay for their meals.

Staff also got priority with containers, i.e. they received shiny new ones, or plates and glass dishes as opposed to metal trays, whereas any bashed object that could conceivably hold food was placed in the patients' trolleys. Different maids and cooks prepared staff and patients' meals, the staff side being allocated a larger quota than the patients' side, perhaps indicating the desire to perform staff preparation more thoroughly.

Ward C contained private patients and they often received the same food as staff, except for those patients on special diets. Patients on this ward got personalised extras, such as individual moulds for jelly, parsley in a small container which could be sprinkled on food if desired, sole instead of haddock and so on. They were also likely to receive 'treats' such as strawberry tarts, while these delights were never offered to other patients. However, it must not be overlooked that much of this personalised treatment may have stemmed from the fact that the food was being served for much smaller numbers. So decisions about the worth and financial contributions of clientele in this instance had a quite dramatic effect, especially for bored patients for whom food could have become the only highlight in the day's dull routine.

Implications for maids

Although the impression may have been given that maids performed 'food-work' routines and engaged in dirty and discriminatory practices with equanimity this was not invariably the case. Although much had become taken for granted they frequently reacted unfavourably towards the job and how it affected them as human beings in general and as women in particular. In a large variety of ways the work had implications for their self conception and their general well-being.

Behaviour in the role of bulk food-producer often conflicted with that of food-producer in the home, and this 'role strain'[3] was felt particularly acutely among newcomers or those whose relatives or friends were also patients. A further element of the maids' problem was that since their products seldom reached the consumer direct, there was no one to praise them. They produced only transient things like cleanness and scraped carrots. In addition the maids saw the work as very hard and the allocation of duties as unfair. The job was also dangerous because of the likelihood of falling on the greasy floors, being burned on the multitude of hotplates and ovens, or being cut by knives or other dangerous equipment. Furthermore maids were subordinate to all others in the kitchen hierarchy, low in power and in status.

It was considered a tough and demeaning job even in comparison with being a maid in other sections of the hospital; other maids did not have to wear the unbecoming caps and aprons in addition to their overalls; they were allowed a greater degree of autonomy in organising their work; and they could increase their status by contact with nursing staff. How lowly kitchen maids were considered in hospital eyes was illustrated by the fact that not only had they to queue silently on Friday lunchtime to be handed their pay abruptly 'like a food ration', but kitchen maids received theirs after all other maids and cooks; consequently they had to stand around longer and their half-hour lunch break was reduced considerably.

Finally, it has been extensively documented that a large portion of kitchen maid work was physically unpleasant. In most occupations there are elements of this dirty work, disgusting, degrading or immoral tasks which the incumbents try to avoid or regulate—for example, by allocating this sort of work to others. In the kitchen cooks' dirty work was allocated to maids.

In sum there were few maids who did not resent the implications of their work for their conception of themselves as clean, attractive, concerned and fairly independent women.

Maids' strategies

As a result of the problems outlined maids utilised a variety of tactics to negate the undesirable effects of the organisational setting, of the dirty, strenuous, repetitive, demeaning and unsatisfying work.

Making adjustments

Maids tried to 'distance themselves' from their position within the kitchen in an attempt to control the definition of themselves in the situation. To indicate that they did not wish to be classed as a 'skivvy', most expressed the forced nature of their work, i.e. 'this is not the *real* me'. To distance themselves from their subordinate position maids attempted to develop a joking relationship with those cooks considered amenable to this approach. A maid might jokingly blame someone else for a mistake or make mock apologies to superiors. For they found that they could be disrespectful to authority if what they said was heavily disguised as a joke. However, such comments were not always accepted as a joke, and negotiation often occurred over whether or not the initial remark or 'insubordination' was merely some fun or whether a message of more serious consequence was intended. As a result, maids had to handle joking carefully in order to avoid disrupting working relationships completely.

Distance from their position as 'skivvy' was also expressed by sullen replies, biting comments after the superior had departed, or, as happened repeatedly in the kitchen because the facilities were available, by loud banging of containers and equipment. Maids often symbolically rejected being ordered around by appearing aloof, walking slowly and taking an extremely long time to perform a task.

Conversational topics were also part of this comprehensive fabric of behaviour which disassociated their role in menial and dirty tasks from their 'real' selves, the good housewives, the interesting people. Talk not only passed time but gave evidence of the lives these women took part in outside work.

Regulating appearance was yet another method used to negate the role. All kitchen maids were forced to wear unattractive nylon caps. The older women with short hair objected to the cap spoiling the style, so they crumpled it into a ball and pinned it at the back. Many of the older maids had their hair styled regularly, and maids and cooks tended to wear a great deal of perfume as if to combat any clinging odours of 'food-work'.

Furthermore, in addition to these distancing tactics, maids worked the system.[4] They would take things from the kitchen as if in compensation for being employed there. They consumed pieces of cooked meat that were lying around; they carefully chose the nicest tomatoes to eat with their toast. Maids would be annoyed if there was nothing for them to pinch; if, for example, all the tomatoes had been used up before breakfast for patients' meals, and not enough remained to take for their own break, an extra box would appear from the larder, with claims that they were bound to need them later.

Taking food out of the premises was far less common, although it would be fair to say that no kitchen maid's family went short of tomatoes; large turnover and ease of handling made them a popular prey. And although there were continual complaints about the shortage of [cleaning] cloths, most of the married women ensured that they had a constant supply of the better ones for private use. They got the most out of the kitchen as if to compensate for being engaged in a rather demeaning job.

Combating monotony

It has been shown that work was not only subordinate and dirty but that several of its aspects were extremely boring, a factor in many low-status occupations. Hence methods of overcoming the tedium were important for doing 'food-work'.

Most maids took a variety of 'smoke-breaks', generally before breakfast, before lunch and before leaving in the afternoon. These were enjoyed in the toilet due to the scarcity of other 'back regions' or 'free places'.[4] The toilet was one of the few areas almost accepted by senior staff as a place of escape from work routines for short periods of time. Unfortunately outside the actual cubicles—in the cloakroom—there were only two chairs, so maids were often found sitting on the cupboards, on the sinks or even on the floor. So the day would be routinely broken up; at about nine o'clock each morning maids asked each other, 'Are you going to the toilet?'; at around nine fifteen the signal was 'It's toilet time'.

'Floor time', the period when respective 'sides' washed the areas of the kitchen allotted to them, also broke the monotony of work like scraping carrots all morning. In addition they had the more illicit 'tea time', taken apart from the regular breaks, and occurring in the vegetable room, another quite secluded region. In addition the older women went to the refectory each Saturday lunch time for a drink (although the break only lasted half an hour) and on Sunday, when the refectory was closed, they drove to a hotel nearby. For these trips they had to remove their working overalls, and in this way they could step out of their role as maids for a short time at least.

Conclusions

This necessarily truncated description of how maids engaged in some aspects of 'food-work' has outlined the dirty, menial and boring routines which came to be accepted as 'maids' work', and the assumptions they made about that work, the materials involved and the recipients of the final product. This occupation had several undesirable, demeaning effects on the maids' conception of self and led to a variety of strategies or adjustments on their part, many of them tolerated by supervision.

What has been described may disturb those who organise catering in medical (and other) institutions, and is highly relevant to debates concerning the generally poor state of hospital meals and the periodic outbreaks of food-poisoning among patients. But it has been made clear throughout the discussion that there were numerous practical factors involved in the behaviour displayed; there would be many 'good' organisational reasons for 'bad' hospital food.

Notes and References

1. For a detailed critique of organisational analyses, see David Silverman, *The Theory of Organisations: A Sociological Framework*, Heineman, London (1971).
2. This 'good'/'bad' categorisation is common in other sorts of occupation. The workers' clientele

is often typified in such a manner. See Raymond Gold, 'Janitors versus tenants: a status-income dilemma', *The American Journal of Sociology,* 57, No. 5, pp. 487–493, (March, 1952) and Raymond Gold, 'In the basement: the apartment-building janitor', in Peter Berger (ed.), *The Human Shape of Work,* Macmillan, New York (1964) for discussion of 'good' and 'bad' tenants.
3. William J. Goode, 'A theory of role strain', *American Sociological Review,* 25, No. 4, pp. 483–496 (August 1960).
4. See Erving Goffman, *Asylums: Essays on the social situation of mental patients,* Penguin, Harmondsworth (1970).

Elizabeth Paterson is a Research Fellow and sociologist at the MRC Medical Sociology Unit, Institute of Medical Sociology, Aberdeen. This article is an edited version of an article originally published in Atkinson, P. and Heath, C. (eds) *Medical Work: Realities and Routines,* Gower, Farnborough, pp. 152–169 (1981).

5.3

Normal Rubbish: Deviant Patients in Casualty Departments

Roger Jeffery

English casualty departments

Casualty departments have been recognised as one of the most problematic areas of the NHS since about 1958, and several official and semi-official reports were published in the following years. The major criticisms have been that Casualty departments have to operate in old, crowded, and ill-equipped surroundings, and that their unpopularity with doctors has meant that the doctors employed as Casualty Officers are either overworked or of poor quality. 'Poor quality' in this context seems to mean either doctors in their pre-registration year, or doctors from abroad.

The reasons for the unpopularity of Casualty work amongst doctors have usually been couched either in terms of the poor working conditions, or in terms of the absence of a career structure within Casualty work. Most Casualty staff are junior doctors and there are very few full-time consultant appointments. Other reasons which are less frequently put forward, but seem to underlie these objections, relate more to the nature of the work, and in particular to the notion that the Casualty department is an interface between hospital and community. Prestige amongst doctors is, at least in part, related to the distance a doctor can get from the undifferentiated mass of patients, so that teaching hospital consultancies are valued because they are at the end of a series of screening mechanisms. Casualty is one of these screening mechanisms, rather like general practitioners in this respect. However, they are unusual in the hospital setting in the freedom of patients to gain entrance without having seen a GP first; another low prestige area similar in this respect is the VD clinic. Casualty has been unsuited to the processes of differentiation and specialisation which have characterised the recent history of the medical profession, and this helps to explain the low prestige of the work, and the low priority it has received in hospital expenditure.

The material on which this paper is based was gathered at three Casualty departments in an English city. These departments would appear to be above average in terms of the criteria discussed above: all were fully staffed; only two of the seventeen doctors employed during the fieldwork period were immigrant; and the working conditions were reasonable. The data presented came from either fieldwork notes or tape-recorded, open-ended interviews with the doctors.

Typifications of patients

Moral evaluation of patients seems to be a regular feature of medical settings, not merely amongst medical students or in mental hospitals. In general, two broad categories were used to evaluate patients: good or interesting, and bad or rubbish. They were sometimes used as if they were an exclusive dichotomy, but more generally appeared as opposite ends of a continuum.

> [CO to medical students] If there's anything interesting we'll stop, but there's a lot of rubbish this morning. On nights you get some drunken dross in, but also some good cases.

In most of this paper I shall be discussing the category of rubbish, but I shall first deal with the valued category, the good patients.

Good patients

Good patients were described almost entirely in terms of their medical characteristics, either in terms of the symptoms or the causes of the injury. Good cases were head injuries, or cardiac arrests, or a stove-in chest; or they were RTAs (Road Traffic Accidents). There were three broad criteria by which patients were seen to be good, and each related to medical considerations.

(i) If they allowed the CO to practice skills necessary for passing professional examinations. In order to pass the FRCS examinations doctors need to be able to diagnose and describe unusual conditions and symptoms. Casualty was not a good place to discover these sorts of cases, and if they did turn up a great fuss was made of them.

(ii) If they allowed staff to practice their chosen speciality. For the doctors, the specific characteristics of good patients of this sort were fairly closely defined, because most doctors saw themselves as future specialists—predominantly surgeons. They tended to accept, or conform to, the model of the surgeon as a man of action who can achieve fairly rapid results. Patients who provided the opportunity to use and act out this model were welcomed. One CO gave a particularly graphic description of this:

> But I like doing surgical procedures. These are great fun. It just lets your imagination run riot really [laughs] you know, you forget for a moment you are just a very small cog incising a very small abscess, and you pick up your scalpel like anyone else [laughs].

For some COs, Casualty work had some advantages over other jobs because the clientele was basically healthy, and it was possible to carry out procedures which showed quick success in terms of returning people to a healthy state.

(iii) If they tested the general competence and maturity of the staff. The patients who were most prized were those who stretched the resources of the department in doing the task they saw themselves designed to carry out—the rapid early treatment of acutely ill patients. Many of the COs saw their Casualty job as the first in which they were expected to make decisions without the safety net of ready advice from more senior staff. The most articulate expression of this was from a CO who said:

> I really do enjoy doing anything where I am a little out of my depth, where I really have to think about what I am doing. Something like a bad road traffic accident, where they ring up and give you a few minutes warning and perhaps give you an idea of what's

happening ... And when the guy finally does arrive you've got a rough idea of what you are going to do, and sorting it all out and getting him into the right speciality, this kind of thing is very satisfying.

Good patients, then, make demands which fall squarely within the boundaries of what the staff define as appropriate to their job. It is the medical characteristics of these patients which are most predominant in the discussions, and the typifications are not very well developed. This is in marked contrast to 'rubbish'.

Rubbish

While the category of the good patient is one I have in part constructed from comments about 'patients I like dealing with' or 'the sort of work I like to do', 'rubbish' is a category generated by the staff themselves. It was commonly used in discussions of the work, as in the following quotes:

> It's a thankless task, seeing all the rubbish, as we call it, coming through.

> I wouldn't be making the same fuss in another job—it's only because it's mostly bloody crumble like women with insect bites.

In an attempt to get a better idea of what patients would be included in the category of rubbish I asked staff what sorts of patients they did not like having to deal with, which sorts of patients made them annoyed, and why. The answers they gave suggested that staff had developed characterisations of 'normal' rubbish—the normal suicide attempt, the normal drunk, and so on—which they were thinking of when they talked about rubbish. In other words, staff felt able to predict a whole range of features related not only to his medical condition but also to his past life, to his likely behaviour inside the Casualty department, and to his future behaviour. These expected features of the patient could thus be used to guide the treatment (both socially and medically) that the staff decided to give the patient. The following were the major categories of rubbish mentioned by the staff.

(i) Trivia The recurring problem of Casualty departments, in the eyes of the doctors, has been the 'casual' attender. For the staff of the Casualty departments I studied, normal trivia banged their heads, their hands or their ankles, carried on working as usual, and several days later looked into Casualty to see if it was all right. Normal trivia treats Casualty like a perfunctory service, on a par with a garage, rather than as an expert emergency service, which is how the staff like to see themselves.

> They come in and say 'I did an injury half an hour ago, or half a day ago, or two days ago. I'm perfectly all right, I've just come for a check-up.'

> [Trivia] comes up with a pain that he's had for three weeks, and gets you out of bed at 3 in the morning.

(ii) Drunks Normal drunks are abusive and threatening. They come in shouting and singing after a fight and they are sick all over the place, or they are brought in unconscious, having been found in the street. They come in the small hours of the night, and they often have to be kept in until morning because you never know if they have been knocked out in a fight (with the possibility of a head injury) or whether they were just sleeping it off. They come in weekend after weekend with the same injuries, and they are always unpleasant and awkward.

(iii) Overdoses The normal overdose is female, and is seen as a case of self-injury rather than of attempted suicide. She comes because her boyfriend/husband/parents have been unkind, and she is likely to be a regular visitor. She only wants attention, she was not seriously trying to kill herself, but she uses the overdose as moral blackmail. She makes sure she does not succeed by taking a less-than-lethal dose, or by ensuring that she is discovered fairly rapidly.

> In the majority of overdoses, you know, these symbolic overdoses, the sort of '5 aspirins and 5 valiums and I'm ill doctor, I've taken an overdose'.

> By and large they are people who have done it time and time again, who are up, who have had treatment, who haven't responded to treatment.

(iv) Tramps Normal tramps can be recognised by the many layers of rotten clothing they wear, and by their smell. They are a feature of the cold winter nights and they only come to Casualty to try to wheedle a bed in the warm for the night. Tramps can never be trusted; they will usually sham their symptoms. New COs and young staff nurses should be warned, for if one is let in one night then dozens will turn up the next night.

> [Tramps are] nuisance visitors, frequent visitors, who won't go, who refuse to leave when you want them to.

> [Tramps are] just trying to get a bed for the night.

These four types covered most of the patients included in rubbish, or described as unpleasant or annoying. There were some other characterisations mentioned less frequently, or which seemed to be generated by individual patients, or which seemed to be specific to particular members of staff. 'Nutcases' were in this uncertain position: there were few 'typical' features of psychiatric patients, and these were very diffuse. 'Smelly', 'dirty' and 'obese' patients were also in this limbo. Patients with these characteristics were objected to, but there was no typical career expected for these patients: apart from the one common characteristic they were expected to be different.

Rules broken by rubbish

In their elaboration of *why* certain sorts of patients were rubbish, staff organised their answers in terms of a number of unwritten rules which they said rubbish had broken. These rules were in part consensual, and in part ideological. These rules, then, can be seen as the criteria by which staff judged the legitimacy of claims made by patients for entry into the sick role, or for medical care. These are rules inductively generalised from accounts given by staff.

(a) Patients must not be responsible, either for their illness or for getting better: medical staff can only be held responsible if, in addition, they were able to treat the illness.

The first half of this rule was broken by all normal rubbish. Drunks and tramps were responsible for their illnesses, either directly or indirectly. Tramps are responsible for the illnesses like bronchitis which are a direct result of the life the tramp has chosen to lead. Normal overdoses knew what they were doing, and chose to take an overdose for their own purposes. Trivia *chose* to come to Casualty, and could be expected to deal with their illnesses themselves. All normal rubbish had within their own hands the ability to effect a complete cure, and since there was little the Casualty staff could do about it, they could not be held responsible to treat the illnesses of normal rubbish. Comments which reflected this rule included,

I don't like having to deal with drunks in particular. I find that usually they're quite aggressive. I don't like aggressive people. And I feel that, you know, they've got them-selves into this state entirely through their own follies, why the hell should I have to deal with them on the NHS? So I don't like drunks.

I think they are a bloody nuisance. I don't like overdoses, because I've got very little sym-pathy with them on the whole, I'm afraid.
[Q: Why not?]
mm well you see most of them don't mean it, it's just to draw attention to themselves, you see I mean they take a non-lethal dose and they know it's not lethal.

The staff normally felt uncertain about the existence of an illness if there was no therapy that they, or anyone else, could provide to correct the state, and it would seem that this uncertainty fostered frustration which was vented as hostility towards these patients. One example of this was in the comments on overdoses, and the distinctions made between those who really tried to commit suicide (for whom there is some respect) and the rest (viewed as immature calls for attention). This seems to be behind the following comments:

It's the same I'm sure in any sphere, that if you're doing something and you're treating it and—say you're a plumber and the thing keeps going wrong because you haven't got the right thing to put it right, you get fed up with it, and in the end you'd much rather hit the thing over the . . . hit the thing with your hammer. Or in this case, to give up rather than go on, you know, making repeated efforts.

(b) Patients should be restricted in their reasonable activities by the illnesses they report with.

This rule has particular point in a Casualty department, and trivia who have been able to delay coming to the department most obviously break this rule. This is implicit in the comments already reported about trivia. However, there is another aspect to this rule, the requirement that the activities being followed should be reasonable, and the obvious offen-ders against this rule are the tramps.

If a man has led a full productive life, he's entitled to good medical attention, because he's put a lot into society.

[Tramps] put nothing in, and are always trying to get something out.

Obviously the Protestant Ethic of work is alive and well in Casualty departments.
(c) Patients should see illness as an undesirable state.

The patients who most obviously offend against this rule are the overdoses and the tramps. The overdoses are seen to want to be ill in order to put moral pressure on someone, or to get attention. Tramps want to be ill in order to get the benefits of being a patient—a warm bed and warm meals.

(d) Patients should cooperate with the competent agencies in trying to get well.

The major non-cooperative patients were the drunks and the overdoses. Drunks fail to cooperate by refusing to stay still while being sutured or examined, and overdoses fight back when a rubber tube is being forced down their throats so that their stomachs can be washed out. These are both cases where patients *refuse* to cooperate, rather than being unable to cooperate, as would be the case for patients in epileptic or diabetic fits. Similarly, they refuse to cooperate in getting 'well' because they cannot be trusted to live their lives in future in such a way that would avoid the same injuries.

In general, then, patients had a duty to live their lives in order to avoid injury, to remain well, and patients who did not do this were not worth helping. These four rules seemed to cover the criteria by which normal rubbish was faulted. It can be seen that each of them required quite fine judgement about, for example, whether a patient was uncooperative by choice or because of some underlying illness.

Punishment

Rubbish could be punished by the staff in various ways, the most important being to increase the amount of time that rubbish had to spend in Casualty before completing treatment. In each hospital there were ways of advancing and retarding patients so that they were not seen strictly in the order in which they arrived. Good patients, in general being the more serious, could be seen immediately by being taken directly to the treatment area, either by the receptionist or by the ambulanceman. Less serious cases, including the trivia, would go first to a general waiting area. Patients there were normally left until all serious cases had been dealt with. Sometimes staff employed a deliberate policy of leaving drunks and tramps in the hope that they would get annoyed at the delay and take their own discharge.

The other forms of punishment used were verbal hostility or the vigorous restraint of uncooperative patients. Verbal hostility was in general fairly restrained, at least in my presence, and was usually less forthright than the written comments made in the 'medical' notes, or the comments made in discussions with other staff. Vigorous treatment of patients was most noticeable in the case of overdoses, who would be held down or sat upon while the patient was forced to swallow the rubber tube used. Staff recognised that this procedure had an element of punishment in it, but defended themselves by saying that it was necessary. However, they showed no sympathy for the victim, unlike cases of accidental self-poisoning by children. Drunks and tramps who were uncooperative could be threatened with the police, who were called on a couple of occasions to undress a drunk or to stand around while a tramp was treated.

Punishment was rarely extended to a refusal to see or to treat patients. The staff were very conscious of the adverse publicity raised whenever patients were refused treatment in Casualty departments, and they were also worried by the medico-legal complications to which Casualty departments are prone, and this restrained their hostility and the extent of the delay they were prepared to put patients to. A cautionary tale was told to emphasise the dangers of not treating rubbish properly, concerning a tramp who was seen in a Casualty department and discharged. A little later the porter came in and told the CO that the tramp had collapsed and died outside on the pavement. The porter then calmed the worries of the CO by saying 'It's all right, sir, I've turned him round so that it looks as though he was on his way *to* Casualty.'

Roger Jeffery is a Lecturer in Sociology in the Department of Sociology, University of Edinburgh. This article is an edited version of one that was originally published in *Sociology of Health and Illness*, 1(1), 90–108 (1979).

5.4

Nurses, Midwives and the Public: Images and Realities. Report of the Briggs Committee on Nursing

Inherited and New Images and the Modern Nurse and Midwife

As is true of many other professions, nursing retains an inherited image which belongs to the late nineteenth century. 'The lady with the lamp' or 'the ministering angel' and similar visions linger in the mind. The familiar association of the nurse with pain, suffering and death and the tendency to place her (almost always 'her' rather than 'him') within the setting of a hospital impede an understanding of the great variety of jobs nurses actually do. The midwife has a quite different and contrasting image associated with the 'happy events' within the family's own history. She seems to have little to do with the care of the sick, and she has her own recognised place in society.

Florence Nightingale had much to do with the creation of the inherited image. She did not create it alone, of course, nor was she responsible for all aspects of it. We have noted the following further features of the inherited image of the hospital nurse which seem to be determined by history:

(a) it groups together doctors and nurses not as partners but as people in charge on the one hand and their 'handmaidens' on the other. In the process of providing care the doctor needed a skilled helper, and in the inherited image (still treasured by some) the nurse figures as such—a person who is strictly ancillary;

(b) at the same time, it is widely appreciated today that even this kind of historical grouping was not achieved without friction, that nurses had to fight, sometimes ruthlessly, for their status. The fact that the nurses were for the most part women and the doctors for the most part men was of the essence of the drama;

(c) there has been a class element in the traditional picture. After Florence Nightingale, enough nineteenth-century nurses from the higher social classes figure in the picture to provide a theme in itself—the theme of 'vocation', a theme, of course, with an older history leading back to the middle ages. The nurse was seen as living apart, thinking in terms not of money but of service, and evolving her own distinctive code. The adjective usually applied to her was 'dedicated';

(d) the essence of the code—to use a phrase of the most recent historian of nursing, Brian Abel-Smith[1]—was 'the search for perfectionism and the attempt to achieve it by discipline'. The hierarchies were thought of as authoritarian, and the image of the matron remains today as one of the most powerful of all popular nursing images.

In thinking of the future, it seemed important to us to clarify the relationship between present and past. We began, therefore, by listing some of the main groups of people with whom we were directly concerned in the early 1970s when we used the term 'nurse'; they can be thought of within a framework both of work and grade:

(a) in hospitals, which have their images as much as the people who work in them, we listed senior administrative and teaching staff in nursing and midwifery, Nursing Officers, ward sisters, midwifery sisters, staff midwives, staff nurses, senior enrolled nurses and enrolled nurses, unregistered students and post-registration students, midwives in training and pupil nurses. All these groups fall within the profession or intend to join it: the grades are very different from nineteenth-century grades, but there is a strong sense of status and some of the grades are distinguished by their uniforms;

(b) we also identified nursing assistants and auxiliaries who have had no professional training. Patients may call them 'nurse' and they enable service to the patient to be maintained and improved, not least at night, but they are outside the profession. They are unevenly distributed but their numbers have risen markedly in recent years;

(c) in the community, functions are not always separated in the same formal way as they are in hospitals and there are overlapping combinations of duties between health visitors, district nurses and midwives. Yet we found it necessary to distinguish between senior community nurses concerned with administration and teaching, health visitors, district nurses who may be either registered or enrolled, domiciliary midwives and a wide range of others, including school and clinic nurses. There are also ancillary staff supporting professional nurses in this field.

It says much for the pull and power of nineteenth-century attitudes that some of the most basic of them have survived vast changes in medical and social history, thereby confusing images and contemporary realities. Part of the reason for their persistence lies in the long life and continuity of buildings. Thus, while the design of new hospitals has been transformed, there are sufficient old ones, particularly out-of-date mental hospitals, to influence the attitudes both of staff and of the general public. The era of custodial care is not dead, particularly in some hospitals for the mentally handicapped, where there is serious overcrowding, where there are genuine shortages of trained staff, where the ratio of older to younger nurses is high and where there is an acute shortage of domestic and supporting staff. In dealing with such hospitals, indeed, and with the nursing staff working in them, we cannot avoid considering the legacy of history.

Current attitudes and policies may be even more strongly influenced by twentieth-century mass media of communication which often succeed in both looking backwards to Victorian Britain and looking forward to the age of integration:

(a) books and mass-circulation magazines for girls and women frequently deal with 'timeless' and 'universal' nursing themes: they are read by large numbers of people, of whom only a few will eventually become nurses. A study of such books and magazines suggests that nursing is thought of as a drama, a drama with a sequence starting with the initial inexperience of the novice nurse and ending either with the achievement of effective control or, less frequently, with disaster. The education of the nurse figures as much in such picaresque writing as the ultimate disposition of her duties. Romantic relationships are basic to the drama: they include relationships centring on jealousy, rivalry and malice as well as virtue rewarded and true love. The juxtaposition of youth and death is also a part of the pattern.

There is also a more realistic vein in some girls' magazines, particularly those which deal with future careers in documentary or semi-documentary fashion. These point to the variety of careers in nursing and midwifery (and the effort needed to pursue them) and by no means concentrate exclusively on the drama. They provide an important medium of information as well as of interpretation. We recommend that these magazines should be made known and their cooperation obtained in providing further and more detailed information relating to nursing and midwifery as a career;

(b) television series and films seek to create, often successfully, the sense of a separate hospital world of its own with characters and shifting patterns of relationships. In this respect they are like comic strips. Again it is the drama and the romance which predominate, with great emphasis being placed on the romantic relationships of nurses both with doctors and with patients.

Serialisation implies concentration on moments of tension, real or contrived. The use of actors and actresses, seen regularly in television series as nurses and doctors over long periods of time, produces a new set of associations diverging sharply, if sometimes only superficially, from the inherited images.

At the same time television also includes documentary films, many of which take as their starting point the divergence between the inherited or contrived image and the 'reality' and can play a helpful and constructive part in keeping both the general public and potential entrants informed. The 'problem' aspects of nursing are usually picked out in documentaries, usually sympathetically;

(c) newspapers include a great deal of material, often fragmentary and personalised, about nurses and midwives, not only news material but photographs and feature articles, and sometimes combinations of news, photographs and feature articles, as in the 'Nurse of the Year' contest sponsored by the *Daily Express*. In two sample weeks in 1971 which we studied in detail there were on each occasion more than 100 references to nurses in the press, most often in local newspapers dealing with individual careers or with social occasions, including prizegivings, in the hospital. The national press always has a regular coverage of nursing. Press references cover an immense variety of themes, not least accident and emergency procedures, ethical questions centring on nursing, petty discipline and, very regularly, uniforms, while during recent years questions of pay and protest have loomed large. Like radio and television, the press has made much also of the 'lure' of nursing employment overseas, particularly in the United States and Canada, pointing both to the pay and to the 'glamour'. Most of the comment is highly favourable to British nurses and nursing, as is the case in unsolicited letters from correspondents, but contrasts are sometimes drawn for effect—with stress on the power motivations of nurses not on their compassion: and with talk not of 'ladies of the lamp' but of 'dictatorial automatons'. 'They're the ones who make hospitals into institutions' was one of the most sweeping comments of 1971.

Public images influence recruitment: they also predetermine attitudes at critical moments in the health history of individuals and families. Yet the surface should not be mistaken for the substance, and in any searching analysis of contemporary attitudes attention should be paid not only to images of nurses but to shifting conceptions of dependency, institutionalisation, discipline and, above all, life and death. These conceptions are related both to expectations and aspirations concerning the National Health Service as a whole, and they should never be ignored by either strategic planners or by 'managers'.

They should remember also that new generations of nurses and midwives share some of the attitudes of their own generations more than they share the attitudes of an older generation of nurses and midwives. One of the purposes of our opinion survey was to judge how far this was true. We noted considerable variation in the age pattern as between different types of nursing. In mental handicap hospitals, for example, 26 per cent of staff were over the age of fifty-five (as against 8 per cent in acute hospitals and 12 per cent in all hospitals). Age proportions matter, and there is a tendency among some of the younger nurses we interviewed to feel that they are being expected to undergo too long and painful a process of initiation before they are fully welcomed into the profession. Senior nurses felt happier about the current situation than students and pupils. A majority of hospital nurses and midwives agreed that 'senior nurses often forget what it was like to be a junior nurse' and the more junior the nurse, the more likely she was to hold this view, and to hold it strongly.

In her study[2] *Threshold to Nursing* (1969) Dr MacGuire drew upon a number of earlier research reports which showed that about a quarter of all adults in one survey considered nursing to be a 'first choice' of career for girls leaving school and saw nursing as the hardest but the most worthwhile of four jobs—nursing, teaching, secretarial work and clerical work in banking—and second to teaching in its demands on 'intelligence'. Adults had a more favourable image of nursing than girls aged sixteen to twenty-four, and two out of three in the general population would have been willing to encourage a daughter to take up nursing. Dr MacGuire also noted evidence that about a third of women and girls developed an interest in nursing at some time of their lives, with the years thirteen to sixteen providing the peak age range for such interest. About one-sixth developed a strong interest. By contrast a small minority of boys of school age interested themselves in nursing. Educational attainment but not social class, family size or geographical location affected interest in nursing. Hours and pay were seen as deterrents; it was felt that there was more 'discipline' than was necessary; and change in the profession (for example, in pay, grades and conditions) was underestimated. Information about nursing conditions was frequently wrong. The need for personal suitability was stressed. Little was known by potential recruits about specialisation, age of entry, educational entry requirements (which were over-estimated), career structure or the difference between registered and enrolled nurses. It was felt that it was difficult to become a nurse.

Most male nurses, Dr MacGuire concluded, came to nursing as their second career after an unsuccessful attempt at another career and for many it was a positive shift to a more worthwhile job. Psychiatric nursing offered a field where, largely for reasons of history, the image of nursing work as 'women's work' did not hold.

The Image Formally Presented to the Recruit

We have carefully examined samples of current recruitment literature, including advertisements and other relevant material, in relation to this evidence and to that presented in our own surveys:

(a) emphasis is now placed in national recruitment brochures on the variety of jobs in nursing and midwifery. In the four brochures on nursing it is stressed that 'every day is different' and 'every patient is different and needs a different kind of approach'. In the *Mentally Ill* brochure a nurse says 'you can't say this is like any other form of nursing. It isn't'.

(b) the subtitle of the most recent brochures on *Nursing the Mentally Handicapped* and *Nursing the Mentally Ill* is 'A profession for people who care'. The brochure on general nursing has as a title '*Someone Special*'. In the *Community Nursing* brochures a key phrase is 'The personal quality which really does count for something is initiative';

(c) emphasis is placed on teamwork in all four brochures rather than on individual vocation, though the sense of 'worthwhileness' is still underlined;

(d) all the brochures are personalised: they deal with individual career profiles, some stressing the youth of the nurses being described, others the benefits of 'maturity' and 'experience'. 'The younger generation of nurses certainly contribute their own quota of verve and zest to the job, but the mature nurse brings a very special kind of help to many patients.'

(e) it is not assumed that all entrants thought of being nurses from childhood. One of the girls, an enrolled nurse, says 'some girls have wanted to be nurses ever since they were children, but it never entered my head until I saw an advertisement in a paper': it was her third job;

(f) all deal with educational methods ('up-to-date' and 'carefully balanced') and conditions of living (agreeable). Discipline is said to be 'sensible' (with 'very good reasons behind the rules');

(g) it is recognised that different nurses have different objectives within the profession; 'I would like to carry on with further training' contrasts sharply with 'I've no desire to climb up the promotion scale because I enjoy my present work so much';

(h) it is recognised finally that the profession is changing. 'Even in the short time I've been in mental nursing, things have changed.' There is a 'continual willingness to try out new ideas'. 'This is a job where you are always learning something new because nursing and medical techniques are constantly being developed or reviewed.' 'The very nature of the work,' it is said of the midwife attached to group practice, 'demands the use of modern equipment, such as the gas and oxygen machine and resuscitators . . . Many midwives are now carrying radio transceivers to summon help when it is needed.'

One of the main reasons for national campaigns is the prevalence of a strong feeling, not least among nurses and midwives, that nurses and midwives are 'born not made', perhaps the most stubborn of all the stereotypes. Even trainees themselves often stick to the stereotypes. After one of them had recently seen a recruiting film she commented 'If a girl or boy has decided to become a nurse nothing will change her or his mind . . . If the person doesn't know what career to follow, the film was of no help.'

We agree with a comment made to us in the evidence of the National Association of Leagues of Hospital Friends that 'contrary to the image presented by the national news media, there is a large and growing awareness among young people . . . of the obligations which the fortunate members of the community owe to the less fortunate, and a desire sincerely felt, if sometimes inadequately expressed, to do something to discharge these obligations'. Emphasis in recruiting on the need for 'care' in a complex society and the changing patterns of provision of care is in our view fully justified. Nursing and midwifery live up to the most profound of their claims: they make nurses and midwives feel that, whatever the privations, they are doing 'something special' and inwardly rewarding.

Students in training and to a lesser extent people working in the profession will ask key questions in the light of their own experience about the kind of recruitment material described. They are bound to treat this material critically, and we believe that their criticisms should be taken into account. Is what has been said about 'rules' borne out in practice? Is there really 'teamwork' and 'a sense of community'? Is the sense of 'worthwhileness' realised? New recruits, in particular, will contrast what they observe from experience with what they have been told, and will do this on their own or in the group of students with whom they are involved in training.

The Voices of Nurses

Such criticisms, which seem to us to reflect clearly the views of the profession in the making, are borne out by more detailed accounts which have been published or submitted to us as a Committee concerning the daily life of the nurse as it is actually lived:

(a) answers to our questionnaires suggested that dissatisfaction with work, hours, shifts and promotion prospects tended to be less prevalent than we expected, yet:

   (i)   when nurses and midwives who cooperated in our postal survey were given a list of different categories and grades of staff, ranging from messengers to doctors and including clerical workers, social workers, other professional staff and less qualified nurses, and asked to say whether during the last week they had carried out work which ought in their view to have been carried out by one of the other categories, 66 per cent of registered and enrolled nurses ticked off at least one item on the list;

   (ii) a quarter of hospital nurses and midwives and nearly a third of community nurses and midwives had worked 'unofficial' unpaid overtime during the previous week and between a quarter and a third of all nurses and midwives had had less than two full days off in the previous week;

   (iii) while there was less concern with questions of promotion than might be expected our interview survey showed that a considerable number of nurses and midwives (39 per cent) feel strongly that the criteria for promotion are wrong—length of service, in particular, rather than ability, while a further 25 per cent share this feeling to some extent;

(b) turning carefully and critically from our questionnaires to the unsolicited letters sent to us and bearing in mind that many, perhaps most, could be expected to come from people with criticisms to offer, we found some of the same points made more strongly. The letters dwell mainly on the extent of 'non-nursing duties' ('sheer drudgery') and the inadequacy of both personal and organisational relationships. The single greatest cause of complaint was the attitudes and behaviour of nurses themselves, and in the words of one critic 'there seems to be a complete disregard for the human being beneath the nurse'. 'Training,' says another, 'tends to destroy initiative, discretion, common sense and dampens the enthusiasm which most nurses have to get to know and look after ill people';

(c) we noted, for example, the comments and criticisms of student nurses, among them one, representative of many, who stayed for only nine months and failed to complete her training. Her comments were on the obverse side of the coin from those presented through the recruiting media. Living conditions were not good. Rules were not sensible. There was too much harshness over trivia and lack of perspective. The preliminary training course was not stimulating, but exhausting. Communications were poor. Questions were not welcomed. The typical day was too long. There was too little time for real care. Everything was institutionalised. There seemed to be an almost perverse desire to 'preserve the [unfavourable] image at all costs'. Others complained, however, from a quite different angle, that 'nursing procedures' had to be undertaken 'without adequate demonstration and supervision'. 'Sisters and staff nurses are too busy to do more than distribute cursory directions with minimal teaching of procedure. The more conscientious and idealistic the student nurse is, the more likely she is to be troubled by this lack of teaching';

(d) from the other side a nurse administrator concerned with the allocation of student nurses wrote that she found 'students remarkably understanding and helpful even when refused a request if told why'. She added that 'the tensions due to medical advancement are greater than when we were students' and that 'some sisters are threatened by a knowledgeable student, or the one who uses initiative which is appreciated in an emergency only'.

We do not subscribe to all these personal opinions, some of which are flatly contradicted by more general evidence submitted to us, for example in reply to our opinion questionnaires. From the questionnaires it emerged that most nurses and midwives seem willing to shoulder the burden of responsibility imposed upon them: only a third of hospital nurses and midwives and a fifth of community nurses and midwives agreed with the statement that 'too much responsibility for difficult decisions about the care of patients is left to nurses'. There is a different side to nursing and midwifery, therefore, from that expressed by nurses or midwives with grievances before or after training. We note that after initial difficulties some of which seem to us to be a necessary part of the process of becoming a nurse, nursing offers to many people 'enjoyment and satisfaction' in a way that few other professions do. 'I've never met a nurse who can't find something to moan about,' one of them writes. 'Yet, whenever I am asked if I enjoy nursing...I say, yes, it's a wonderful life. Compared with chasing after money, it is. Compared with the rat race of office life it is. Compared with living in luxury on a Pacific Island it probably isn't. But, then, who gets that chance?'

Relevant criticisms, justifiable or not, often focus attention on critical relationships at work. Some point to the difficulties which the part-timer can experience, others to the fact that 'staff nurses are not trusted'. Almost all direct attention to the key role of the ward sister. 'Any senior nurse who has worked on a particular ward or department for some time and has confidence in her own technical ability, can break slightly from the traditional inflexibility of nursing and mould her own work among both patients and juniors, with initiative, discretion and sensitivity. The ward or departmental sister is the key person there: her powers vary according to the administrative policy of the hospital; they are likely to be greater in matters concerning patients than in matters concerning the nursing staff. Her own personality is important in creating the atmosphere most conducive to happier nurses and patients . . . The sister often has considerable control over the off-duty, she can rarely dictate the hours of the shifts worked, but often arranges the weekly off-duty schedule and can deal sympathetically, or not, with requests for special off-duty. . . . Most important of all, she has the power to affect the morale of the whole ward, more even than it is affected by the nature of disease cared for in that ward. Her own behaviour in a crisis determines the confidence that the nurses have, not only in her, but in the knowledge that were something unexpected to occur while they were treating a patient she would support them; such confidence generated to the junior nurses is easily felt by patients as well. A ward sister needs to be perceptive to notice the nurse under stress, or the nurse who is disturbed by an event or a particular patient. In dictating her own priorities, she can affect the welfare of both patients and staff: should tired nurses go for their tea breaks or tidy the sluice? is she content if the patients are comfortable or must they look neatly arranged? are the most ill patients in a position where not only can the nurses see them easily, but so too can young, newly arrived patients? It is the ward sister who must always be available to patients, their relatives and the nurses for advice and reassurance in all problems; then she alone can combine the roles of all members of the medical team to present a clear pattern of treatment and progress that they can all understand. She should attempt to know each patient's family so that from her explanations and reassurance they are able to appear less anxious. Fear of the unknown is probably the greatest fear of patients, relatives and nurses, and the ward sister is in the best position to dispel those fears. The respect which all sisters should command, should not be the awesome respect of a subordinate, but a respect based upon the ward sister's competence and skill in nursing and management.

We conclude our brief comparison of images and realities with three basic points:

(a) there is an immense variety in the practice of different hospitals and local authorities, such a variety that it is almost impossible to generalise. If good practices in the best hospitals and local authorities were to be adopted more generally there would be immediate and in some cases striking improvements;

(b) individual disillusionment often sets in most quickly in relation to practical matters, particularly hours of work, days off duty, shift working, night duty and the duty rota. Yet not all the 'images' of discontent are backed by facts. For example, in response to a statement in our questionnaire that nurses were asked to undertake too much night duty, it was found that a large majority of nurses and midwives disagreed. From a list of eleven suggestions for improving conditions less night duty was the least popular.

(c) when nurses and midwives were asked what were their first and second priorities for improved conditions only two items attracted the attention of more than a small minority—the length of the working week and pay.

After examining together all the criticisms and hopes of improvement, we wish to stress that unless sympathetic care within nursing and midwifery administration is shown to nurses and midwives both in training and after they are trained, the wider claims of the profession to rest on individual care will ring hollow. Care starts with the relations between nurses and nurses. So, too, does sympathetic understanding on which all care is based.

References

1. Abel-Smith, B. *A history of the nursing profession,* Heinemann, London, p. 241 (1966).
2. MacGuire, J. M. *Threshold to Nursing: a review of the literature on recruitment to and withdrawal from nurse training programmes in the United Kingdom* (Occasional Papers on Social Adminstration No. 30), Bell, London (1969).

This article is an edited extract from Chapter 2 of the *Report of the Committee on Nursing* (Chairman: Professor Asa Briggs), Cmnd. 5115, HMSO, London, pp. 23–38 (1972).

Part 6

Experiencing health and disease

Introduction

What does it mean to be healthy or sick? What factors—biological, medical and social—interact to construct the experience of health and disease? Inevitably it will be shaped by individual character traits and the nature of the condition being experienced. But experience will also be influenced by the social situation in which we live and by the formal services, particularly health services, with which we come into contact.

Sickness itself imparts a particular status on the individual involved, but it also carries its own obligations. In the extract from *The Psychology of the Sickbed* van den Berg powerfully yet simply illustrates the experience of sickness as the passage into a world where one can neglect obligations of home and work, where one is actually excluded from everyday 'normality' and where one begins to see the 'familiar' as strange and new. Yet, as he also suggests, the status of sickness may have to be demonstrated—the thermometer confirms that one is 'running a temperature', inability to eat means one must 'really be sick'.

Though minor illnesses such as 'flu or a cold are conditions with which we are all familiar, we tend to forget that we acquire our knowledge of these conditions and our way of coping with them through others around us. This process can be a powerful determinant of our experience of illness, as the extract from Sally Macintyre and David Oldman, 'Coping with migraine', demonstrates. Both authors are migraine sufferers, yet the ways in which they acquired knowledge about the condition—how it was identified and treated—present a stark contrast. For Oldham, the experience was 'normalised' by another who had herself experienced migraine. For Macintyre, whose migraine was 'alien to everyone else's experience', the process of identification and treatment was more problematic, involving professional medical help and resulting in greater anxiety. Contrary, however, to popular and perhaps professional opinion, Macintyre and Oldman consider that experiencing illness without having any contact with the medical profession is quite typical.

Both the process by which knowledge is acquired and the nature of the knowledge itself are relevant to understanding: this is particularly true of the experience of disability. Though the event that leads to a disability may be tragic, Ann Shearer, in her book *Disability: Whose Handicap?*, argues forcefully that the experience of disability need not be. But the attitudes and behaviour, rules and regulations which people with disabilities meet every day produce a picture of disability as 'a last personal tragedy'. Through their encounters with family and friends, the public and professionals, their own understanding of their disability is constructed against a backcloth of concepts of normality. In this way, society actually creates handicap where none need exist.

The experience of old age is also to a large extent socially constructed. Increasing age inevitably means increasing frailness. But the experience of isolation, segregation and lack of human contact which Ellen Newman describes in the extract from her diary *This Bed My Centre* are not inevitable. Nor are such experiences confined to the elderly in nursing homes. Those living alone may similarly feel that they are being treated as 'no longer average human beings'. Social attitudes and behaviour can also powerfully influence the experience of bereavement and the way people cope after the death of someone close to them. In their book, *Life after Death*, Ann Bowling and Ann Cartwright describe the range of problems facing the elderly widowed. Formal and informal support may also be important determinants of experience, and the role of the GP was a central focus of the Bowling and Cartwright study. However, the extract we have included here focuses specifically on caring for a dying spouse, highlighting practical problems, the experience of support and the restriction which such caring responsibilities can impose.

The often profound influence of formal health services in the experience of health and disease is an important theme running through much of the literature in this field. The extract from *Aliens and Alienists* by Roland Littlewood and Maurice Lipsedge provides a dramatic illustration of the processes involved. They describe the interface between two often very different perceptions of the world when psychiatrist and immigrant patient meet. Given the status, authority and power vested in the medical profession this may have catastrophic implications for the immigrant patient. In this case, both racial discrimination and cultural differences influence this interaction. Sometimes assumptions about the way social factors influence attitudes and behaviour towards health care are wrong, as the paper by Bronwen Earthrowl and Margaret Stacey suggests. It appears that parents from different social classes have similar expectations for their children when in hospital though economic reasons may prevent them being fulfilled.

The personal experience of health and disease and of formal health-care is therefore shaped by a multitude of factors. The articles included in this part do not aim to provide an exhaustive account of these—rather they illustrate the range of factors which may be influential and the processes which are at work.

6.1

The Meaning of Being Ill

Jan H. van den Berg

If we wish to realize what it means to be ill, we should begin by trying to remember what happened when a short, passing, but positively uncomfortable, illness made us stay in bed for a few days. What will come back to us might be something like the following report.

Report by the Father of a Family

After a restless and disturbed sleep, I wake up in the morning, not feeling too well. I get out of bed, however, intending to start the day in the usual manner. But soon I notice that I cannot. I have a headache; I feel sick. I notice an uncontrollable urge to vomit and deem myself so incapable of facing the day that I convince myself that I am ill. I return to the bed I just left with every intention of staying there for a while. The thermometer shows that my decision was not unreasonable. My wife's cautious inquiry whether I would like something for breakfast makes the reason much clearer. I am *really* ill. I give up my coffee and toast, as I give up everything the day was to bring, all the plans and the duties. And to prove that I am abandoning these completely I turn to the wall, nestle myself in my bed, which guarantees a comparative well-being by its warm invitation to passivity, and close my eyes. But I find that I cannot sleep.

Then, slowly, but irrevocably, a change, characteristic of the sickbed, establishes itself. I hear the day begin. From downstairs the sounds of household activities penetrate into the bedroom. The children are called for breakfast. Loud hasty voices are evidence of the fact that their owners have to go to school in a few minutes. A handkerchief has to be found, and a bookbag. Quick young legs run up and down the stairs. How familiar, and at the same time how utterly strange things are; how near and yet how far away they are. What I am hearing is the beginning of my daily existence, with this difference, though, that now I have no function in it. In a way I still belong completely to what happens downstairs; I take a share in the noises I hear, but at the same time everything passes me by, everything happens at a great distance. 'Is Daddy ill?' a voice calls out; even at this early moment, it has ceased to consider that I can hear it. 'Yes, Daddy is ill.' A moment later the door opens and they come to say goodbye. They remain just as remote. The distance I measured in the sounds from downstairs appears even greater, if possible, now that they are at my bedside, with their fresh clean faces and lively gestures. Everything about them indicates the normal healthy day, the day of work and play, of street and school. The day outside the house, in which 'outside' has acquired a new special meaning for me, a meaning emphasizing my exclusion.

I hear that the day has begun out in the street. It makes itself heard; cars pull away and blow their horns, and boys shout to one another. I have not heard the sounds of the street like this for years, from such an enormous distance. The doorbell rings; it is the milkman, the postman, or an acquaintance; whoever it is I have nothing to do with him. The telephone rings; for a moment I try to be interested enough to listen, but again I soon submit to the inevitable, reassuring, but at the same time slightly discouraging, knowledge that I have to relinquish everything. I have ceased to belong; I have no part in it.

The world has shrunk to the size of my bedroom, or rather my bed. For even if I set foot on the floor it seems as if I am entering a *terra incognita*. Going to the bathroom is an unfriendly, slightly unreal, excursion. With the feeling of coming home I pull the blankets over me. The horizon is narrowed to the edge of my bed and even this bed is not completely my domain. Apart from where I am lying it is cold and uncomfortable; the pillow only welcomes me where my head touches it. Every move is a small conquest.

Change of the Future and the Past

The horizon in time too is narrowed. The plans of yesterday lose their meaning and their importance; they have hardly any real value. They seem more complicated, more exhausting, more foolish and ambitious than I saw them the day before. All that awaits me becomes tasteless, or even distasteful. The past seems saturated with trivialities. It appears to me that I hardly ever tackled my real tasks. Future and past lose their outlines; I withdraw from both and I live in the confined present of this bed which guards me against the things that were and those that will be. Under normal circumstances I live in the future, and in the past as far as the future draws upon it to prescribe my duties. Apart from a few special moments I never really live in the present, I never think of it. But the sickbed does not allow me to escape from the present.

Normally I am not aware of my body; it performs its tasks like an instrument. Now that I am ill, I become acutely aware of a bodily existence, which makes itself felt in a general malaise, in a dull headache and in a vague nausea. The body which used to be a condition becomes the sole content of the moment. The present, while always serving the future, and therefore often being an effect of the past, becomes saturated with itself. As a patient I live with a useless body in a disconnected present.

Everything gets an 'actual' meaning, and this is quite a discovery for us who are pledged to the future. The telephone, rather than conveying the message from the person at the other end of the line, makes me aware of the fact that, as a frozen appeal, it rings with a new sound through a house which has become remarkably remote and strange. The blankets of my bed, articles so much devoted to utility that they used to disappear behind the goal they served, so that in my normal condition I could not possibly have said what colour they are, become jungles of colored threads in which my eye laboriously finds its way. The sheets are immeasurable white plains with deep crevasses, steep slopes and insurmountable summits; a polar landscape to the paralyzed traveller that I am.

The wallpaper which I only noticed vaguely, if I ever saw it at all, has to be painfully analyzed in lines, dots, smaller and larger figures. I feel an urge to examine the symmetrical pattern, and to see in it caricatures of people, animals and things. It is as if I am taking a Rorschach-test, immensely enlarged. Hopeless and nightmarish interpretations urge themselves upon me, particularly when I am running a fever. And I feel I am going mad when I find a spot that cannot be made to fit into the structure which took me such pains to evolve.

After a few days I begin to hate the oil painting on the wall. For by this time I have acquired a certain freedom to change the caricatures of the wallpaper; I can replace the configuration I created by another one when I am bored with it. But the figures in the painting, the people, the animals, the houses and the trees, resist every attempt in this direction. The hunter, about to shoot the flying duck, remains aiming motionlessly, while I have judged his chances a hundred times. And the duck, which would probably manage to reach a hiding place if it is quick enough, defies all dangers as it comfortably floats over the landscape where the sun forgets the laws of cosmography in an eternal sunset. 'Oh! please, hurry up' I say, exasperated, and even if I am amused at my own words, I do ask the next visitor to please be kind enough either to turn the picture to the wall or to remove it altogether.

Professor van den Berg is Head of the Faculty of Social Science at the University of Leiden. This is an edited extract of the first chapter from his book *The Psychology of the Sickbed* published by Humanities Press Inc., New Jersey (1981).

6.2

Coping with Migraine

Sally Macintyre and David Oldman

The main emphasis in the following accounts is on the acquisition of our knowledge of migraine. In these two accounts we introduce the idea of knowledge as developing in a series of discrete *stages* concerned with experiencing the complaint, identifying it as migraine, and finally acquiring a repertoire of methods for coping with it. All migraine sufferers pass in turn through these stages. The forms of the repertoire of coping may change over time through a series of *phases*, each phase characterised by an emphasis on one or another cell in a typology of treatments. Shifts between these phases do not have any necessary sequence.

Sally Macintyre's Account

The first stage of my career as a migraine sufferer we characterise as being an anomic stage. My first migraine attack, which I distinctly remember, occurred when I was twelve. During the following five years I had further attacks ranging in frequency from every six weeks to six months. I was unable to name, predict or account for these experiences, and did not possess the appropriate vocabulary with which to describe them to others. I did not know what these attacks were or what they implied. Was I 'just tired', developing a serious illness, about to have a stroke, epileptic, or mad? I had no means of predicting attacks and I had no means of establishing how best to cope with them when they happened. They were thus inexplicable, unpredictable, not amenable to rational means of coping, and apparently alien to everyone else's experience.

The second stage was an identificatory stage, occurring when I was seventeen and lasting for several months. The trigger for this stage was my collapsing in public during an attack. Having been trying for five years unsuccessfully to explain to others that I had 'funny turns', this public manifestation forced a recognition of this account and the process of diagnosis was set in motion. After a number of diagnostic tests arranged by my GP I was admitted to a hospital in London for investigation. The whole of this identificatory stage was characterised by negative diagnosis, i.e. identifying and eliminating what I had *not* got. Thus, the tests I underwent were designed to examine the possibilities of a brain tumour (skull X-rays, angiogram, radioactive tracing tests), epilepsy (EEGs) and other CNS disorders (reflex tests, lumbar puncture). I was finally told, 'Well, you'll be relieved to hear that you haven't got a brain tumour after all—it's only migraine.'

Immediately after the diagnosis my emphasis was on the physicalist/ameliorative aspect of migraine. I accepted myself, and was so accepted by others, as a basically normal person who periodically experienced transient physical disturbances. These disturbances were regarded as being separable from me as a social being with a particular biography, personality and social environment: I was merely a host for occasional physical disturbances. The propensity to attacks was regarded as a morally neutral matter, a definition which I suspect was enhanced by the fact that the diagnosis was conducted through the high technology and high prestige of a neurological department, rather than, for example, a psychiatric department. Coping consisted of handling the attacks, once they occurred, with Cafergot-Q, and learning how to recognize the onset of an attack and how to judge the most efficacious dosage. My knowledge about these techniques derived only secondarily from my GP, mainly stemming from personal experience and trial and error.

On arrival at university my attention shifted to the 'personal/social' and 'preventive' cell. The student health service doctors were oriented towards patients as 'social beings in their total environment'. Rather than providing repeat prescriptions of Cafergot-Q, these doctors recommended recognition and avoidance of stressful situations, a reduction in ambition and competitiveness, and mild sedation at the onset of an attack. The prevailing etiological theory was that migraine was typical of over-conscientious, neurotic and intelligent women; role conflicts (e.g. degree versus marriage); and stressful life events (exams). I was redefined from a blameless, passive host to an active producer of migraines. I learnt and developed strategies for coping with the problem of being a 'migrainous person', mainly by stressing the assumed flattering correlations (conscientious, intelligent, sensitive), avoiding situations in which an attack would be disruptive, and exploiting the definition of myself as neurotic.

This phase of regarding migraine as a personal attribute reached a crisis when I moved to another university for a year and registered with the student health service there. My new GP believed that migraine was the result of deep-seated personality conflicts. When I declined to enter a course of psychoanalysis he refused to provide any further advice or chemotherapy. He variously informed me that my migraine resulted from my not having a boyfriend, sublimating my desire for children for postgraduate studies, and having over-strong internalised guilt and achievement-strivings. When I became depressed lest all these analyses were true, the migraine was attributed to depressive tendencies. These theories were to me highly unwelcome and on one level I rejected them. On another level I suspected that they might be true.

During this time I experienced an attack while on the top of a London bus, and found the experience of social and mental incompetence in such a situation to be deeply disturbing. I developed a fear of having an attack, which after a few months developed into acute anxiety states about travelling by public transport, eating in restaurants, attending seminars and other public meetings. My GP felt that my agoraphobia confirmed his previous character analysis of me, and attempted to refer me to another psychiatrist. When I was unable to keep the appointment, my plea that agoraphobia had prevented me from travelling across London was rejected as a rationalisation.

An acquaintance commented on my rather sorry state at this time, and when I explained the situation arranged for me to see her GP husband. He prescribed Valium. I began to conquer the phobias, started to eat properly again, found the frequency and severity of migraine attacks reduced, and ceased feeling panicky about the possibility of having attacks. I sought out information about the physical correlates of attacks, learned to stop eating certain foods, and wore dark glasses in bright sunlight. Over exams the GP put me on the Pill, which I found made a great improvement in the attacks previously correlated with the two days before a period. I thus moved out of the 'personal/social' phase back into a 'physicalist' phase, but this time one with the main focus on prevention.

Having obtained what to me was satisfactory evidence that physical prophylaxis 'worked', I totally rejected the psychoanalytic interpretations of my previous GP, which I had in any case found injurious to my self-image.

When I moved to another part of the country I registered with a group practice and discovered that the practitioners espoused widely differing theories about migraine and its proper treatment. While registered with one doctor I continued regularly to consume Valium with his approval. He was interested in migraine, would discuss various new theories about it and tried out some of the new prophylactic drugs on me. When he left and I applied to another doctor for a repeat prescription I was scolded for taking dihydroergotamine and was refused further prescriptions. The next doctor spent six months weaning me off Valium; the fourth partner in the practice said that he himself was a sufferer, and found that Valium was the best way of managing it.

I registered with a new practice, and informed the new GP of the regimen I preferred. I now regard myself as an 'expert' patient, knowing exactly what I want and using the GP partly as a resource to supply me with those drugs that I want, but which are on prescription.

David Oldman's Account

The first significant point about my own career as a migraine sufferer is that I cannot remember my first attack. Fairly regular attacks began somewhere around the age of nine, but the anomic and identificatory stages took up no more than an hour or two of my life. My mother had experienced frequent attacks during childhood and adolescence and was presumably able to normalise my first encounter with the complaint. I have a dim recollection of my mother prescribing by her actions what became for me the standard organisation of an attack—bed, a darkened room, hot-water bottle, bowl within easy reach for the attacks of vomiting, and Lucozade as the only liquid I could tolerate. So, from the start I not only had the complaint identified, but was also given the elements of a therapeutic routine which changed little for twenty years.

The imposition of identification and routine has not necessarily been as helpful as one might expect. If it is done early in life it may prove very hard to alter, and may take on a ritualistic quality which may even hamper the possibilities of more effective prevention and relief. I sweated my way through every attack in childhood surrounded by at least two hot-water bottles and never quite managed to convince myself that I suffered less when chilled—a 'fact' to which I now subscribe. More seriously, on four occasions in thirty years of attacks I have been caught in situations in which it was impossible to withdraw from ongoing social routines. In three cases I was able to get by, with much distress but not necessarily any more than I would normally have felt in the comfort of my own bed. Indeed, on the two occasions when I started an attack on top of a Scottish mountain, the effort of walking at least six miles to safety distracted me from the pain. Occasionally I have wondered whether withdrawal during an attack is either necessary or beneficial.

The very imposition of routine during my school years contained the seeds of liberation. My attacks were then almost invariably associated with the relief of tension *after* two classes of event—exams and rugby matches. The frequency and unpredictability of rugby matches made them loom largest in the production of migraine. I suddenly found myself in a position of control, for when I left school I stopped playing rugby and reduced my migraines to two attacks in five years!

Over the past thirteen years, during which period I have been regularly employed, residentially stable and suitably married, my relationship with the medical profession has been one in which I am invited to speculate on the causes and consequences of migraine as a 'normal' member of society—indeed, one of rather high status. Provided that I remain within the boundaries of legitimate migraine pharmacology I can discuss the effects of drugs and even request some rather than others. My current diet of dihydro-ergotamine and Migril resulted from an egalitarian discussion with my GP. The fact that I top this up with Stemetil and Valium for an actual attack is unknown to him, and is only possible by 'borrowing' these drugs from friends and relatives.

These ways of coping are not merely the result of achieving a 'normal' social status in the lay sociology of the GP, but are also a result of a definite attempt on my own part to 'medicalise' migraine given that, over the last thirteen years, I have lost the power to correlate my attacks with features of my own life style. I get about three attacks a year and if they correlate with anything at all, it is with quite major events such as moving house or changing jobs—not aspects of one's life that can be stepped around. I now have no way of avoiding migraine—I can only treat the attacks.

So far, then, my career as a migraine sufferer has been a prolonged attempt to find improved physical methods of preventing, and particularly treating, attacks. My 'way of life' has never seemed amenable to change in ways that would affect my migraines. As a child I had no power over my social routines; as an adult my routines have been regarded as too desirable to warrant change. The only development in my methods has been an increasing awareness that I could dictate the physical treatments and, at the same time, an increasing divergence from accepted and acceptable pharmacology.

Discussion—The Development of Personal Theories of Migraine

The most striking difference between our two accounts is the different length of time it took us to pass through the anomic and identificatory stages—5½ years compared with at most a few hours. We attribute this to the respective absence and presence of fellow-sufferers or 'wise' persons in our immediate social environments. We suggest that it is not surprising that migraine 'runs in families', if the quickest identifier is a fellow-sufferer. Subsequent to her own diagnosis, Macintyre 'identified' classical migraine in her brother and sister.

When fellow-sufferers are available as identifiers, symptoms may rapidly be interpreted and named as being migraine, and we suggest that the learning process may be a didactic one of imparting received wisdom both about etiology and coping. In the absence of a pool of fellow-sufferers such symptoms may have to be interpreted by the medical profession. Such medical identification may rely more on the negative diagnosis described above—the successive elimination of alternative and more serious diagnoses—and may present the sufferer with fewer practical recipes for coping. Given this lack of practical advice or the outlining of etiological theories, the sufferer may then more actively search for knowledge from which to construct useful theories, and his knowledge may differ from that of a sufferer socialised by fellow-sufferers.

Another consequence of our differing experiences of identifying migraine is that it appears that Macintyre found the 'anomic' stage deeply disturbing and that this has left a greater residue of anxiety about the topic than that experienced by Oldman, with his relatively unproblematic and matter-of-fact introduction to migraine, mediated by 'wise' family members.

In general, Macintyre's experience more closely approximates the models of illness behaviour posited by medical sociologists than does Oldman's—an initial period of disorganised symptomatology, a 'trigger' for seeking medical help, diagnosis and treatment offered by the medical profession, and reappraisal of doctors' actions.[1,2,3] We suspect that it is Macintyre's experience which is atypical, and that the experience of illness behaviour, diagnosis and coping, without contact with the medical profession, is a more ubiquitous and frequent phenomenon than is often implied in the medical sociological literature.

References

1. Rosenstock, I. M. 'Why people use health services', *Milbank Memorial Fund Quarterly*, Vol. LXIV, No. 3, Part 2 (1966).
2. Mechanic, D. *Medical Sociology: A Selective View*, Free Press, New York (1968).
3. Stimson, G. and Webb, B. *Going to See the Doctor: The Consultation Process in General Practice*, Routledge and Kegan Paul, London (1975).

Sally Macintyre is Director of the MRC Medical Sociology Unit at Glasgow University. David Oldman is a Medical Sociologist at Aberdeen University. This is an edited extract from a chapter with the same title which originally appeared in the book *Medical Encounters*, edited by A. Davis and G. Horobin and published by Croom Helm, London (1977).

6.3

Disability: Whose Handicap?

Ann Shearer

If the onset of a disability can seem to signal the end of everything that people value and enjoy, it need not. In *Journey into Silence*, Jack Ashley recounts his experience of becoming totally deaf. He remembers the realization that he was wholly excluded from the conversation of his wife and brother-in-law as they drove him home from hospital as 'one of the greatest shocks of my life'. When he first tried to get back to work, to a job in which quick understanding and discussion are essential, he realized that he was unable to participate at all. 'I was cut off from mankind, surrounded by an invisible, impenetrable barrier. I could see people clearly, but they belonged to a different world—a world of talk, of music and laughter.' He had to give up aspirations of reaching the top of his career ladder. But his old life was not destroyed. He is still a Member of Parliament, working energetically in the interests of people with disabilities.

Then again, disability can bring a narrowing of life and its pleasures. A woman in her seventies who has severe arthritis reckons herself lucky to have had a full and interesting life, and to have plenty to occupy her still. But she adds: 'I dare not indulge in nostalgia. I dare not remember how I once walked miles with a long, swinging stride.'

For some people, what is present does not amount to a life at all. A middle-aged woman, chairbound by arthritis, has a good job and her own house. But, she says:

> None of what goes on in the real world seems relevant to me, everything I see or hear about concerns activities from which I am barred. In fact, I am disconnected from life, because I am no longer a living human being. I think that there is only one solution, and that is termination of this non-life which is a burden and an embarrassment to the community and is cruel to the sufferers.

For others again, disability is a fact of life, not death, a fact to be lived with in all its complexity. A young woman with a progressive neuro-muscular disease remembers her capitulation to sticks and a wheelchair.

> The previous 'active' year had been spent in such a haze of effort, pain and weakness that when I finally could not try any more, the resultant inactivity was a relief. Then the full horror of frustration and dependence hit me and I went through a few months of self-pity and expecting others to make life easier for me. I finally came through with the realization that life was going to be tough but that I had to cope with it myself, keeping my dependence on others down to a minimum and making my life as interesting as possible within the confines of disability.

There is nothing in these glimpses of living with disability to say that it must be 'tragic'. The *event* that leads to disability may be; the life that stems from it need not, for each individual will bring to it his or her own quota of individual beliefs, abilities and strengths. Each of us lives in our own way with what is normal for us.

Yet the contention that disability is a lasting personal tragedy can be drummed home every day. Pick up a professional journal and you can read about a young man who is 'suffering' from Down's Syndrome. Pick up a newspaper and you can read an article about the British Voluntary Euthanasia Society which features a young man who was determined to kill himself and only failed because his battery-powered wheelchair obstinately stuck within inches of the river bank. Pick up that same newspaper a week later and you can read a letter from a professional counsellor who contends that, however dire and depressing people feel their lives to be, they can always make some choices—unless, that is, they are 'physically handicapped or under lock and key'.

The literature on the psychology of disability can make contention fact. We can learn that the birth of a child with a disability is a tragedy not only for that child, but for its family. Hannah Mussett writes in *The Untrodden Ways* about her daughter Lucy, who has Down's Syndrome. 'There is in life sometimes, suffering so great as to make us for ever resist the imagining, and where a babe new-born is already destined to live to this, there does not seem to me to be any justification for denying it the mercy of a swift and painless death.' She recounts her own anguish as she struggles between her desire to kill the child and the social pressures which, she feels, compel her to cherish it; she lays bare her own torn instincts and the damage that is done to family life by Lucy's presence. 'Show me a handicapped child and I'll show you a handicapped family.'

But if literature on physical disability can seem to produce a catalogue of sorrows, there is the experience of individuals to challenge its inevitability. In *Does She Know She's There?*, Nicola Schaefer describes her feelings on learning that her daughter Catherine, her first child, has profound disabilities, both mental and physical. 'This is a lousy blow we've been dealt, but what's the point of moaning and moping? I'll accept and enjoy Catherine for what she is and take things step by step and not worry about the future for the time being.'

The literature as well as the experience of countless parents shows that life with a child with a disability is very far from unmitigated horror. That along with the sorrow and the strains comes at least the usual quota of delight and enjoyment. So why the assumption of continuing 'tragedy'? The obverse, the notion that disability need not be tragic, is a dangerous one to our Western societies. If people can enjoy life when they so obviously fall short of that elusive 'norm' towards which we all, consciously or unconsciously, strive, then what is our striving worth? If they, in their obvious 'imperfection', may actually seem within touch of what we recognize as happiness and fulfilment, then what imperfections in us are blocking our way? If they, in their possible economic 'uselessness' nevertheless have a sense of their own worth, then what of the values of materialism? Paul Hunt, who himself lived and died with muscular dystrophy, makes the point in *A Critical Condition*:

> Severely disabled people are generally considered to have been unlucky, to be deprived and poor, to lead cramped lives. We do not enjoy many of the 'goods' that people in our society are accustomed to . . . If the worth of human beings depends on a high social status, on the possession of wealth, on a position as a parent, husband or wife—if such things are *all-important*—then those of us who have lost or never had them are indeed unfortunate. Our lives must be tragically upset and marred for ever, we must be only half alive, only half human . . . But set over against this common sense attitude is another fact, a strange one. In my experience even the most severely disabled people retain an ineradicable conviction that they are still fully human in all that is ultimately necessary. Obviously each person can deny this and act accordingly. Yet even when he is most depressed, even when he says he would be better off dead, the underlying sense of his own worth remains.

The challenge is not a comfortable one. The 'norm' demands that people whose disabilities are obvious and severe must be at least 'sad' and even 'tragic'. And if that defence breaks down in the face of individual reality, it is ready with its own flip-side. The reaction to people who break out of the mould becomes: 'Aren't they wonderful?'

So in the United States there is an award for the Handicapped Person of the Year. In Britain, the Spastics Society has been making its special achievement award since 1972. In 1978 it went to a man who, despite his very severe disabilities—he is unable to eat unaided, dress himself or walk, and his speech is impaired—has set up a cultural centre for people with disabilities, a playgroup for handicapped children and a telephone club which has 500 members.

Just as it is not in any way to deny the reality of individual tragedy to question the myth of its inevitability, it is not in any way to belittle individual achievement to point out that 'Aren't They Wonderful?' is in its way as pernicious as its reverse. What it does is to confirm the rule by singling out the apparent exception. As Paul Hunt says: 'The "unfortunate" person is assumed to have wonderful and exceptional courage . . . This devalues other people by implication, and leaves the fit person still with his original view that disablement is really utterly tragic.' This is as true if the person singled out for praise is the person who lives with someone with a disability. If their mothers, wives or husbands are 'wonderful' for coping, where does that leave the people who have the disability?

It leaves them with a problem. And the question that needs to be asked is how far that problem is their own and how far they are carrying it for other people. People who have a disability must live with it; it is their 'normality'. How they live with it will have to do not just with their individual qualities, but with the situation they find themselves in; they are not somehow 'different' from anyone else in that , either. And while disability is a 'given', the handicaps that come from the behaviour of other people and the attitudes that lie behind it are not ineradicable.

The assumptions can throw up powerful barriers between people as they go about their lives. 'Aren't you wonderful?' may be easier to live with than the gush of uneasy sympathy that comes with 'Aren't you sad?', and even seductive in its flattery. But it is no nearer who you are. A woman who was born without a right forearm is tired of hearing how 'wonderful' she is to cope. She is more than irritated by the consequence of this attitude, which is that she isn't 'allowed' to have any problems at all.

Attitudes and the behaviour that follows them don't affect just individuals. They affect whole groups of people. As they move about their community, people with physical disabilities meet not just a barrage of physical barriers in the shape of steps and unadapted spaces, but a whole host of rules and regulations as well. The thinking behind many of these hardly stands up to scrutiny. Why does 'safety' demand that a blind person is accompanied in theatres and cinemas, when he or she is the one person who could give lessons to the rest of the audience on what to do if the lights fuse? What is so 'safe' about the ruling that people in wheelchairs must transfer into ordinary theatre seats, when in any situation that called for speedy reaction they would lose vital time in transferring back to the chairs that can propel them as fast as other people's legs may do them? There is little that is rational in the regulations. But perhaps there is little that is rational in the attitudes behind them. If people with disabilities are 'sad', if their situation is 'tragic', what use have they for the pleasure of life?

It is in the responses to the claims of people with severe disabilities to the full range of sexual and emotional relationships that perceptions of them as less than fully human find their touchstone. In *The Invalid Mind*, Judith Thunem, who has had severe rheumatoid arthritis since she was in her late teens, has this to say:

In his encounter with society, the invalid rarely meets active dislike or disgust. But if he ventures into the world of love, such feelings are not so far off. It happens, on occasion, that a disabled person falls in love with a normal member of society. Sometimes it even happens that this love is reciprocated. It is interesting to observe the different reactions to such— one is tempted to say—a social outrage. One gets the impression that the invalid has more or less committed an indecent act. He isn't supposed to have such feelings. And the 'normal' partner in such a crazy adventure—well, he is hardly considered normal at all. He ought to have his head examined. Some people seem to feel offended at the thought that a 'disabled' person feels the same way as a 'normal' person does. This reaction is not apparent when invalids marry one another. As long as they keep to themselves society doesn't really mind. The invalid may marry another of his kind, and live happily or unhappily ever after. Society doesn't greatly care whether he is happy or unhappy as long as society isn't troubled. A wall is raised between the 'normal' world and the world of the disabled—a wall invisible and hard and cold as unbreakable glass.

The 1970s have brought their own sexual revolution. 'Sex and disability' has become something of a boom industry. Where once there was silence and shuffling, there are conferences, reports and advice centres. [Yet] in some curious way, the avowals of the new liberalism, in their insistence on technique in isolation from social context, somehow confirm that people with disabilities are not far from 'animals' after all. As one man said: 'The aids and the advice are fine and good. But I can't even get to the places where I might meet someone—and even if I could I wouldn't have enough money to buy them a drink.' 'For the able-bodied, normal world,' says Paul Hunt:

> we are representatives of many of the things that they most fear—tragedy, loss, dark and the unknown. Involuntarily we walk, or more often sit, in the valley of the shadow of death. Contact with us throws up in people's faces the fact of sickness and death in the world, which in themselves are an affront to all our aspirations and hopes. A deformed and paralysed body attacks everyone's sense of well-being and invincibility. People do not want to acknowledge what disability affirms—that life is tragic and we shall all soon be dead. So they are inclined to avoid those who are sick or old, shying from the disturbing reminders of unwelcome reality.

References

Ashley, J. *Journey into Silence*, Bodley Head (1973).
Hunt, P. 'A Critical Condition', in Hunt P. (ed.) *Stigma: The Experience of Disability*, Geoffrey Chapman (1966), pp. 145–59.
Mussett, H. *The Untrodden Ways*, Verry (1976).
Schaefer, N. *Does She Know She's There?*, Futura (1979).
Thunem, J. 'The Invalid Mind' in Hunt P. (ed.) *Stigma: The Experience of Disability*, Geoffrey Chapman (1966), pp. 47–53.

Ann Shearer is a freelance writer and journalist specialising in health and social services. This is an edited extract culled from several chapters of her book *Disability: Whose Handicap?*, published by Basil Blackwell (1981).

6.4

This Bed My Centre

Ellen Newton

Prince Edward's, and three months of intensive care, comfort and humour, had got me on my feet. Sister calls me. Not unsteadily I go inside. This must be my GP coming to tell me when I can go. 'Miss Newton.' Pause. Then, 'Mrs Zachary's blood pressure has gone up pretty high.'

'Your sister feels she can't stand the strain of your long illness.'

But why didn't she tell me herself? Why must she leave it to him to tell me?

'We've decided it will be best for you to live in a nursing home where you will get the expert care you need.' *We've decided*. Clever, downright Sister Mead could have told this highly qualified young doctor that they might at least have given me a small voice in their decision to wrap up my life forever. [. . .]

'It will be better if you do not go home,' he says. Home is your peculiar treasure. For your GP it is just another address. You are no longer an average human being, alive with joys and doubts and fears. Hope is not for you, either. From today you are a Patient.

'We've arranged for you to go straight from here on Thursday to Haddon—the nursing home where we've booked you in.' [. . .]

Haddon: Four a.m. Not light yet. Day has already begun. If you are bedded down with the birds it may be that a biological clock tends to wake you with the birds—if not before.

Almost daylight. The hall has become a noisy thoroughfare. A nurse drags a heavy, acrid-smelling bag past my door, down the steps and probably into the laundry which seems to be under the spread of iron roof a few steps from my window.

Breakfast—no comment. [. . .]

There's a hint of sun today in my small wedge of sky, but it does not touch my room. The sense of segregation is so palpable, you feel as if at any moment you will be tightly enclosed in a cocoon of isolation. Except for the milkman, before dawn, there's no sound of traffic passing by. Everything is negative. You never hear young people singing, speeding recklessly home from late parties, or even the stereophonic calls of philandering tomcats. Never the sound of children's voices, laughing and calling to each other as they race down the street. Only spasmodic screeching a few doors away, that would send cold shivers down anyone's spine. It's like living in space. But it has its own grim kind of permanence, for we are all here for the term of our unnatural lives. Unless you are 'away with the fairies', the lasting anguish of being uprooted from your own kind must destroy you. And there's no speaking of it to anyone.[. . .]

This afternoon, in watery sunshine, five of us are wheeled out on to the grass and grouped in a tight half circle immediately opposite the front door. One is blind. Three are deaf, with modern hearing-aids, which they carefully keep out of action. All but one are unsmiling and completely withdrawn. My attempts at communication meet no response. Pity, and a sense of complete frustration wrack me. They have put me next to Miss Alice, with neatly coiled white hair and forget-me-not blue eyes. She smiles at me. Perhaps she lip-reads a little. The sky has quickly clouded over. She looks up, smiles and says, 'The good Lord Jesus sends us the weather.' She repeats this phrase every few moments. Of them all, she alone seems to live happily in some unseen world of her own. She might even manage a simple jigsaw puzzle, or enjoy watching TV if there were room, or any opportunity for it. All the others stare, hard-eyed, into space. [. . .] The tragedy of this sad assortment at Haddon is that almost everyone has ceased to be a person. Nothing seems to touch the emptiness of lives so far away from even the fringe of ordinary human values. If only one could do something about it. [. . .]

Night came early to Haddon. Eerie calls and cries of protest, then loud and frequent instructions from hostile inmates, who must surely have been stone deaf, were met with patient exhortations. After about an hour, suddenly the battle ended. All seemed to have been sedated and bedded down. But this was no easy peace. A bell rang. A dozen others joined in chorus. Various demands were trumpeted over and over.

Later, the light outside my door went out. Then silence—at last. It was music—after what had gone before. [. . .]

Pain can be endured. But the laceration of one's spirit and senses in this place is quite another thing. Only a saint could bear this. A saint is what I'm not.

Ellen Newton was born in Australia, in 1896; she worked as a freelance writer, broadcaster, and short-story writer. In her 70s, suffering from angina, she spent six years in a series of nursing homes, years she laboriously recorded in her secret diary. At the age of 81 she discharged herself from hospital. With the help of her family, she found a small flat where she still happily lives and prepared her diaries for publication. *This Bed My Centre* was published by Virago (1980).

6.5

Caring for the Spouse who Died

Ann Bowling and Ann Cartwright

This article is based on a study of experiences and attitudes of over 360 elderly widowed men and women, their general practitioners and their relatives, friends and neighbours.

The last illness

Widowhood is occasionally a sudden event with no prior warning, but more usually, especially among older people, it is the climax of a period during which life has revolved around caring for a sick spouse. It is the final stage of the role of wife or husband. Indeed, for women, eventual widowhood can realistically be regarded as a normal part of the process of ageing.

Two-fifths of the widowed said the death was expected as far as they were concerned. An illustration of such a death is:

> He was treated for two years with gastro-enteritis and pains in his back. He had primary cancer in his stomach and spleen—he had them removed but it had gone too far. The doctors gave him two months but I kept him alive by nursing him for eighteen months, and they sent me no nursing help at all.

Coping with illness over a long period may make the surviving spouse tired and, if they do not get adequate support, resentful. But it can give them an opportunity to prepare for the changes ahead. One widower commented that he had few problems now as he had had time to prepare himself for the death and adjust to new roles:

> No problems really. If she'd gone suddenly it would have been much more of a blow.

Expected deaths were more common if the cause was cancer, 56 per cent; for bronchitis, or other respiratory diseases, 53 per cent; whereas it was 34 per cent for deaths from other causes. And, as might be predicted, the death was more often expected if the person had been ill for a long time. Roughly a third were ill for less than a year, a third for between one and five years, and a third for longer.

It was not only the length but also the nature of the illness which contributed to the distress of both the person who died and the surviving spouse. A symptom which gave rise to much concern and anguish for their relatives was confusion. Just under a third, 30 per cent, of the deceased were said by the widowed to have been mentally confused before they died. Almost two-thirds, 63 per cent of the widowed whose spouses were mentally confused found this 'very distressing', and 12 per cent found it 'fairly distressing'.

He used to have brain storms, at least that's what I'd call them because he tried to strangle me a couple of times and he said he was going to poison me.

He used to lose his way home, and one day he moved all the dandelions from the side alley and planted them in the front garden. He didn't know. I had bad nerves and I used to lean on him, but when he became so ill I had to be the one to do everything.

Two-fifths of the widowed said the deceased had other symptoms or problems which they themselves had found distressing. These included pain, depression, sleeplessness, incontinence, inability to move, vomiting, loss of appetite, difficulty breathing or talking, and difficulty eating or feeding.

He couldn't hold his knife to eat. Things kept shooting off his plate. Vomiting all the time. He was all dirty and my daughters used to clean him up, all sick and blood.

So widowhood for most, three-quarters, was preceded for a period of six months or more when their spouse was ill, and this was often accompanied by distressing symptoms. What help did they get during that time?

Just over half, 53 per cent, of the deaths in our sample took place in hospital. In addition, 44 per cent of those dying at home were admitted to hospital at some time during the last year of their lives. Just over two-fifths, 42 per cent, had ten or more consultations with a general practitioner in the year before they died, and almost three out of ten, 29 per cent, had ten or more home visits.

Nearly half of all those who died had needed help while at home with dressing or undressing and a similar proportion with bathing, while two-fifths had needed some help at night. A relatively high proportion of those dying from cancer, 80 per cent, and those whose deaths were ascribed to pneumonia or influenza, 79 per cent, had needed some sort of help while at home. And Table 1 also shows the heavy demands of those who had been confused.

Table 1 Care at home by whether or not the person had been mentally confused at all before death

	Mentally confused before death		All deaths
	Yes	No	
Type of care given:	%	%	%
Dressing and undressing	65	38	46
Getting in or out of bath	64	39	47
Washing or shaving	53	35	41
Being lifted	65	34	43
Getting to lavatory	60	32	41
Help or care at night	61	33	42
Other care of this sort	28	15	19
None	18	42	35
Number of deaths (=100%)	106	252	359

In over a third of instances where any help was given, 38 per cent, the widowed person had done everything, and in a further third, 39 per cent, they had helped mainly. For 17 per cent the care was equally shared between the widowed and others, and for 6 per cent the care was given mainly or entirely by people other than the widowed. There was no difference between the widows and the widowers who said this care had fallen mainly or on them. Apart from the spouse the main person who gave help when it was needed was a relative, 31 per cent, a professional person, 25 per cent, and a friend or neighbour, 6 per cent. A fifth of the widowed felt that their spouse or they themselves could have done with more help; help with lifting being the most frequent need, by one in eight.

The burden on those widowed who had cared mainly or entirely for their spouses often seemed considerable:

> He had a stroke three years ago. It left him paralysed and he never spoke afterwards. He was like a baby. I managed to look after him all the time. He was able to use the one leg if I helped him to . . . I would get him out into the sun sometimes. It was a struggle but I did it. In fact I dropped him several times when I had to lift him, he was ten stone!

Attitudes to care

The widowed were asked what they felt about the care and treatment their spouse had from their general practitioner before their death and then to sum up whether this care was 'very good', 'fairly good', or 'not very good'. We have already noted that 8 per cent had no contact with a general practitioner in the year before their death. For the others, in two-thirds the care was felt to be 'very good', a quarter of the widowed described it as 'fairly good', and a tenth as 'not very good'.

We asked the widowed whose spouses died at home whether they would rather the person had been in hospital or whether they were glad he or she had died at home. The majority, 91 per cent, said they were glad their spouse had been at home when he or she died:

> I'm glad he was in his own home and I was there.

Among the five who said outright that it would have been better if the person had been in hospital were two who were somewhat critical of their general practitioners.

> They didn't bother with him. I don't suppose they could do much for him. They were very nice, but they're busy aren't they? I didn't dare send for him. He came once and said 'There's nothing I can do for him'. We couldn't lift him. He was a dead weight—even the nurse said it was too much. It used to be terrible. She said he ought to be in hospital in a special bed. He had terrible back sores. They did their best to get him into hospital.

Restrictions on the surviving spouse

Some of the widowed had been under a great deal of strain in caring for their ill spouse. The following examples are of widows who cared for their husbands entirely on their own. They both said the could have done with help:

> He wasn't able to get into a bath. I used to have to wash him all down. He couldn't even stand in the shower for that length of time. I had to lift him up the bed. He used to pull the door and hang onto the door-handle and I'd help him up.

> I was exhausted when he passed away after looking after him. The nurse promised to bring me a stool so I could put it on the bath. She kept promising but they never came. They sent a night commode but that was only suitable for a lady. My husband was fifteen stone, he couldn't sit on it.

Also, many of those who said no help, or no more help, was needed with caring for their husband or wife went on to say that this was because they would not have accepted help from anyone other than the widow or widower.

> He didn't want to be exposed to the nurses, he was a modest sort of man.

> He didn't want anyone else to do things for him—it's private and personal. I used to rush my shopping so I could get back to him. I had not had a full night's sleep for eighteen months.

Similarly, one of the familiars commented that the deceased had preferred his spouse to help with nursing care as he found personal help from others embarrassing:

> He would get embarrassed, with me being his daughter, and wouldn't let me help except at the very end. The night he died he let me clean him. He said 'Fancy you having to do this'. Ten minutes later it was the end.

Even when professional nursing care was given the widowed sometimes commented that it was inadequate because it was hurried or infrequent. In one case the nurse came just fortnightly to bath the deceased, and in another the nurses visited but asked relatives to help as they had such little time:

> We had a very hard time. My daughter and I had to help him with everything at the end—eating and everything. My daughter helped so much with him—she washed him, cleaned him. The nurses came every day but they were often in a rush so they often used to ask my daughter to take over.

We asked the widowed if they had given up or done less of anything during the time of the deceased's illness. Thirty-six per cent had not, more, 53 per cent, had given up something, and 11 per cent had done less of something. The activities they cut down on were: visiting friends or relatives for 45 per cent of all the widowed; going out to other social activities, 46 per cent; going on holiday, 41 per cent; entertaining people at home, 31 per cent; going to work, 12 per cent. Restrictions on other activities were mentioned by 10 per cent. Many of those who said their activities were not, or only a little, restricted, said this was because they had no outside activities to be disrupted. For example:

> Social wise we never went out anyway, so that didn't matter.

The strain imposed by caring for the dying spouse was greater when the surviving husband or wife was not robust. The proportion who said their activities had been severely restricted increased from 21 per cent of those who rated their own health as excellent or good, to 31 per cent of those who rated it as fair, and 44 per cent of those who regarded it as poor. It was not that those in poor health were more likely to have given up visiting relatives or friends, or entertaining people at home, but that they apparently became too exhausted to do even ordinary activities. One widow said:

> I was an ill person over eighty with a heart complaint and yet they sent a dying man home to me with no help at all. I had a bed downstairs for him but he was always messing it. He had no control over his legs. When he fell I had a twelve stone man to lift— and I've got a heart condition! I was so tired my ankles were enormous at night. I had to sleep in the chair in the end as I was too tired to go up and down stairs.

Restrictions on the activities of the spouse were rather greater for cancer deaths than for others. Thirty-six per cent of the widowed whose spouse had died of cancer said their activities had been severely restricted compared with 23 per cent of other deaths. At the same time the longer the illness the more likely it was to restrict the spouse's activities; 53 per cent of those whose spouse was ill for less than six months had been restricted in some way, compared with 65 per cent when the illness lasted between six months and two years, and 76 per cent for longer illnesses.

The more restricted their lives had been the more likely the widowed were to wish something could have been done differently. The proportion wishing this rose from 18 per cent of those who were not restricted to 33 per cent of the severely restricted.

> I couldn't go far. I couldn't go anywhere—just down the road, shopping. I couldn't leave him for any length of time. It made me confused and ill at times—looking after him for so long. For the past few months I had to carry him to the bathroom.

> I didn't go out—it caused my blood pressure. I used to like a drink at the pub but I couldn't leave her, or ask anyone to stop in whilst I went for a drink. You can't do that can you?

In addition to restrictions on physical activities, the widowed often mentioned the mental strain they suffered in the period before the death:

> It was nerve-racking—living with the knowledge that he could die any day. When he was choking I was on my own and there was no-one to help me—I never saw a nurse. I had to be awake at night because of the choking. I wasn't given any advice as to what to do for him. [Died from cancer of the stomach.]

In some of these cases an element of relief at the death was expressed. One woman who died of multiple sclerosis was described as mentally confused and depressed. She had been ill for twenty years and her husband had retired early to look after her:

> Friends and relatives would come in and see her sitting there in her chair, all clean and cheerful, she always had a smile for them, they didn't realize what I had to do to keep her like that. I think the doctor and the nurse realized that I was on the edge of a break-down myself. She kept calling at night, I never got no sleep.

The widowed often seemed to accept the burden of caring that had been placed on them as their duty. Two widows said:

> It was like living in a vacuum really, it was all unreal, but I would not have had it any other way.

> When you marry someone it is for life so it was my place to look after him.

The feeling that they themselves, not only professionals, had done all they could, and that their husband or wife had been well looked after, may help reduce feelings of guilt after the death. As one widow said:

> The only thing that goes through my mind is 'Did I do everything to help, did I do enough?' It keeps going through my mind.

Almost a quarter of the widowed, 24 per cent, said their spouse's ill-health had affected them financially. This proportion was higher for widows, 28 per cent, than widowers, 18 per cent. Although no differences were found with place of death or length of illness, deaths from cancer and bronchitis had more effects on finances than other deaths, 32 per cent in comparison with 21 per cent. It was pointed out earlier that cancer deaths also imposed the most restriction on the spouse's activities.

Those classified as working class were more likely to say they had been affected financially, 26 per cent, than those classified as middle class, 15 per cent. Forty-three per cent of those who said they were affected financially received no financial help. Altogether, 23 per cent received supplementary benefit before the death and 9 per cent received a disability pension, 9 per cent an attendance allowance, and 10 per cent received help from a relative or other sources. One widow whose husband was chronically ill with bronchitis for twelve years and whom she nursed intensively for about six months was discouraged from claiming the attendance allowance by her general practitioner. She said the doctor told her:

It wasn't worth it, he wouldn't be here long enough.

As 26 per cent had said their activities were severely restricted and 19 per cent said they were fairly restricted because of the deceased's illness, probably more than the 9 per cent receiving an attendance allowance were eligible for it. Those who were affected financially mentioned the cost of extra food, clothes, and heating as being the main problems:

> I had to keep getting him trousers, the others were falling off him. I had to get baby foods, Complan, and the nurse told me to get Ovaltine. The gas bill was high, we had to burn that night and day, same as the lights.

It is clear that the care of dying people at home often imposes severe physical, financial, and psychological strains on their relatives. Wives and husbands generally take on this task willingly but often they do it unaided when appropriate help and support could mitigate the physical hardship, the social isolation, and the mental distress.

The authors of this article are both medical sociologists. Ann Bowling was formerly a Research Officer and Ann Cartwright is Director at the Institute for Social Studies in Medical Care in London. This is an edited extract from a chapter in their book *Life After Death: A Study of Elderly Widowed*, published by Tavistock (1982).

6.6

Ethnic Minorities and the Psychiatrist

Roland Littlewood and Maurice Lipsedge

The meeting between psychiatrist and patient does of course involve two people who have their own particular expectations. If the situation is familiar to them, they will probably make an effort to live up to the other person's expectations.[1]

The psychiatrist is likely to regard psychiatric illness as he does physical illness. He also has less clear expectations of how the patient is likely to behave and what, in different societies, the limits of normality and abnormality are. In addition to his background and training, the psychiatrist's attitude to the minority patient will be formed by his own personal problems, conscious or unconscious racist assumptions and the particular setting in which the two meet. He is, amongst other things, an employee of the state and responsible to it for maintenance of its beliefs and disposal of its funds.

Patients too have their expectations: to be sick in our society offers us freedom from many social obligations and from responsibility for the illness, but it presumes a desire to get well and a motivation to ask for medical help.[2] The extent to which a patient sees himself as ill and in need of treatment varies with his culture. What may be endured in India requires therapy in New York. What is insane behaviour in Barbados may not be in Jamaica. Acceptance of the role of a mental patient depends on our beliefs about the nature of mental illness and whether any stigma is associated with it. Psychiatrists are rare in developing countries and admission to a mental hospital is an uncommon—perhaps unheard of—event. There is one psychiatrist in Britain for every twenty thousand people compared with one for over a million in India and one for four million in Nigeria. The immigrant family may be hesitant about agreeing with a doctor who tells them that their relative is mentally ill. They may not even see the problem as a medical one: the patient may come from a rural community in which all Western medicine is regarded with distrust. Many societies carry out similar religious healing ceremonies for both physical and emotional distress and do not make our customary separation between the two.

The immigrant patient may well see the psychiatrist as a doctor rather than specifically as a psychiatrist. Not burdened with our folk-lore about psychiatrists (and endless cartoons of bearded doctors sitting next to patients on couches), he looks for themes familiar to him from his experiences with other doctors and hospitals: the ward with its rows of beds and quiet discipline, the uniformed nurses and white-coated doctors; authority, certainty, a minimum of questioning and immediate treatment. Ironically these are the very aspects of medicine which psychiatrists are discarding, in the belief that they may actually perpetuate psychological difficulties.[3] As psychiatry has sought to relinquish the magical symbols of medicine, many of these have been confusingly adopted by other professions: porters, clerks and domestic staff may now wear the clinical white coat.[1]

A common mode of arrival of immigrant patients at a hospital is to be brought in by police, often at night.[4] Does the psychiatrist see himself as an ally of the police or the patient, or perhaps of both? Is his overriding reaction to dispose of the problem as soon as possible and get back to bed?

To observe another person is always to some extent to diminish their individuality—especially in a hospital interview. For the patient the stress of the interview is increased when the doctor starts by talking privately with the police who are waiting on the ward, taking them aside, reading the admitting form and glancing periodically at the patient. If he then dismisses the police, greets the patient, shakes his hand and talks to him as if he is about to explain this embarrassing situation, the doctor will soon find himself in a difficult position. The patient sees a friend and confides his denunciation of the police to him while the doctor listens patiently. The psychiatrist is then startled by a request from the patient to return home. He feels irritated—the patient has taken advantage of his kindness. With the police gone, the nurses will be reluctant to help him to restrain a person he may now believe to be in urgent need of medical attention; their looks suggest he has made a fool of himself and wasted their time; he cannot persuade the increasingly anxious patient even to continue to talk to him. The patient begins to realize that the doctor has not really been sympathizing with him and that he has other plans. The doctor changes: his tone becomes hectoring and tense, and he provides increasingly unpleasant arguments for the patient to stay.

In the end the patient is sedated wth the help of the nurses or dishonestly promised that he will be allowed home in the morning. In either case, he feels betrayed—he is not going to be so trusting again. Since his attempt at understanding the patient produced an unsatisfactory result, the psychiatrist also decides not to waste time talking next time. No more messing about—in future he will sedate the patient straight away. He rationalizes this by saying that it is not fair to the patient to deceive him and that it is easier anyway to talk the next morning, when he will be able to listen to a comfortably sedated patient with their respective roles clearly defined and his own anxieties diminished.

The immigrant brought to a psychiatric ward by the police will regard the whole business with suspicion, if not panic. He is puzzled by the doctor's insistence that he is there to *help*. The doctor's behaviour does not bear this out. If the patient is in the hospital because of behaviour associated with unusual religious experiences, he may wonder whether the doctor thinks these are 'genuine experiences'. If the doctor says they are, he is placating the patient, who realizes he is lying—why otherwise would he keep the patient in hospital? If the doctor ventures a medical explanation of the phenomenon the patient knows he has no chance of a fair hearing—the doctor will continue to try to persuade him to accept his own interpretation.

However sympathetic he may be initially to a patient who is anxious to spread the news of his divine mission, the psychiatrist will soon change. He must observe the patient and 'take a history' in accordance with the expectations of medical practice and the watching nursing staff. He tentatively suggests the patient is ill. If the patient disagrees, wakes the other patients or throws things about the ward, the doctor writes down 'no insight' and moves, reassured, into his more rewarding decision-making role.

Whatever interest doctor and patient may take in each other, the confrontation is limited by time. The interview is limited to a few key questions. The doctor wants to know whether the voices talk among themselves or talk directly to the patient. Such a question seems irrelevant to the patient. He is initially concerned with whether they are going to harm him. Why is the black patient feeling so suspicious? Maybe the police and the hospital are behaving in this extraordinary manner because they have a grudge against him. How widespread is this conspiracy? How much will it be wise to say to the doctor? The psychiatrist is meanwhile looking for such 'first-rank symptoms of schizophrenia' as whether the patient experiences his thoughts being controlled by external influences. If these are found, the patient's own explanation of his situation can again be dismissed. He is now firmly told he is sick and must have some medicine; patient and doctor have achieved their definitive roles.

The patient is told he must stay in hospital, he is asked to strip and the doctor examines him physically. The psychiatrist may be unsympathetic and harsh and he may make the wrong diagnosis, but by tradition he must on no account miss any physical illness. Further reduced to an object, the patient lies there as the doctor applies various instruments and listens and peers. The doctor gives instructions and leaves; the patient tells the nurses his age, address and occupation and accepts sedation for the night. The black patient may be reassured by the fact that the nurses, who are frequently black themselves, accept without question the medical definition of his experience. Often he is not.

Until both doctor and patient can agree on common grounds, there is unlikely to be a basis for friendship or even an acceptance of help. At present this tension is resolved only when the patient accepts the doctor's view of the situation and entirely rejects his own. Over the next few days responsibility is gradually withdrawn from the patient: for his liberty, his clothes and his beliefs.[3,5,6] His most popular move will have been to present a typical symptom to the doctor, resulting in swift and standard procedures to deal with his condition and a lessening in uncertainty for the staff. His further progress depends on the rapidity with which he accepts the new concepts and opportunities open to him.

An immigrant patient who has had many admissions to mental hospitals will have been given repeated explanations that he is not entirely responsible for his actions. The doctor should not then be surprised to find that the patient will not take any further responsibility for his problems and that he now passively expects the doctor to find him a job and accommodation and to solve his various domestic difficulties. The psychiatrist is confirmed in his belief that one of the effects of mental illness is a long-term loss of initiative and motivation. Unless he offers the unlikely option of psychotherapy, the psychiatrist now steps back and explains that medicine is not the solution to all problems but only those accepted by the patient as divine intervention, spirit possession or sorcery. Psychiatry thus deals with that part of the immigrant's experience associated with his original society but not with those related to problems in Britain—discrimination, housing and unemployment. It de-Caribbeanizes and de-authenticates him. While depriving the patient of much of his tradition, it does not seem to offer much in return. [. . .]

If we take class and age differences into account, are there any differences in treatment offered to blacks and whites in Britain? No one has yet looked at this methodically. Although less likely than the British-born to see a GP for psychiatric reasons, West Indian men are more likely to be admitted to psychiatric hospitals.[7] Psychotic black patients are twice as likely as British-born and white immigrants to be in hospital detained involuntarily, 'sectioned' under the Mental Health Act.[8,9] Four out of ten of them in one study were involuntary patients at some point in their admission.[4] Asian-born patients in Britain are also more likely to be involuntary patients in psychiatric hospitals and less likely to refer themselves.[10] A study of the use of psychiatric facilities in a London hospital over a three-week period suggested that immigrant patients, both black and white, are particularly likely to refer themselves to hospital as emergencies but they are less likely than the British-born to attend appointments booked for them.[11] Black patients are more likely than white patients to see a black member of the psychiatric team and to see a junior rather than a senior doctor. When differences in diagnosis are allowed for, they are still more likely to receive the powerful phenothiazine drugs and to receive electro-convulsive therapy. A large proportion of Jewish patients receive convulsive treatment; this is, however, related to a greater incidence of depression among Jews.

Racialism in psychiatric treatment may occur in many forms. Overt discrimination in Britain is rare, perhaps because of the considerable number of psychiatrists and psychiatric nurses who are themselves members of ethnic minorities. Members of minorities are less likely to get the more 'attractive' type of psychiatric care such as individual or group therapy because they are regarded as not meeting the 'ideal' criteria for psychotherapy (including the type of problem or middle-class mode of describing their feelings) which are traditionally associated with the best response to this type of therapy in Europe. What is particularly lacking is the commitment of psychotherapists to work with ethnic minorities.

Between a white doctor and a black patient the colour difference may be either exaggerated or it may be ignored. Exaggeration is likely to lead to stereotypes of 'West Indian psychosis' and neglect of individual emotional difficulties unrelated to discrimination. A sympathetic doctor may see his patients as so scarred by racialism as inevitably to be a passive victim with no secure identity and little self-respect; he may then bend over backwards to support him, to avoid any guilt the patient brings out in *him*. Underestimating the difference in culture by the white psychiatrist leads to an avoidance of the problems of discrimination and to a lack of sensitivity in understanding non-medical approaches to emotional difficulties.

The meeting of a white patient with a black psychiatrist produces a *status contradiction* for the doctor. Patients and relatives have to reconcile their rather different attitudes to immigrants and to doctors. In our experience they are often patronizing, feel they are getting second-class treatment and complain to a white psychiatrist that a black doctor cannot understand them or even has too many problems of his own to be helpful.

Status contradiction also occurs with black patient and black psychiatrist. The mutual awareness that both are immigrants is usually concealed beneath class and professional differences. The patient regards the doctor as really 'white', while the psychiatrist, often from quite a different society from the patient, agrees with his white colleagues that psychotherapy with a working-class patient (not of course a *black* patient) is rather unrewarding. The patient suspects that an English doctor might have helped him more. Neither recognize themselves in the other.

Racism is neither a science nor a disease but a set of political beliefs which legitimates certain social and economic conditions. It is pointless to ask which is primary—prejudice, or exploitation. They developed historically together, each validating the other.

References

1. Goffman, E. *The Presentation of Self in Everyday Life*, Allen Lane, London (1959).
2. Parsons, T. *The Social System*, Routledge and Kegan Paul, London (1952).
3. Wing, J. K. and Brown, G. W. *Institutionalism and Schizophrenia*, Cambridge University Press (1970).
4. Lipsedge, M. and Littlewood, R. 'Compulsory hospitalisation and minority status' 11th Biennial Conference of the Caribbean Federation for Mental Health, Gosier, Guadeloupe (1977).
5. Goffman, E. *Asylums*, Penguin, Harmondsworth (1968).
6. Scheff, T. J. *Being Mentally Ill*, Aldine, Chicago (1966).
7. Cochrane, R. 'Mental illness in immigrants to England and Wales. An analysis of mental hospital admissions', *Social Psychiatry*, **12**, 23–35 (1977).

8. Lipsedge, M. and Littlewood, R. 'Transcultural psychiatry'. In *Recent Advances in Psychiatry*, 3rd edn, Churchill Livingstone, London (1959).
9. Rwegellera, G. G. C. 'Mental illness in Africans and West Indians of African origin living in London', M.Phil. thesis, University of London (1970).
10. Pinto, R. T. 'A study of psychiatric illness amongst Asians in the Camberwell area', M.Phil. dissertation, London University (1970).
11. Littlewood, R. and Cross, S. 'Ethnic minorities and psychiatric services', *Sociology of Health and Illness*, 2, 194–201 (1980).

Roland Littlewood is a psychiatrist and a Research Fellow at the Institute of Social Anthropology at Oxford University. Maurice Lipsedge is a Consultant in Psychological Medicine at Guy's Hospital, London. This is an edited extract of pages 25–28 and 65–66 from their book *Aliens and Alienists, Ethnic Minorities and Psychiatry*, published by Penguin (1982).

6.7

Social Class and Children in Hospital

Bronwen Earthrowl and Margaret Stacey

It has often been suggested that there are cultural factors associated with social classes which lead to differences of attitude and belief and to variations in behaviour above and beyond those solely derived from economic differentials. With regard to patterns of child rearing, marked differences have been suggested between middle and working classes,[1] and some middle class conviction is periodically expressed, e.g. by the National Association for the Welfare of Children in Hospitals, and by some hospital personnel, that working class parents do not understand the social and emotional needs of their children in hospital.

In a survey of 1,368 children discharged from Welsh hospitals after a short period of illness in 1972 these suggestions were not upheld. Although some class differences occurred in the routes whereby children reached hospital and some hints also that those in higher economic classes used the hospital services differently from those in lower classes, few differences were found in attitudes about the needs of the child in hospital, and the only major differences to emerge among the classes were associated with economic differences.

The children's mothers, or mother substitutes, were interviewed within five or six weeks of the child's discharge. Respondents were assigned to social classes on the basis of the occupation of the head of the household, with the classification of occupations being taken from the National Readership Survey. Six social classes are distinguished by this method:

A   Upper middle class
B   Middle class
C1 Lower middle class
C2 Skilled working class
D   Semi-skilled and unskilled working class
E   Those at the lowest level of subsistence

In this study, because of the low numbers involved at the extremes of the scale, classes A and B have been aggregated, as have classes D and E.

Previous hospital experience and pattern of admission

There was some evidence to suggest that children from the higher social classes had more previous experience of hospital than those from lower classes, but examination of the data indicates that this experience derives more from attendance at out-patient clinics and visits to in-patients than from actual in-patient stays. Table 1 indicates that middle class children do, in fact, have fewer in-patient stays and data collected for siblings showed a similar pattern. Mapes and Dajda[2] report a greater referral rate by lower socio-economic groups to the general practitioner and Carstairs a greater use of hospital by these groups in general.[3] The higher experience rate of our sample children in classes A and B remains unexplained, but appears to relate to a higher accident rate, as the following table suggests.

Table 1 Previous hospital experience × social class

	Social Class					
Previous hospital experience	AB	C1	C2	DE	Total	
	%	%	%	%	%	N
No previous experience	15	25	23	29	24	335
Some previous experience	85	75	77	71	76	1,033
(a) in-patient stay	38	29	45	42	41	559
(b) out-patient visit	64	57	59	51	56	769
(c) visit to in-patient	48	43	33	34	37	500
TOTAL %	100	100	100	100	100	
N	155	194	522	497		1,368

Table 2 also suggests that middle class children generally have an above-average proportion of planned admissions and a below-average proportion of emergency admissions, unlike classes C2 and DE where these findings were reversed. Satisfactory explanations for class differences in patterns of consultation do not yet seem to be available, the present state of knowledge being usefully reviewed in Cartwright and O'Brien,[4] who conclude that the middle class make more use of preventive services and may receive better and more sympathetic care.

Table 2 Type of admission × social class

	Social Class					
	AB	C1	C2	DE	Total	
Type of admission	%	%	%	%	%	N
Accident	29	18	16	20	19	264
Emergency	21	31	43	39	37	512
Planned admission						
readmission	51	50	39	40	43	581
Unplanned admission	0	1	1	1	1	11
TOTAL %	100	100	100	100	100	
N	155	194	522	497		1,368

Attitudinal differences

Admission to hospital finds any child in a strange and bewildering setting. Children admitted as accidents and emergencies, while already having suffered the shock of sudden illness, were found to have the least prior experience of hospital (67 per cent of accident cases and 69 per cent of emergencies had either stayed in or visited a hospital before in comparison with 83 per cent of planned admissions). A view is from time to time expressed by members of the middle class that the emotional and social needs of the child patient are not understood by working-class parents. This view was not supported by the present survey which found little variation in the views of parents from different social classes about the importance of explaining hospital to children where possible or of maintaining regular contact with them during their hospital stay. The proportion from the different classes who tried to explain various aspects of hospitalization to their children before admission are similar, although running in the direction of most explanation being given to those in higher classes. Despite the explanations, there was little reported difference concerning the child's understanding of the facts, as the parents perceived that understanding.

About three-quarters of the 1,217 mothers who travelled to hospital with their children when they were admitted were very or quite satisfied with the information they were given, although there were slight variations by social class in the direction of those in classes AB and C1 being more satisfied than those in classes C2 and DE. When the same question was asked of all the 1,368 respondents about the information they received during their child's stay in hospital, no social class differences were apparent. Nor among those parents (733 out of 1,368) who were not able to discuss their child's case with a doctor were there any differences by social class in the proportions who would have liked to have such a discussion. Overall 53 per cent did not discuss their child's case with a doctor and 56 per cent of these would have liked to do so.

Beliefs which respondents held as to the harm caused to a child in hospital through lack of regular visiting are indicated in Table 3, class C1 exhibiting greatest concern.

Table 3 Beliefs held about harm caused through lack of regular visiting

| | Social Class | | | | | |
| | AB | C1 | C2 | DE | Total | |
Harm caused	%	%	%	%	%	N
A great deal	58	71	56	60	60	817
Some in some cases	41	25	37	31	34	460
Not much	0	4	4	5	4	55
None	1	1	3	3	2	33
Don't know	0	0	0	*	*	3
TOTAL %	100	100	100	100	100	
N	155	194	522	497		1,368

*=less than 0.5%

Class AB respondents tended to give the child's age and personality as the most important factors determining harm, perhaps reflecting psychological findings being more available to them, whereas respondents from other classes laid greater stress on the need for a mother's love and regular visitors. Whatever the reason, however, considerable effort was made by respondents from all classes to maintain regular contact and little difference was noted with regard to the importance of frequent visiting. In the event, 92 per cent of AB respondents and 77 per cent of DE respondents visited daily (cf. 84 per cent C1 and 88 per cent C2). This difference is likely to have an underlying economic cause and is discussed in Section D below.

Social distance

Considerable information is available to suggest that the social distance between doctors and their patients (in this case their patients' parents) leads to differential satisfaction with communication in the hospital and also that differential information is given.[5]

Despite the commonly expressed feeling that parents should be able to obtain information from an authoritative source when they require it, effective channels of communication do not always seem to be available. A quarter of respondents from the main sample who went with their children to hospital when they were admitted were dissatisfied with the information they were given regarding the children's treatment. It may well be that some of these parents were given information which they did not take in or failed to understand because they were distressed at the time, but many were given no information at all. Nor was the situation remedied later. During the hospital stay over a quarter (27 per cent) of all main sample respondents were still dissatisfied with the information, and, as mentioned previously, over half (53 per cent) of all respondents stated that their child's treatment was not discussed with them, although 57 per cent of these would have welcomed an opportunity for discussion.

Satisfaction with information received tended to be higher among middle class respondents than among working class respondents, although care is obviously needed in interpreting variations in satisfaction as the information itself is bound to vary. It has been found, for example, that manual-worker respondents are less likely to receive information from doctors as opposed to other staff members and less likely to have spoken to the doctor in charge of the case (although they considered this to be as important as did non-manual category workers and their wives).[5] Seventy-two per cent of the non-manual category in the Stacey sample (1970) were satisfied with the information they received in hospital in comparison with 62 per cent of the manual category and it is suggested that the lower satisfaction related not only to social distance, but also to the ability to understand what is being said. Cartwright[4] suggests, too, that working class people may be more diffident about expressing criticism and possibly less articulate about difficulties in communication. Satisfaction with information given to the child himself (Do you think your child was given enough information about what was happening to him?) showed no marked variation among classes.

The pattern which emerged regarding the availability of information about the child's treatment also emerged with regard to more general information about facilities in the hospital. In line with other studies, working-class respondents were found to be less likely to ask for information in a situation of uncertainty than were middle-class respondents. For example, 28 per cent of those who had had some refreshment when they accompanied a child to hospital had asked what facilities were available. Within this category, however, the proportion asking for information declines sharply with social class (50 per cent AB, 43 per cent C1, 20 per cent C2 and 23 per cent DE).

Differential use of facilities was also noted. Class AB respondents were most likely to use the hospital staff canteen (41 per cent cf. 13 per cent C1 and 23 per cent C2 and DE), whereas class DE respondents were most likely to be given food on the ward (52 per cent cf. 32 per cent AB, 26 per cent C1 and 38 per cent C2). Class C respondents made proportionately more use of visitors' canteens (39 per cent C1 and 32 per cent C2 cf. 18 per cent AB and 13 per cent DE).

Although only 17 respondents actually stayed overnight at the hospital (3 AB, 9 C1, 3 C2 and 2 DE), as many as 239 (15 per cent of the sample) reported that there had been occasions when they had not been allowed to do so, although they had wanted to. Present evidence suggests that it is likely that working class parents will feel less able to ask to stay in what they may consider to be unfavourable circumstances than will middle class parents. Indeed, fewer such instances of a refused request were reported by respondents from classes AB (11 per cent cf. 19 per cent C1, 16 per cent C2 and 18 per cent DE), perhaps because class AB respondents may have felt themselves to be on a better footing to argue the point with hospital staff.

Economic factors

One might predict that, of all the problems associated with having a child in hospital, those involving expenditure would be most likely to be associated with social class because this is associated with differences in income level. Furthermore, if the child's hospitalization necessitates the household head taking time off work, this is likely to hit working class families more severely than middle class. Cartwright[6] found that during a spell in hospital, only 20 per cent of working class heads of household received full wages in comparison with 77 per cent of those from middle classes. In addition, only 12 per cent of middle class heads of household received no money at all from their employer in contrast to 55 per cent from the working class. As a result, 52 per cent of working class respondents felt they had encountered moderate or severe financial strain, but this feeling was shared by only 9 per cent of middle class respondents.

The major economic problem caused by a child in hospital involves obtaining and paying for transport, but expenditure on other necessary items such as special clothing, toys, food and drink for the child is also important.

Transport

The transport system in Wales today presents many very real problems for patients travelling to visit a child in hospital. The policy of centralization of the hospital services involves an increase in the distance between home and hospital in many cases, with a consequent increase in cost. It has been suggested that the cost involved is the major deterrent to parental visiting.[6] However, cost and distance are not the only factors. Existing public transport facilities result in a disproportionate length of time being spent on travel in some areas, while in others withdrawal of bus and rail services have made travelling to hospital almost impossible without a private car. As 39 per cent of all survey respondents had no car, and 31 per cent had children hospitalized at least ten miles from home, the frequency with which transport problems were reported is not surprising. Such problems are severe enough when parents are travelling on their own, but must surely be exacerbated when taking the child home after discharge. Not unexpectedly problems in this context arose more frequently when public rather than private transport was used (18 per cent of those using public transport reported difficulty in comparison with 4 per cent of those using the household car and 7 per cent using a friend's or relative's car).

Despite official recommendations that parents should be allowed to visit their children in hospital whenever possible, little has been done to ease the financial burden which this must place on many families. The present situation with regard to financial aid for visitors to patients in hospital has been described by Ryan and Thomas[7] and by

Browse,[6] and is seen to consist of inadequate subsidies for those in need and inadequate information about what subsidies are, in fact, available. Practical attempts to alleviate this situation have been made. Such attempts are seen to be very necessary in the light of the finding that 16 per cent of respondents found obtaining transport to visit very or quite difficult and 27 per cent found similar difficulty in meeting the cost. Table 4 indicates the greater severity of problems among lower class respondents. Only 3 per cent of respondents from social classes AB reported any difficulty in obtaining transport to visit and 7 per cent in paying for it. The corresponding proportions from class C1 were 7 per cent and 8 per cent respectively, but for classes C2 and DE they were considerably higher; 17 per cent of respondents from C2 and 25 per cent from DE found obtaining transport very or quite difficult while 22 per cent from class C2 and as many as *46 per cent from classes DE* found payment very or quite difficult.

Table 4 Reported transport difficulties × social class

| | Social Class | | | | Total | |
Problem	AB %	C1 %	C2 %	DE %	%	N
Obtaining transport						
Very/quite difficult	3	7	17	25	17	231
Not very/not at all difficult	97	89	83	73	82	1,120
Don't know	0	4	*	1	1	17
TOTAL %	100	100	100	100	100	
Paying for transport						
Very/quite difficult	7	8	22	46	27	371
Not very/not at all difficult	93	88	77	52	72	978
Don't know	0*	4	1	1	1	19
TOTAL %	100	100	100	100	100	
N	155	194	522	497		1,368

*=less than 0.5%

In view of the extent of reported difficulties experienced by respondents from the lower social classes, particularly with payment for transport, it may well be that many persons might qualify for financial assistance if made aware of their rights. Only 1 per cent of respondents, however, reported being given any information by the hospital about claiming social security benefit. The giving of information by the hospital showed no meaningful variation with social class, but information from other sources was more commonly given to respondents from classes DE. Very few respondents actually claimed benefit.

Expenditure on other items
Respondents were questioned about the amount of money which they had spent on various items for the child throughout his stay, for example, special clothing, toys, food and drink. No systematic differences emerged with social class with the possible exception that working class parents found it necessary to buy special clothing for the child to wear in hospital rather more frequently than was the case with middle class parents. This finding ties in with an overall picture showing parental care and concern to be spread evenly throughout the classes, but involving a greater sacrifice for those of lower socio-economic status.

Conclusions

Despite suggestions which have been expressed to the contrary, attitudes concerning the appropriate care and treatment of a child in hospital do not appear to differ significantly between social classes. The survey has shown that there is some correlation between the social class of the child's family and the route by which he reaches hospital and also between social class and the use made of the hospital services. But social class differences in attitudes to the needs of a child in hospital or to the importance of visiting are few.

Differences occur in two ways. The first is that working class parents appear to be treated differently by hospital staff, which results in them finding out less about their child's treatment and the facilities available, and to some extent, therefore, using facilities less. The second set of differences are economically based. The major variations which occurred were, as one might expect, a consequence of the differential availability of resources. The lower occupational groups have fewer cars, have greater difficulty both in obtaining and in paying for transport, and are more likely to suffer a loss of income if the household head absents himself from work to ease the home situation or to be with the child in hospital. If respondents from lower social classes visit their children less, it is not because they believe less in maintaining contact, but because of the greater problems involved for them. There were respondents who did not visit through a belief that the child was happy in hospital and would be upset at the sight of his parents, but such a belief was not class related. If lower class children get a less good deal in hospital, it is not because of any lack of willingness or understanding on the part of their parents as a class. They and their parents encounter greater economic problems and experience differential treatment from some hospital staffs.

References

1. Newson, J. and Newson, E. *Infant Care in an Urban Community*, Allen & Unwin (1963).
2. Dajda, R. and Mapes, R. 'The general household survey as a source of information'. In *The Sociology of the National Health Service*, Stacey, M. (ed), Sociological Review Monograph, **22** (March 1976).
3. Carstairs, V. and Paterson, P. E. 'Distribution of hospital patients by social class', *Hlth. Bull.* **XXIV** (3) (July 1966).
4. Cartwright, A. and O'Brien, M. 'Social class variations in health care and in the nature of general practitioner consultations'. In *The Sociology of the National Health Service*, Stacey, M. (ed), Sociological Review Monograph, **22**, University of Keele (March 1976).
5. e.g. Stacey, M., Dearden, R., Robinson, D. and Pill, R. *Hospitals, Children and Their Families*, Routledge & Kegan Paul, London (1970). Cartwright, A. *Human Relations and Hospital Care*, Institute of Community Studies Series, Routledge & Kegan Paul, London (1964).
6. Browse, B. 'The Fares Enquiry', NAWCH Report.
7. Ryan, T. M. and Thomas, E. J. 'Repayment of travelling expenses to hospital', *The Hospital and Health Services Review* (August 1972).

Margaret Stacey is Professor of Sociology at the University of Warwick and Bronwen Earthrowl was a research assistant at the University College of Swansea in Wales. The data on which the paper was based were collected for the Welsh Hospital Board and the original, longer, article appeared in *Social Science and Medicine*, 11, 83–88 (1972).
Since this article was published more work in this field has been undertaken and this is summarised in the *Black Report on Inequalities in Health* published in 1982. An extract from this is included in Part 7 of this Reader.

Part 7

Prospects and Speculations

Introduction

Every age, as René Dubos has remarked, seems to construct its own version of the past, in which a special place is reserved for an arcadia of health and happiness. This age has concentrated more on speculating on the future: as utopia, where disease will be conquered and ill-health banished. Many ways of reaching this utopia are on offer, ranging from a whole-hearted embrace of high technology to the rejection of orthodox scientific medicine, and from vesting the state with sweeping powers of intervention and control to placing maximum influence in the hands of patients or 'consumers'.

The prospect of reaching utopia, however, or even the striving after it, has never commanded universal enthusiasm. Fear or scepticism about the future also has its own tradition. The articles in this part are intended largely to reflect the range of views among utopian enthusiasts—the 'onwards and upwards' school of thought—but the sceptical perspective is also represented. This part begins with an extract from an 'enquiry into the future of the three enemies of the rational soul' by the radical biologist J. Desmond Bernal, the three enemies being 'the World, the Flesh, and the Devil'. Bernal's speculations are unashamedly extravagant: 'For I dipt into the future, far as human eye could see, saw the Vision of the World, and all the wonder that would be.' In 'The Flesh', Bernal pushes to its extreme the view of the body as an increasingly troublesome appendage to the 'cerebral mechanism'. The future brain, literally removed from the body and attached to a complex array of artificial mechanisms providing sensory information and communication, is seen in this 'long view' as no more than a small, logical, evolutionary step. The final vision, of brains communicating so intimately that the individual ceases to exist as an entity and is subsumed in a 'compound mind', is one in which time, space, life and death are transformed by applied scientific knowledge. Bernal's concluding comment, of an aetherial consciousness, 'ultimately perhaps resolving itself entirely into light', has an unmistakeable tongue-in-cheek air. It is, however, uneasily echoed by the position at which contemporary physics seems to have arrived.

Bernal's visions of the future may be viewed as science fiction but, as Bruce Durie, a science journalist, observes, breakthroughs in scientific medicine, and in particular in medical technology, seem to be an almost weekly event. Organ transplantation, body scanning, and artificial devices, such as pace-makers and hip joints, are only a few examples of many innovations that were until recently science fiction but that are now almost commonplace. Genetic or bio-engineering, to judge by the commercial and industrial interest, might well hold fabulous potentialities for further innovations. At this rate, Bernal's mechanised person may seem less and less far-fetched. Moreover, the pursuit of high-technology medical solutions has developed a powerful momentum, fuelled by the behaviour of physicians and the incentives they have to innovate, by the commercial interests of large corporations, by the expectations of the public, and not least by the momentum of current research programmes.

Nothing has attracted more faith in a technological solution than looking for a cure for cancer, as is well illustrated in the review of the work of the American National Cancer Chemotherapy Program by Emil Frei III, a professor of medicine and Director of the Boston Cancer Institute. The article is striking in demonstrating the truly astonishing range of compounds which have been screened as potential anti-tumour drugs: chemical synthetics, fermentation products, plant products and marine animal products. In all some 700,000 compounds have been examined in this programme of research to produce a mere handful with any established anti-tumour activity. However, a careful reading of the article reveals the very limited success of many of these chemotherapies when subjected to universal trial, and the high incidence of toxic side-effects.

There are grounds for doubting whether technology can be relied upon to provide the miracle breakthroughs that some advocates claim. Moreover, there have been increasing doubts about the historical importance of medicine and medical technology in improving health, and these have prompted some fresh thinking about future policies. If public health measures, improvements in nutrition, and increased standards of living contributed so much to rising health status in the past, perhaps it would make sense to look to these factors rather than to 'hi-tech' medicine in the future also.

A recent comprehensive statement of what future health policy might flow from recognising the limitations of medical intervention is provided by the 'Black Report' on health inequalities in the UK. This report, which was commissioned by a Labour Government in 1977 and presented its findings to a Conservative Government in 1980, takes its name from Sir Douglas Black, the then chief scientist at the DHSS, who chaired the small Working Group which prepared it. Starting from a statistical examination of the depth and tenacity of social class differences in health, the Black Report proceeded to an analysis which attributed these inequalities to wider material inequalities in society. As the extract included here demonstrates, the Report's policy recommendations were accordingly focused on ways of reducing these social and economic inequalities, for example, by comprehensive income redistribution. By framing health policy recommendations in a context not confined to health services (although these were not neglected), the Report moved into territory previously uncharted by official government health-policy working groups. In doing so, however, it sparked off a major public debate in which the Government took the role of chief antagonist. A flavour of this debate is provided by the comments and correspondence, carried by the medical press, which accompany the extract.

As these comments on the Black Report show, a major issue in the debate over its recommendations concerned the cost of implementing them. Ironically, costs are also an emerging issue in the future role of high technology. It is not surprising, therefore, that cost containment has become a dominant theme in debates over future policy for one health-care system that is more open to high-technology innovation than any other—the American one. Alain Enthoven, a leading American health economist, is quite as critical of current American health policy as is the Black Report of UK health policy. But his diagnosis and recommendations are very different. Enthoven's concern is that a great deal of American health-care is of little tangible benefit to patients, but is nevertheless provided because the structure of the insurance system gives patients, on the one hand, no incentive to choose economical forms of care and physicians, on the other hand, every incentive to supply expensive ones. His proposal, a 'consumer choice health plan', is to introduce more competition between health-care providers, and more choice for health-care consumers, so that both groups have incentives to seek out less costly care. Enthoven's proposals are based on an assessment of the balance of interests: as he notes, his proposals are likely to be nobody's first choice but could well be the second choice of many, if and when structural reform is forced by the cost crisis.

The proposals of Enthoven and of the Black Report differ radically, but do share a reliance on legislative change to initiate and enact new health policy. In contrast, the 'alternative medicine' movement is comprised of many different elements with a common bond in the emphasis on the role of the individual, and the rejection of health policies imposed from above, whether of a technological or social nature. Alternative medicine, as Ruth West's survey makes clear, embraces a rich diversity of traditions, some of classical origins which pre-date scientific medicine, and other, more recent, off-shoots of orthodox practice. A unifying characteristic, however, is an adherence to an alternative *philosophy* which stresses the capacity to heal from within. Indeed, the criticisms of the effectiveness of much orthodox medical practice which she reports among followers of alternative medicine have echoes in the proposals of, for example, the Black Report. There the similarities end, however, for the essentially individualist response of most alternative medicine is far removed from the collectivist response of the Black Report's 'wider strategy'.

The guide to occupational cancer prepared by the British trade union GMBATU is based on a recognition of the importance of collective action by workers in identifying the risks that face them and taking action to remove them. As such, it marks an innovative mixture of non-reliance on the good-will of legislators, employers or health services to present, detect or treat ill-health, and of collective, rather than individual, 'self-help'. Indeed, the GMBATU guide, by its very existence, illustrates that legislation, factory inspectors, safety executives, and other products of past health policy may not be effective, and cannot substitute for well-informed and well-organised groups monitoring their health and environment, insisting on their legal rights, and campaigning for improved conditions. The guide also exemplifies the degree to which medical terminology and health problems can be 'demystified' and made widely accessible, given sufficient determination and imagination.

The visions of the future offered in the extracts in this part may vary widely, but they have in common an optimism that dissatisfactions with the present can be redressed. It was noted earlier, however, that there exists another tradition, of ambivalence towards the future. Nowhere, perhaps, is this awareness of the losses and gains of systematic social intervention and control more elegantly stated than in Aldous Huxley's *Brave New World*. The Central London Hatchery and Conditioning Centre, the mass incubation of Alpha and Epsilon Workers, build up a picture of the future which is in the mainstream of science-fiction nightmare. To dismiss it as such, however, would be to miss the point. Huxley clearly states the *benefits* which can be perceived in such a system: conditioning provides the 'secret of happiness and virtue—liking what you've *got* to do'. The message may be unpalatable, but the co-existence of gain and loss lies at the heart of the ambivalent attitude over the future which Huxley expresses. The choices he presents reflect the one, and perhaps only, theme uniting high-tech enthusiasts, proponents of alternative medicine, social reformers and utopian speculators.

7.1

The Flesh

J. Desmond Bernal

In the alteration of himself man has a great deal further to go than in the alteration of his inorganic environment. Man has altered himself in the evolutionary process, he has lost a good deal of hair, his wisdom teeth are failing to pierce, and his nasal passages are becoming more and more degenerate. But the processes of natural evolution are so much slower than the development of man's control over environment that we might, in such a developing world, still consider man's body as constant and unchanging. If it is not to be so then man himself must actively interfere in his own making and interfere in a highly unnatural manner. Biologists are apt, even if they are not vitalists, to consider [evolution] as almost divine; but after all it is only nature's way of achieving a shifting equilibrium with an environment; and if we can find a more direct way by the use of intelligence, that way is bound to supersede the unconscious mechanism of growth and reproduction.

In a civilized worker the limbs are mere parasites, demanding nine-tenths of the energy of the food and even a kind of blackmail in the exercise they need to prevent disease, while the body organs wear themselves out in supplying their requirements. On the other hand, the increasing complexity of man's existence, particularly the mental capacity required to deal with its mechanical and physical complications, gives rise to the need for a much more complex sensory and motor organization, and even more fundamentally for a better organized cerebral mechanism. Sooner or later the useless parts of the body must be given more modern functions or dispensed with altogether, and in their place we must incorporate in the effective body the mechanisms of the new functions. Surgery and biochemistry are sciences still too young to predict exactly how this will happen. The account I am about to give must be taken rather as a fable.

Take, as a starting point, the perfect man such as the doctors, the eugenists and the public health officers between them hope to make of humanity: a man living perhaps an average of a hundred and twenty years but still mortal, and increasingly feeling the burden of this mortality. Sooner or later some eminent physiologist will have his neck broken in a super-civilized accident or find his body cells worn beyond capacity for repair. He will then be forced to decide whether to abandon his body or his life. After all it is brain that counts, and to have a brain suffused by fresh and correctly prescribed blood is to be alive—to think. The experiment is not impossible; it has already been performed on a dog and that is three-quarters of the way towards achieving it with a human subject. But only a Brahmin philosopher would care to exist as an isolated brain, perpetually centred on its own meditations. Permanently to break off all communications with the world is as good as to be dead. However, the channels of communication are ready to hand. Already we know the essential electrical nature of nerve impulses; it is a matter of delicate surgery to attach nerves permanently to apparatus which will either send messages to the nerves or receive them. And the brain thus connected up continues an existence, purely mental and with very different delights from those of the body, but even now perhaps preferable to complete extinction. The example may have been too far-fetched; perhaps the same result may be achieved much more gradually by using of the many superfluous nerves with which our body is endowed for various auxiliary and motor services. We badly need a small sense organ for detecting wireless frequencies, eyes for infra-red, ultra-violet and X-rays, ears for supersonics, detectors of high and low temperatures, of electrical potential and current, and chemical organs of many kinds. We may perhaps be able to train a great number of hot and cold and pain receiving nerves to take over these functions; on the motor side we shall soon be, if we are not already, obliged to control mechanisms for which two hands and feet are an entirely inadequate number; and, apart from that, the direction of mechanism by pure volition would enormously simplify its operation. Where the motor mechanism is not primarily electrical, it might be simpler and more effective to use nerve-muscle preparations instead of direct nerve connections. Even the pain nerves may be pressed into service to report any failure in the associated mechanism. A mechanical stage, utilizing some or all of these alterations of the bodily frame might, if the initial experiments were successful in the sense of leading to a tolerable existence, become the regular culmination to ordinary life.

But this is by no means the end of [man's] development, although it marks his last great metamorphosis. Apart from such mental development as his increased faculties will demand from him, he will be physically plastic in a way quite transcending the capacities of untransformed humanity. Should he need a new sense organ or have a new mechanism to operate, he will have undifferentiated nerve connections to attach to them, and will be able to extend indefinitely his possible sensations and actions by using successively different end-organs.

The carrying out of these complicated surgical and physiological operations would be in the hands of a medical profession which would be bound to come rapidly under the control of transformed men. The operations themselves would probably be conducted by mechanisms controlled by the transformed heads of the profession, though in the earlier and experimental stages, of course, it would still be done by human surgeons and physiologists.

It is much more difficult to form a picture of the final state, partly because this final state would be so fluid and so liable to improve, and partly because there would be no reason whatever why all people should transform in the same way. Probably a great number of typical forms would be developed, each specialized in certain directions. If we confine ourselves to what might be called the first stage of mechanized humanity and to a person mechanized for scientific rather than aesthetic purposes—for to predict even the shapes that men would adopt if they would make of *themselves* a harmony of form and sensation must be beyond imagination—then the description might run roughly as follows.

Instead of the present body structure we should have the whole framework of some very rigid material, probably not metal but one of the new fibrous substances. In shape it might well be rather a short cylinder. Inside the cylinder, and supported very carefully to prevent shock, is the brain with its nerve connections, immersed in a liquid of the nature of cerebro-spinal fluid, kept circulating over it at a uniform temperature. The brain and nerve cells are kept supplied with fresh oxygenated blood and drained of de-oxygenated blood through their arteries and veins which connect outside the cylinder to the artificial heart-lung digestive system.

The brain thus guaranteed continuous awareness, is connected in the anterior of the case with its immediate sense organs, the eye and the ear—which will probably retain this connection for a long time. The eyes will look into a kind of optical box which will enable them alternatively to look into periscopes projecting from the case, telescopes, microscopes and a whole range of televisual apparatus. The ear would have the corresponding microphone attachments and would still be the chief organ for wireless reception. Smell and taste organs, on the other hand, would be prolonged into connections outside the case and would be changed into chemical testing organs, achieving a more conscious and less primitively emotional role than they have at present. The remaining sensory nerves, those of touch, temperature, muscular position and visceral functioning, would go to the corresponding part of the exterior machinery or to the blood supplying organs. Attached to the brain cylinder would be its immediate motor organs, corresponding to but much more complex than, our mouth, tongue and hands. This appendage system would probably be built up like that of a crustacean which uses the same general type of arm for antenna, jaw and limb; and they would range from delicate micro-manipulators to levers capable of exerting considerable forces, all controlled by the appropriate motor nerves. Closely associated with the brain-case would also be sound, colour and wireless producing organs. In addition to these there would be certain organs of a type we do not possess at present— the self-repairing organs—which under the control of the brain would be able to manipulate the other organs, particularly the visceral blood supply organs, and to keep them in effective working order. Serious derangements, such as those involving loss of consciousness would still, of course, call for outside assistance, but with proper care these would be in the nature of rare accidents.

The remaining organs would have a more temporary connection with the brain-case. There would be locomotor apparatus of different kinds, which could be used alternatively for slow movement, equivalent to walking, for rapid transit and for flight. On the whole, however, the locomotor organs would not be much used because the extension of the sense organs would tend to take their place. Most of these would be mere mechanisms quite apart from the body; there would be the sending parts of the television apparatus, tele-acoustic and tele-chemical organs, and tele-sensory organs of the nature of touch for determining all forms of texture. Besides these there would be various tele-motor organs for manipulating materials at great distances from the controlling mind. These extended organs would only belong in a loose sense to any particular person, or rather, they would belong only temporarily to the person who was using them and could equivalently be operated by other people. This capacity for indefinite extension might in the end lead to the relative fixity of the different brains; and this would, in itself, be an advantage from the point of view of security and uniformity of conditions, only some of the more active considering it necessary to be on the spot to observe and do things.

The new man must appear to those who have not contemplated him before as a strange, monstrous and inhuman creature, but he is only the logical outcome of the type of humanity that exists at present. Although it is possible that man has far to go before his inherent physiological and psychological make-up becomes the limiting factor to his development, this must happen sooner or later, and it is then that the mechanized man will begin to show a definite advantage. Normal man is an evolutionary dead end; mechanical man, apparently a break in organic evolution, is actually more in the true tradition of a further evolution.

A much more fundamental break is implicit in the means of his development. If a method has been found of connecting a nerve ending in a brain directly with an electrical reactor, then the way is open for connecting it with a brain-cell of another person. Such a connection being, of course, essentially electrical, could be effected just as well through the

ether as along wires. At first this would limit itself to the more perfect and economic trans-
ference of thought which would be necessary in the cooperative thinking of the future. But
it cannot stop here. Connections between two or more minds would tend to become a
more and more permanent condition until they functioned as dual or multiple organisms.
The minds would always preserve a certain individuality, the network of cells inside a
single brain being more dense than that existing between brains, each brain being chiefly
occupied with its individual mental development and only communicating with the others
for some common purpose. Once the more or less permanent compound brain came into
existence two of the ineluctable limitations of present existence would be surmounted. In
the first place death would take on a different and far less terrible aspect. Death would still
exist for the mentally directed mechanism we have just described; it would merely be postponed for three hundred or perhaps a thousand years, as long as the brain cells could be
persuaded to live in the most favourable environment, but not for ever. But the multiple
individual would be, barring cataclysmic accidents, immortal, the older components as
they died being replaced by newer ones without losing the continuity of the self, the
memories and feeling of the older members transferring themselves almost completely to
the common stock before its death. And if this seems only a way of cheating death, we must
realize that the individual brain will feel itself part of the whole in a way that completely
transcends the devotion of the most fanatical adherent of a religious sect. It is admittedly
difficult to imagine this state of affairs effectively. It would be a state of ecstasy in the literal
sense, and this is the second great alteration that the compound mind makes possible.
Whatever the intensity of our feeling, however much we may strive to reach beyond ourselves or into another's mind, we are always barred by the limitations of our individuality.
Here at least those barriers would be down: feeling would truly communicate itself,
memories would be held in common, and yet in all this, identity and continuity of individual development would not be lost. It is possible, even probable, that the different individuals of a compound mind would not all have similar functions or even be of the same
rank of importance. Division of labour would soon set in: to some minds might be delegated the task of ensuring the proper functioning of the others, some might specialize in
sense reception and so on. Thus would grow up a hierarchy of minds that would be more
truly a complex than a compound mind.

The complex minds could, with their lease of life, extend their perceptions and understanding and their actions far beyond those of the individual. Time senses could be altered:
the events that moved with the slowness of geological ages would be apprehended as
movement, and at the same time the most rapid vibrations of the physical world could be
separated. As we have seen, sense organs would tend to be less and less attached to bodies,
and the host of subsidiary, purely mechanical agents and perceptors would be capable of
penetrating those regions where organic bodies cannot enter or hope to survive. The
interior of the earth and the stars, the inmost cells of living things themselves, would be
open to consciousness through these angels, and through these angels also the motions of
stars and living things could be directed.

The new life would be more plastic, more directly controllable and at the same time
more variable and more permanent than that produced by the triumphant opportunism of
nature. Bit by bit the heritage in the direct line of mankind—the heritage of the original life
emerging on the face of the world—would dwindle, and in the end disappear effectively,
being preserved perhaps as some curious relic, while the new life which conserves none of
the substance and all the spirit of the old would take its place and continue its development. Such a change would be as important as that in which life first appeared on the
earth's surface and might be as gradual and imperceptible. Finally, consciousness itself
may end or vanish in a humanity that has become completely etherialized, losing the

close-knit organism, becoming masses of atoms in space communicating by radiation, and ultimately perhaps resolving itself entirely into light. That may be an end or a beginning, but from here it is out of sight.

J. Desmond Bernal was a writer, physicist and communist. He was involved, until his death in 1971, in the politics of science. The extract 'The Flesh' included here is drawn from *The World, the Flesh and the Devil: An Enquiry into the Future of the Three Enemies of the Rational Soul*, first published in 1929 by Cape, London, and republished by Indiana University Press, Bloomington.

7.2

High Technology Medicine

Bruce Durie

This article sets out to explore how high technology will mesh with medicine in the future, and some of the options that present themselves. It is intended to be a less-than-critical paean of praise for the bright new future engendered by the steady march of progress into (some would say all over) our lives, and the place of biomedical science in this. As such it does not discuss the nature of scientific advance, the ethics of applying science to the human condition, nor even attempt to introduce the concepts of cost : benefit or risk : benefit ratios, except obliquely.

What HiTech medicine means

It is easy to find criticisms of applied science, especially in the ethical and moral minefield of human medicine, just as it is easy to accept wholeheartedly (as does the man in the street) that science is A Good Thing, and that we have a right to expect solutions for all human ills.

Mankind has a tendency to believe in magic and the wisdom of his betters—hence religion, patent medicines, slimming cures and the aesculapean authority worn by many medical practitioners. Be that as it may, this article takes the view that high technology will have a beneficial and an increasingly important role to play in medicine from henceforth.

It is practically impossible to extrapolate from present technology to its future applications, not least because much is synergistic—the unexpected fusion of two or more disparate fields of research into one new technique or discipline. It is also interesting to see how techniques can be replaced by wholly different solutions to the same problems—polio vaccine, a prophylactic measure now enshrined in public policy in Britain, has all but done away with the iron lung; gastric freezing, a common treatment for ulcers in the 1960s, is now hardly practised, partly because other surgical practices have supplanted it, partly because drugs have arrived which treat the condition; CAT scanning has almost become routine in some centres for the investigation of headaches.

First a definition: high technology medicine, for the purposes of this article, means the direct application to the patient of state-of-the-art, sophisticated, and above all expensive technologies. An electronic stethoscope might fulfil the first two of these criteria but not the last—not in the same way as a cyclotron costing millions.

The definition adopted here is a pragmatic one: HiTech medicine is the application of the most recent advances in the basic sciences, and in other applied sciences (such as engineering and materials science) to the diagnosis, alleviation, palliation and/or cure of human medical problems. As such, it embraces what has come to be known as the New Biology (genetic engineering, recombinant DNA technology, improved industrial production methods for biochemicals and drugs) and disciplines like particle physics (as in the CAT Scanner), electromagnetics and radio frequency engineering (in NMR Scanners), laser optics (used in surgery and ophthalmics), computers (practically everywhere). It is by definition expensive.

What does HiTech medicine have to offer

A society is only as advanced as its applied science, and one measure of human contentment is the degree to which its health care needs are met. High technology medicine is seen as a basic right by the general population, who often judge the quality of the care being offered by the sophistication of the technology involved. And since, in the context of medicine, it is the white-coated professionals who condition society's expectations, they cannot really be expected not to deliver what they have promised. To do so would destroy part of their credibility as deliverers of the modern miracle.

But one of the paradoxes of human existence is that satisfying a need does not necessarily generate contentment, but dissatisfaction. So it is not enough to point to the successes of medicine, for example in eradicating smallpox—what about eradicating the common cold? Typhoid, diphtheria and tuberculosis have been all but eliminated, but what about flu? Hip replacements are fine but what about fully-automated artificial limbs?

The potential for HiTech medicine is to find solutions for these very problems—better vaccines, improved drugs with more specific actions and therefore fewer side effects, the elaboration of human biochemicals (such as hormones) by recombinant DNA technology, the application of microchips to muscular and neural control (as in spinal injuries), new solutions to infertility, including 'test tube babies'—are all addressable by the application of new technology to medicine.

Many advances in medicine have come historically from better diagnostic methods, and here technology plays a part. Improved visualisation of the interior of the body and even the identification of specific chemicals by non-invasive means is now possible, which in turn leads to safer treatments in appropriate cases. The technology of immobilised enzymes has meant complex chemical tests on a simple plastic reagent strip—and with multiple tests on one strip—so that a biochemical profile of a patient can be built up by one single test performed on the spot by the GP rather than within the week by three separate labs, each miles away.

Advances in screening—such as in cervical cytology for the early diagnosis of cancer, and the identification of those at risk of heart disease by analysis of blood components and the characteristics of cell surfaces—may mean better preventive medicine and therefore reduced mortality, greater quality of life and less medical care needed subsequently.

These approaches are expensive initially. The investments by pharmaceutical companies in genetic engineering are huge, and previously undreamt of; one CAT Scanner will cost £1 million or more. However, the savings come later. Every heart attack prevented is a saving to the state in hospital time. Every cancer caught early and treated with radiation and drugs is an operation avoided and possibly a life saved or lengthened.

To take some historical examples: had there been no investment in the esoteric field of blood cell surface chemistry, the basis of transfusion compatibility and blood groups would not have been elucidated and the success of surgery would be far lower than it is now, thanks to adequate cross-matching and a well-organised blood-collection service. Had there been no investment in the chemical synthesis of obscure steroids derived from the Mexican yam, there would not now be the safe and effective combined oral contraceptive pill.

If the pharmaceutical industry did not risk spending, at current prices, some £20 million and fifteen years on evaluating 10,000 compounds in order to find one marketable drug, most of the great advances in modern medicine would not have been made, since not only do drugs have the desired effect, they also have side effects, which may be of themselves desirable. No one knew that slight chemical modifications to the side-chain of pethidine (originally intended as an atropine-like drug, but now used for its morphine-like pain-killing properties) would lead to the whole class of butyrophenones, the anti-psychotic medications which have largely emptied the mental hospitals of schizophrenics.

The moral is: the steady march of progress is inevitable, and a desirable thing in its own right, but there are spin-offs, themselves beneficial which cannot be foreseen, and therefore HiTech medicine should be stimulated, encouraged and nurtured for its own sake.

Examples of HiTech medicine

1 Better Scanning
The CAT scanner

Computerised axial tomography (CAT) is essentially an X-ray technique, but which gives a picture of a 'slice' through the body rather than a flat image. The X-rays are beamed through the body from different angles, and at each angle, a computer records the information of the image and uses this to reconstruct a picture of a 'slice' of the patient.

The CAT scan has replaced more dangerous and distressing techniques, such as pneumoencephalography, where air is blown into the ventricles of the brain so that certain features—tumours, abscesses, etc.—are shown up, and at a lower radiation exposure than the standard X-ray. Against this, the CAT scanner is still an invasive technique—it not only irradiates the patient, but in most cases it requires the injection of a contrast medium, a dye which shows up outlines of tissues, and to which some patients can abreact.

CAT scanning rarely gives information that could not be got by other methods, although the computer-generated visualisation of a body slice gives more *useful* information than a planar X-ray and may do so quicker and with less patient distress.

Nuclear magnetic resonance scanning (NMR)

Even less invasive than CAT scanning, since it uses no radiation, but just as expensive and even less widespread, is NMR. Its great advantage is the need for no radiation or contrast media. The basis of NMR is radio emission. Certain molecules subjected to a sufficiently strong magnetic field will align themselves with the field—like tiny compass needles. When the field is switched off, the alignments collapse, but the energy is dissipated as radio waves, which are indicative of the chemistry and the environment of the molecule.

Most NMR scanning concentrates on water, a prosaic but ubiquitous substance. So, for example, the signal from water complexed with proteins is different to that generated from water in a free form. This gives the possibility of spotting tumours and other abnormalities, including, say, the earliest stages of multiple sclerosis in nerves. In fact, NMR may replace analytical biochemistry as we know it, since all the body's components could in theory be measured by their NMR signals, and a single pass through an NMR scanner may eventually be a complete health screening programme.

2 Bioengineering

Bioengineering essentially means taking specially synthesised lengths of DNA, or segments of genes from other organisms, and inserting them into the genome of a lower organism (generally a bacterium) in such a way that the inserted 'gene' is expressed, that is, produces a protein. Thus, the gene for human insulin can be excised from the appropriate human cells in tissue culture and inserted in multiple copies into the bacterium *E. coli*, which is then grown in a fermentation vat and produces insulin as one of its products. The insulin is harvested, purified, and formulated in a form which diabetics can inject. The advantages to this approach are:

* the insulin is human, rather than isolated from the usual sources (pig or cattle);
* there is no reliance on a supply of pig pancreas from which to isolate porcine insulin;
* the quality and composition of the insulin can be standardised.

Similarly, human growth hormone (hGH) is now produced by bacterial fermentation. Now, for the first time, all children suspected of lacking hGH can be screened for their response to the hormone, and if warranted, treatment can be started early enough to normalise their height, and thus avoid the psycho-social consequences of remaining forever of abnormally short stature.

But between true dwarfs and those of normal height, there is a spectrum of hGH deficiency. With the availability of bioengineered hGH, any child growing at a rate considered slow compared to his or her contemporaries can be 'normalised', and therefore realise their true potential rather than suffer the stigma of being shorter than average. After all, if shortness is a hormone deficiency analogous to hypothyroidism, why should it not also be treated?

The lessons learned from bioengineered insulin and growth hormone will be used to advantage in producing other human proteins. As the technology advances, insertion of human genes into cells other than bacteria will become routine—yeast, other mammalian cell culture lines and even human cells themselves. This raises the possibility of gene transplantation.

Where an individual lacks a gene product (a hormone, or an enzyme, say) or makes an abnormal one (such as a haemoglobin subunit which does not carry oxygen correctly, as in thalassaemia), it may be possible to culture the appropriate stem cells, include the correct gene, add the cells back to the body in such a way that they will 'take' and therefore start producing the correct gene product. Combined with improved ante-natal screening for birth defects and metabolic abnormalities, the implication is a future free of inheritable diseases, which in theory could only take a generation or so to accomplish.

3 Hybridomas and cloning

Analogous techniques are already available to turn human cells into factories for antibodies and other proteins. The characteristic feature of cancer cells is that they are immortal, and will grow forever in the right conditions. If a certain antibody were wanted—say against a leukaemic cell—it is possible to stimulate a patient's lymphocytes to make that antibody, isolate the appropriate lymphocyte and culture it (since all the cells are identical, i.e. from one clone, this is a monoclonal culture) and subsequently fuse these cells with cancer cells. The resulting hybrid cell (called a hybridoma) is then an immortal anti-leukaemia cell antibody producer—a factory in other words. It would be possible to inject a small culture of this cloned cell line back into a patient, and the antibodies would clear any leukaemia cells from the body.

4 Prostheses

The microchip has been described as a 'swift idiot', but the swifter they become, the cleverer they appear to be. Microchips are now being used to replicate the functions of muscular reflexes, to reproduce the actions of a damaged nerve tract. Victims of spinal accidents may have the power of motion returned to them, controlled by a microprocessor.

Ever more sophisticated pacemakers for the heart and the phrenic nerve (which controls the diaphragm and therefore breathing) will help those with cardiac and respiratory difficulties. Neural prostheses implanted in the brain could take over the functions of diseased or excised tissue, and the cure for Parkinson's disease may eventually be to remove or inactivate the substantia nigra, and have its functions taken over by a chip.

A neat application of microprocessors to the cure of the disabled is the Possum, which allows any possible movement to be translated into commands, instructions and simple mechanical actions. But an implanted Possum-like microprocessor, neurally controlled, could restore such functions as motor control and speech.

Allied to this is the better understanding of materials and surfaces which is making implanted prostheses which are non-antigenic and wear-proof. Better and longer-lasting heart valves, mechanical hearts and kidneys, joints and even whole replacement bones are not far off.

5 In vitro fertilisation

Each month seems to being a new advance in help for infertile couples, from better fertilised egg implantation techniques to banks of frozen embryos by which the technically infertile can plan a whole family. Given the complete failure of tubal surgery to correct infertility, these techniques seem to hold most promise, and may eventually be cheaper than hormone treatments, which have the disadvantage of occasionally promoting multiple births.

But this technology need not be restricted to the infertile. Individuals could deposit their eggs and sperm (or even a fertilised embryo) in a bank, be sterilised, and lead lives free from the worries of pregnancy and contraception until such times as the decision was taken to start a family. With the element of chance taken away, there would be much closer control over population growth and the spacing of children in families, such that a couple could decide to delay their first childbirth until middle age. In addition, chromosomal defects could have been screened out of the stored eggs and sperm.

6 Heart Transplants

The need for human donors is the major limiting factor on heart transplants, and the main factor in survival is not the surgery—which is fairly straightforward—but the acceptance or rejection of the graft. The main consideration in matching a donor heart to a recipient is that the blood groups be compatible—this is more important than the tissue type matching.

Before long, monoclonal antibody technology will have solved most of the remaining problems of graft–host incompatibility, by providing masking antibodies to prevent this happening. It is likely that every individual will carry a 'credit card' bearing all the necessary information on their health status, including blood groups, tissue types, etc., thus making a computer match of donor and recipient faster and more accurate.

But perhaps humans are not the ideal donors in any case. It has been proposed that, calf heart being of the right size and characteristics, herds of cattle could be kept which are chimaeras for human blood groups—in other words, their blood is compatible with human serum. Knowing a heart disease victim would benefit from a transplant, the appropriately matched heart could be ordered 'off the shelf' or even grown to order for an operation three years hence.

7 Better drugs

Rather than spend tens of millions and over a decade screening 10,000 or more synthesised substances in the hope of finding one fit to market, the pharmaceutical industry is coming to realise that the way forward is to understand the physiology of the system to be influenced, identify the crucial receptor or enzyme to modify, act on or inhibit, and use computer-generated 3-D representations of molecular structure to design a drug with the required actions. A new class of antihypertensives, the angiotensin converting enzyme (ACE) inhibitors, was developed in this way. Increased understanding of receptor pharmacology itself has led to the design from scratch of drugs for conditions which were previously not treatable this way—cimetidine, an anti-ulcer drug, has decimated the number of operations for gastric ulcers, for example.

8 Lasers for surgery

There are already over 200 lasers in over 170 NHS hospitals in the UK, spanning all fields of medicine. Lasers fall into three main categories. The CO_2 laser, whose light is absorbed by water, and therefore by tissue, but without damaging the surrounding tissues, is essentially a bloodless scalpel, which is mostly used in laryngology (where the surgeon can operate *through* the trachea without cutting it) and gynaecology. The argon laser, whose blue–green light is absorbed by red, i.e. blood, is used to control bleeding from ulcers, in ophthalmology, careful brain surgery and to remove unsightlingly 'port wine stains' from the skin. The neodymium YAG laser light is in the low infra-red, and can be transmitted via flexible fibre-optics, and is used to kill tumours in the lung, gut, brain and bladder wall.

An advance on this is to 'tune' lasers by generating the light through a dye, and marking the operative site—such as a tumour—with a photoreactive dye which absorbs it. The implications of lasers in surgery are that operations, even for major tumours, could become quick, safe, bloodless, anaesthetic-free procedures, possibly performed by a technician-nurse in an out-patient clinic. This itself could practically do away with surgical wards altogether.

The Future

Any speculative gaze into the future of medicine sounds to the lay person like a cross between a scientist's wish fulfillment, science fiction and Shangri-La. The future cannot really be discussed without reference to the social implications of applying HiTech medicine, and the generation of funds to pay for it.

But what is clear is that not only will HiTech bring to medicine ways to deal with its present problems better, it will bring within the scope of medicine diseases which are simply not addressable today. Coupled to better, faster and more reliable diagnostic methods applied earlier or even routinely, the future looks very rosy indeed.

Bruce Durie trained as a biochemist before becoming a full-time medical and science journalist. He is currently Director of Moving Finger, a medical mass media and technical information company. This article has not previously been published.

7.3

The National Cancer Chemotherapy Program

Emil Frei III

In 1955 the US Congress authorized $5 million for the National Cancer Institute (NCI) to establish a Cancer Drug Development Program. This remains a major program at NCI. It was and continues to be of concern both within the scientific community and the lay press. It is timely, therefore, to review the program with respect to progress, perspectives, and problems.

Factors that influenced the initiation and large-scale support for the program include the following.

1. The need for systemic [whole body] treatment for cancer. Advances in surgery and radio-therapy have been such that curative treatment can be delivered to many patients whose tumor has not spread beyond the local and regional lymph-node-bearing areas. Of the 785,000 new patients with cancer annually in the United States, 30 per cent fall into this category. Cancer prevention and early detection techniques may improve these figures, and priority has been given to such research. For the 550,000 patients whose disease has spread beyond the local or regional area, major advances in treatment, and particularly curative treatment, require systemic therapy. This includes chemotherapy, hormone therapy for endocrine-dependent tumors, and immunotherapy.

2. The observation in 1943 that nitrogen mustard, a congener of the war gas sulfur mustard, was capable of producing tumor regression in patients with lymphoma and the discovery, in 1947 and 1955, respectively, that the folic acid antimetabolites produced temporary remissions in childhood leukemia and a cure in patients with choriocarcinoma.

3. The development of the science of pharmacology and its application to a variety of areas, including, for example, the highly successful programs of screening and development of antibiotics for the control of infectious diseases and the 'crash' program for the development of antimalarial compounds during World War II.

4. The development of transplantable animal tumors and therefore the potential for quantitative drug assessment.

5. The control of infectious diseases and the emergence of cancer as the second major cause of death in the United States (after cardiovascular diseases).

The drug development program has undergone changes and refinements over the past 27 years.

A linear array system was organized for new drug development, which included the following stages: (i) the acquisition of new compounds, (ii) screening*, (iii) production and formulation*, (iv) toxicology*, (v) phase I clinical trials*, (vi) phase II clinical trials, and (vii) phase III and IV clinical trials.

The key decision points in the linear array, where rather precise criteria must be met before a drug can advance from one stage to the next, are indicated by the asterisks between the various stages of drug development. An affirmative decision for a particular drug at each point commits large amounts of the division's resources to the development of that drug.

The Acquisition of New Compounds

Drug development begins with the selection and acquisition of agents for screening. From 1955 to 1975 up to 40,000 agents per year were selected for screening, largely on an empirical, random basis. After 1975 the number of compounds was reduced to less than 15,000 per year by the more rational development of agents. This was made possible by prior experience and particularly by further developments in medicinal chemistry, pharmacology, and tumor biology.

The 700,000 compounds and extracts that have been acquired and screened by the National Cancer Chemotherapy Program since 1955 may be broadly categorized as follows.

Chemical synthetics.
These include some 350,000 compounds, most of which were acquired empirically in the early years of the program. Only a minority of the agents fall into identifiable classes of antitumor drugs. These include the alkylating agents and antimetabolites.

The prototype alkylating agent is nitrogen mustard, which was discovered during World War II. Ten thousand alkylating agents have been synthesized in an effort to improve their antitumor activity, on the one hand, and to lessen toxicity on the other. These studies have resulted in the development of alkylating agents with substantially greater stability that can be given by mouth, a major practical advantage.

A large number of analogs of metabolites (antimetabolites) known or thought to be important to the survival of tumor cells have been synthesized. Of the antitumor agents with established clinical activity, six are antimetabolites.

The heavy metals have recently been emphasized in the chemical synthetic area. In experiments conducted for an entirely different purpose, it was observed that a platinum coordination compound released from electrodes in electrolysis experiments produced morphologically distinct antibacterial effects. These complexes were isolated and tested for antitumor activity experimentally, and *cis*-diamminedichloroplatinum II (cisplatin) was subsequently shown to have substantial activity in a variety of human tumors. Twenty-five hundred additional platinum and other heavy metal coordination compounds have been synthesized. Several of the newer platinum compounds have less nephrotoxicity [cause kidney damage] experimentally than the parent compound and are being evaluated in clinical trials.

Fermentation products.
Approximately 200,000 fermentation products have been acquired by the National Cancer Chemotherapy Program. With the demonstration that highly effective antibiotics for infectious disease were produced by soil fungi, these began to be screened for antitumor activity in cancer cells in culture. In the past ten to fifteen years, several antibiotics with

major clinical activity have been identified. These include the anthracyclines adriamycin and daunorubicin, which were discovered in Europe, and bleomycin, mitomycin C, and other antibiotics discovered and developed largely in Japan.

Plant products.

One hundred and twenty thousand plant extracts have been prepared from 35,000 different species obtained largely through the US Department of Agriculture from worldwide sources. Some were selected because of folklore evidence that they had medicinal value. The extracts were screened and, if positive, sent to chemists supported by NCI contracts for isolation and purification. In the early 1960s this area received a major boost with the discovery that products of the periwinkle plant, vincristine and vinblastine, had major, clinically useful antitumor activity. While many new novel alkaloids have been discovered and several have reached clinical trial, the plant product program has been disappointing in terms of identifying active agents and has been scaled down.

Marine animal products.

Sixteen thousand marine and other animal products and extracts have been screened. However, only extracts of a tunicate [sea squirt] have proved to be of interest experimentally, and no such products have reached clinical trial. This area is also being deemphasized.

Biological response modifiers.

In the past several years, NCI has developed a major program relating to biological response modifiers. These include (i) agents that modulate the immune system, (ii) agents that inhibit suppressor cell function; (iii) agents that affect the antigenic potential of tumor cells; and (iv) agents that modulate the state of differentiation of tumor cells.

Screening

In contrast to the situation for infections, experimental models for the selection of agents for clinical trial in cancer were, and continue to be, a major scientific challenge. The development of in-bred mouse strains and of transplantable tumors provided a highly reproducible system for large-scale application (screening). In the 1960s and 1970s, transplanted solid tumors closely resembling the major tumors in man (lung, breast, colorectal) were developed and incorporated into the preclinical evaluation system. Also in recent years, *in vitro* systems for the assay of chemotherapeutic agents against a given patient's tumor have been developed. While this approach is still in the investigative stages, it has major importance for the selection of new agents, as well as the individualization of treatment.

The Clinical Program

Of the large number of compounds that were screened in the past twenty-five years, 150 were judged to be sufficiently and reproducibly active to warrant clinical trial. Of these, 40 have been found to be active in one or more categories of cancer in man.

Initial clinical (phase I) trials with a given new agent are designed to provide evidence of therapeutic effect and to determine the tolerated dose, clinical pharmacology, and qualitative toxicity of the agent. Phase I studies are conducted in patients with advanced cancer known to be refractory to established treatment. Such studies generally require 15 to 30 patients, and if successful are followed by phase II and III studies, which are designed to determine more precisely the presence and magnitude of antitumor activity in a spectrum of categories of human cancer.

Such studies raise the specter of human experimentation. This is particularly true of phase I studies where the physician has very limited information to impart to the patient as to the potential for therapeutic effect and toxicity. It is complicated by the fact that the patient involved has advanced cancer and may 'grasp at straws'. It is a central, complex, and poorly understood ethical issue, which deserves attention here.

A patient for whom there is no known effective treatment has two choices; no further treatment (other than supportive and symptomatic care) or experimental treatment. The emotional overlay in such a setting is major, and it is a situation rife for exploitation, as evidenced by the thriving, overpromising cancer quackery industry. The skill and empathy of the physician is sorely tested. He must know the patient and family, know how they are likely to interpret what he says, and not promote options that he knows are unacceptable. Some patients accept the inevitability of death and reject new treatment, but for many the door of hope cannot be closed. Accepting this, what on the basis of past and current phase I agents can we realistically offer the patient in terms of therapeutic effect?

As above, of the 150 agents introduced into phase I study during the past twenty-five years, 40 were found to have significant activity in one or more human tumors. Therefore a patient participating in a phase I trial has a 25 to 30 per cent (40/150) chance of receiving an active drug. All of the 40 active antitumor agents exhibited some antitumor effects in a variable proportion of patients in a phase I trial. Antitumor effect means substantial tumor regression and symptomatic improvement lasting for one or more months.

It is inappropriate to suggest that a new agent has a chance of being curative in a phase I trial. However, patients who cannot accept that answer will generally not ask the question. Another kind of phase I study involves the novel use of established agents, such as combination chemotherapy. In such phase I studies, cure was achieved in Hodgkin's disease and testicular cancer. Phase I studies may help future patients, but it is inappropriate, in my judgement, for the physician to mention this unless such information is requested by the patient. The patient may choose to discontinue participation in the study at any time.

The patient and family can be assured that the effectiveness and toxicity of the drug *in vitro* and in animals and the intended method of administration (protocol) has been extensively reviewed, both by an Institutional Review Board associated with the patient's hospital and by external review bodies such as those organized by the Food and Drug Administration and NCI. An Institutional Review Board includes lay persons as well as scientists not directly involved in the research under review.

Cancer is a malignant disease and requires vigorous treatment. Surgery and radiotherapy, as well as chemotherapy, are 'toxic'. The toxic potential of the agent, based on preclinical, and usually very preliminary clinical, studies, must be explained to the patient and included in detail in a written consent form. For most patients, some toxicity occurs, which lasts for a few days and is completely reversible. Patients with advanced cancer have a variable symptom complex, which worsens gradually or episodically, and may be falsely attributed to the drug and sometimes cannot be distinguished, even by the skillful physician, from drug toxicity. A review of phase I studies conducted at major cancer centers indicates that 1 to 3 per cent of such patients will die with (but not necessarily of) toxicity.

Unfortunately, tumor regression does not occur in most patients participating in phase I studies. In the end, the major contributions that the physician, nurses, and paramedical personnel have made in such clinical situations are optimal supportive and symptomatic care and, very particularly, the knowledge on the part of the patient and family that their physician is not only an expert in cancer care but cares for the patient. While patients and their families are grateful for whatever success is achieved in this setting, those of us involved in cancer therapeutic research can attest that immediately, and often for long periods after the patient's demise, families remember in a positive way the hope, attention, and care that was provided.

In summary, phase I studies over the past twenty-five years have provided limited but realistic hope to patients and families, particularly where the other choice is unacceptable. Moreover, we can hope that rapid developments in the science of therapeutic research in cancer will lead to the development of agents that are more specific for tumors; that is, that will provide a greater therapeutic effect at a lesser cost in toxicity.

Curative Cancer Chemotherapy

To date, phase I studies have provided some 40 chemotherapeutic agents that have differing mechanisms of action and that exhibit antitumor activity in one or more forms of human cancer. These therapeutic 'tools' provided the opportunity for a major research effort in the therapy of clinical cancer.

The major initial experiments focused on acute lymphocytic leukemia in children, and in a series of clinical trials, the principles and practice of combination chemotherapy were developed. The importance of combination chemotherapy can be appreciated when it is realized that essentially all highly effective and curative cancer chemotherapy involves combinations of effective agents.

Once complete remission was achieved in a high proportion of children with acute lymphocytic leukemia, it was recognized that treatment during remission with chemotherapy was essential and that this must involve chemotherapy agents different from those used to induce remission. As a result, the duration of remission progressively increased.

Highly effective, complete remission-producing chemotherapy, followed by central nervous system 'prophylaxis' and by combination chemotherapy designed to eradicate systemic microscopic disease, has resulted in a cure rate of 50 to 60 per cent in children with acute leukemia. This achievement occurred primarily in the early 1960s, and some of the principles and therapeutic strategies derived from these studies, particularly those relating to combination chemotherapy, were applied to patients with advanced Hodgkin's disease and non-Hodgkin's lymphoma, where cures were also achieved. The development of additional agents during the past ten to fifteen years, has, with the application of some of the aforementioned principles, resulted in the cure of 70 to 80 per cent of patients with disseminated testicular cancer.

Experimental studies clearly indicate that curative treatment with chemotherapy correlates inversely with tumor burden. Thus a given chemotherapeutic agent which was marginally active against advanced gross tumor in the mouse was frequently curative against the same tumor in its early microscopic phase. It was similarly recognized that a major adverse prognostic factor for chemotherapy for most human tumors was gross disease. There are many 'solid' tumors where treatment of the primary tumor with surgery, radiotherapy, or both is highly effective, but relapse occurs because of the presence of clinically undetectable disseminated disease. For example, in patients with breast cancer, where the tumor is limited to the breast (stage 1), the cure rate with local treatment only (surgery, radiotherapy, or both) is in the range of 80 per cent. However, if the tumor has spread to the axillary lymph nodes, surgery and radiotherapy will provide local control, but relapse at distant sites will occur in 70 to 80 per cent of patients because of disseminated disease. 'Adjuvant' chemotherapy is given immediately after treatment of the primary site in those patients at high risk of having disseminated disease. This strategy was used initially, and successfully, in the early 1950s for children with Wilms' tumor, and was subsequently shown to be effective in increasing the cure rate in several relatively rare solid tumors in children.

In the past ten years, this adjuvant treatment strategy has been the subject of a number of clinical trials. In general, that chemotherapy which is most effective against advanced states of a given tumor has been used in the adjuvant setting. Since cancer is a chronic disease, and since adjuvant treatment is evaluated primarily on the basis of time to relapse, it may take a long time to evaluate the effectiveness of an adjuvant study. Breast cancer, the most common cause of death from cancer in women, is important and instructive in this regard. Controlled studies of adjuvant chemotherapy of breast cancer were initiated in 1972. These studies involved initial control of the primary tumor with surgery. Patients with axillary metastases, that is, at high risk of dissemination, were randomly allocated to treatment with chemotherapy or to no treatment. Essentially all studies, particularly those involving combination chemotherapy, have led to a significant decrease in the relapse or failure rate as a result of chemotherapy, particularly in premenopausal women with one to three positive nodes. Although the results of these studies are positive, their full impact must await further follow-up, in view of the chronicity of the disease.

In summary, chemotherapy alone, or in the multimodality (adjuvant) setting, is curative for patients with acute lymphocytic leukemia, Hodgkin's disease, diffuse histiocytic lymphoma, testicular cancer, gestational choriocarcinoma, Wilms' tumor, Ewing's tumor, embryonal rhabdomyosarcoma, and Burkitt's lymphoma. In addition, chemotherapy is probably curative (pending further follow-up) for limited small-cell lung cancer; acute myelogenous leukemia; and, in the adjustment setting, for breast cancer and osteogenic sarcoma.

Curative Cancer Chemotherapy and US Cancer Mortality

A major indicator of curative treatment is the impact on national cancer mortality statistics. In general, for the thirteen diseases mentioned above, there has been a significant reduction in national mortality statistics, and the magnitude of the reduction for a particular disease correlates with the known effectiveness of treatment for that disease as well as the year such treatment was introduced and became widely used. Specifically, the decline in mortality in the United States between 1966 and 1976 for the following diseases has been: Wilms' tumor, 66 per cent; Hodgkin's disease, 39 per cent; pediatric leukemia, 38 per cent; non-Hodgkin's lymphoma, 24 per cent; bone tumors in children, 23 per cent; premenopausal breast cancer, 19 per cent; and for testicular cancer, between 1973 and 1978, 34 per cent. Whereas the number of patients cured annually by chemotherapy was less than 10,000 per year in the United States ten years ago, it is now greater than 40,000. Chemotherapy tends to be more effective and have a greater potential for cure in the younger individual. Thus, when cancer mortality over the past fifteen years was analyzed by age groups, it was found that there has been a 20 to 43 per cent reduction in cancer mortality in the United States in subjects under the age of 45 (Figure 1). Detailed analyses of cancer incident and stage at time of diagnosis over these time periods indicate that the decline is a result of improved treatment, largely improved chemotherapy. This decline is countered by an increase in cancer mortality in older subjects, almost all of which is due to smoking-related cancer, particularly lung cancer (Figure 1). Indeed, when

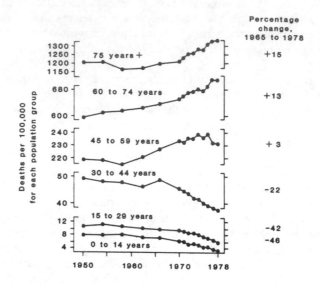

Figure 1 Age-specific cancer mortality trends, 1950–78

smoking-related cancers are subtracted, there has been a slight decline in the incidence of cancer in the United States over the past thirty-five years.

In addition, chemotherapy short of cure can produce substantial tumor regression and symptomatic improvement lasting a number of months in patients with metastatic breast cancer, cervical cancer, head and neck squamous cell carcinoma, insulinomas, ovarian cancer, soft tissue sarcoma, chronic leukemias, and nodular lymphomas. It remains true, however, that chemotherapy has been of limited benefit for some of the major forms of cancer, such as non-small cell lung cancer, melanoma, and gastrointestinal and prostate cancer.

Toxicity

These therapeutic results attest to the efficacy of cancer chemotherapeutic agents. However, some adverse effects on normal organs occur (toxicity). Toxicity commonly relates to organs with a high rate of cell turnover. This includes the bone marrow, gastrointestinal tract, and the hair follicle. The major subjective manifestation of toxicity is nausea and vomiting, which is a significant problem with some 60 per cent of the agents currently used. Chemotherapy-induced damage to the hair follicle may produce temporary loss of scalp hair. Although the above and other toxic manifestations significantly compromise the quality of life while the patient is receiving therapy, they are usually completely reversible. Significant progress has already been achieved in reducing the incidence of chemotherapy-induced nausea and vomiting over the past several years.

In addition to the acute effects of cancer chemotherapy, long-term effects may also occur. These effects include suppression of ovarian function and spermatogenesis, and, with the anthracycline class of drugs, cardiac toxicity. A more ominous late toxic manifestation has been the development of secondary tumors, particularly acute myelogenous leukemia. Some antitumor agents, such as the alkylating agents, alter the structure of DNA, and therefore are mutagenic in bacterial assay systems and carcinogenic in experimental animals. It is not surprising, therefore, that such agents have proved to be carcinogenic in man. However, the generalization that all cancer chemotherapeutic agents are carcinogenic is not true. The dose of, and particularly the duration of treatment with, potentially carcinogenic chemotherapeutic agents correlates strongly with the subsequent development of tumors. An increase in the incidence of secondary tumors, particularly acute myelogenous leukemia, has been observed in several forms of human cancer treated with agents that are potential carcinogens (the latent period for secondary tumor development is generally greater than two years).

In recent years the strategy of clinical trials has included attempts to decrease the risk of carcinogenicity. Thus there is good evidence that four to six months of treatment for many tumors (testicular cancer, Hodgkin's disease, adjuvant-treated breast cancer) is sufficient and that the longer durations of treatment previously used are unnecessary.

The Future

Although the National Cancer Chemotherapy Program has received some criticism, it is, on the basis of any balanced analysis, at least a qualified success. Cure or palliation has been achieved in an increasing proportion of patients, and many problems and prospects previously unperceived have been brought into focus and are the subject of current research. Of particular importance is the evidence that basic and applied science is leading to the development of more effective and less toxic agents in the area of cancer chemotherapy, immunotherapy, and endocrinology. A few areas of research deserve emphasis.

Different clinical therapeutic strategies are under study. Where local control of tumor is difficult to achieve, such as in patients with head and neck cancer, chemotherapy is being used initially with the intent of achieving tumor regression and therefore improving the prospects for definitive treatment with surgery or radiotherapy. This approach has been successful in Wilms' tumor and certain other childhood tumors.

Certain chemotherapeutic agents increase the sensitivity of tumors to radiotherapy. There is a long precedent in cancer chemotherapy to the effect that progress can be achieved by the more imaginative and effective use of established agents.

The biochemical tools today are such that it is possible to determine at a molecular level the mechanism of action of some of our established antitumor agents and therefore the basis of whatever specificity exists against tumor cells compared to normal cells.

There are a number of growth and modulating factors in the microenvironment that regulate the proliferation and behavior of normal cells. Many of these factors may also affect tumor cells. In studies *in vitro*, some of these factors, such as growth factors and lymphokines, have been identified. The first such new agent to reach the clinic has been leucocyte interferon. Since many of the factors are polypeptides it should be possible to produce them by recombinant DNA technology.

Studies of tumor immunology, particularly as a result of monoclonal antibody technology, are providing new knowledge about the pathogenesis, diagnosis, and treatment of cancer. A patient's immune response may be selectively altered by cancer and can be selectively manipulated by such antibodies. Monoclonal antibodies alone or complexed with highly cytotoxic chemotherapeutic agents (immunotoxins) are in early, phase I, clinical trials.

Finally, advances in tumor biology should provide an increasing number of future biochemical 'targets' for treatment.

Emil Frei III is Professor of Medicine at Harvard Medical School, Boston, and Director and Physician-in-Chief of the Sidney Farber Cancer Insititute, Boston, Mass. The article of which this extract is an edited version was published in *Science*, 217, 600–606 (13 August 1982).

7.4

Inequalities in Health: The Black Report and Reactions to it

Introduction

'Inequalities in Health', or 'The Black Report', was published in August 1980 by the Department of Health and Social Services. In their report, the research working group document inequalities in the health of different social classes in Britain, explore how these might be explained and make recommendations for action. The extract which follows focuses primarily on recommendations for action outside the NHS, though detailed consideration was given to action within the health service. The publication of the report, its findings and its recommendations were the subject of great controversy, which continues today, a flavour of which is given both in the journal extracts which follow The Black Report Recommendations and in the extract from the Pelican edition of the Report published in 1982. For reasons of space this material has had to be severely edited.

Foreword by Patrick Jenkin

The Working Group on Inequalities in Health was set up in 1977, on the initiative of my predecessor as Secretary of State, under the Chairmanship of Sir Douglas Black, to review information about differences in health status between the social classes; to consider possible causes and the implications for policy; and to suggest further research.

The Group was given a formidable task and Sir Douglas and his colleagues deserve thanks for seeing the work through, and for the thoroughness with which they have surveyed the considerable literature on the subject. As they make clear, the influences at work in explaining the relative health experience of different parts of our society are many and interrelated and, while it is disappointing that the Group were unable to make greater progress in disentangling the various causes of inequalities in health, the difficulties they experienced are perhaps no surprise given current measurement techniques.

It will come as a disappointment to many that over long periods since the inception of the NHS there is generally little sign of health inequalities in Britain actually diminishing and, in some cases, they may be increasing. It will be seen that the Group has reached the view that the causes of health inequalities are so deep-rooted that only a major and wide-ranging programme of public expenditure is capable of altering the pattern. I must make it clear that additional expenditure on the scale which could result from the report's recommendations—the amount involved could be upwards of £2 billion a year—is quite unrealistic in present or any foreseeable economic circumstances, quite apart from any judgement that may be formed of the effectiveness of such expenditure in dealing with the problems identified. I cannot, therefore, endorse the Group's recommendations. I am making the report available for discussion, but without any commitment by the government to its proposals.

PATRICK JENKIN
Secretary of State for Social Services

August 1980

The Black Report

Extracts from Summary

Most recent data show marked differences in mortality rates between the occupational classes, for both sexes and at all ages.

Available data on chronic sickness tend to parallel those on mortality. [. . .] In the case of acute sickness (short-term ill-health) the gradients are less clear.

The lack of improvement, and in some respects deterioration, of the health experience of the unskilled and semi-skilled manual classes (class V and IV), relative to class I, throughout the 1960s and early 1970s is striking. Despite the decline in the rate of infant mortality (death within the first year of life) in each class, the difference in rate between the lowest classes (IV and V combined) and the highest (I and II combined) actually increased between 1959–63 and 1970–72.

Inequalities exist also in the utilization of health services, particularly and most worryingly of the preventive services. In the case of GP, and hospital in-patient and out-patient attendance, the situation is less clear.

We do not believe there to be any single and *simple explanation* of the complex data we have assembled. *In our view much of the evidence on social inequalities in health can be adequately understood in terms of specific features of the socio-economic environment:* features (such as work accidents, overcrowding, cigarette smoking) which are strongly class-related in Britain and also have clear causal significance. Other aspects of the evidence indicate the importance of the health services and particularly preventive services. But beyond this there is undoubtedly much which cannot be understood in terms of the impact of specific factors, but only in terms of the more diffuse consequences of the class structure: poverty, working conditions, and deprivation in its various forms. It is this acknowledgement of the *multicausal* nature of health inequalities, within which inequalities in the material conditions of living loom large, which informs and structures our policy recommendations.

Recommendations

[These have been severely edited but original numbers have been left in the text to help readers to locate them in the original.]

Our recommendations for policy, we have divided into those relating to the health and personal social services, and those relating to a range of other social policies. Three objectives underpin our recommendations and we recommend their adoption by the Secretary of State.

—To give children a better start in life.

—To encourage good health among a larger proportion of the population by preventive and educational action.

—For disabled people, to reduce the risks of early death, to improve the quality of life whether in the community or in institutions, and as far as possible to reduce the need for the latter.

[The group made several recommendations related to resource allocation within the NHS and personal social services.]

Our further health service-related recommendations, designed to implement the objectives set out above, fall into two groups.

We first outline the elements of what we have called a District Action Programme. By this we mean a general programme for the health and personal social services to be adopted nationwide, and involving necessary modifications to the structure of care.

Second, we recommend an experimental programme, involving provision of certain services on an experimental basis in ten areas of particularly high mortality and adverse social conditions, and for which special funds are sought.

District action programme
Health and Welfare of mothers and pre-school and school children
(10) *A non-means-tested scheme for free milk should now be introduced beginning with couples with their first infant child and infant children in large families.* (Chapter 8, p. 142)

(11) *Areas and districts should review the accessibility and facilities of all ante-natal and child-health clinics in their areas and take steps to increase utilization by mothers, particularly in the early months of pregnancy.* (Chapter 8, p. 151)

(12) *Savings from the current decline in the school population should be used to finance new services for children under 5.* (Chapter 8, p. 154 and Chapter 9, p. 182).

(13) *Every opportunity should be taken to link revitalized school health care with general practice, and intensify surveillance and follow-up both in areas of special need and for certain types of family.* (Chapter 8, p. 155)

The care of elderly and disabled people in their own homes
[Several recommendations were made under this heading.]

Prevention: the role of government
Effective prevention requires not only individual initiative but a real commitment by the DHSS and other government departments. Our analysis has shown the many ways in which people's behaviour is constrained by structural and environmental factors over which they have no control. Legislation and fiscal and other financial measures may be

required and a wide range of social and economic policies involved.

(19) *National health goals should be established and stated by government after wide consultation and debate. Measures that might encourage the desirable changes in people's diet, exercise and smoking and drinking behaviour should be agreed among relevant agencies.* (Chapter 8, p. 162)

(20) *An enlarged programme of health education should be sponsored by the government, and necessary arrangements made for optimal use of the mass media, especially television. Health education in schools should become the joint responsibility of LEAs and health authorities.* (Chapter 8, p. 161)

The following recommendation should be seen not only as a priority in itself but as illustrative of the determined action by government necessary in relation to many elements of a strategy for prevention:

(21) *Stronger measures should be adopted to reduce cigarette smoking. These would include:*
a. Legislation should be rapidly implemented to phase out all advertising and sales promotion of tobacco products (except at place of purchase);
b. Sponsorship of sporting and artistic activities by tobacco companies should be banned over a period of a few years, and meanwhile there should be stricter control of advertisement through sponsorship;
c. Regular annual increases in duty on cigarettes in line with rises in income should be imposed, to ensure lower consumption;
d. Tobacco companies should be required, in consultation with trades unions, to submit plans for the diversification of their products over a period of ten years with a view to the eventual phasing out of harmful tobacco products at home and abroad;
e. The provision of non-smoking areas in public places should steadily be extended;
f. A counselling service should be made available in all health districts, and experiment encouraged in methods to help people reduce cigarette smoking;
g. A stronger well-presented health warning should appear on all cigarette packets and such advertisements as remain, together with information on the harmful constituents of cigarettes. (Chapter 8, p. 162)

Additional funding for ten special areas
(23) *We recommend that the government should finance a special health and social development programme in a small number of selected areas, costing about £30 m. in 1981–82.* (Chapter 8, p. 165)

Measures to be taken outside the health services
(26) [. . .] We have been necessarily selective. We have attempted to pay heed to those factors which are correlated with the *degree* of inequalities. Second, we have tried to confine ourselves to matters which are practicable now, in political, economic and administrative terms, and which will none the less, properly maintained, exert a long-term structural effect. Third, we have continued to feel it right to give priority to young children and mothers, disabled people, and measures concerned with prevention.
(27) Above all, we consider that the *abolition of child-poverty* should be adopted as a national goal for the 1980s. We recognize that this requires a redistribution of finan-

cial resources far beyond anything achieved by past programmes, and is likely to be very costly. Recommendations 24–27 are presented as a modest first step which might be taken towards this objective. [. . .]

28. Beyond these initial elements of an anti-poverty strategy, a number of other steps need to be taken. These include steps to reduce accidents to children, to which we have referred (Recommendation 3). Further,

(28) *Provision of meals at school should be regarded as a right* [. . .] *without charge.* (Chapter 9, p. 188)

(29) *A comprehensive disablement allowance for people of all ages should be introduced by stages at the earliest possible date, beginning with people with 100 per cent disablement.* (Chapter 9, p. 191)

(30) *Representatives of the DHSS and DE, HSE, together with representatives of trade unions and CBI, should draw up minimally acceptable and desirable conditions of work.* (Chapter 9, p. 195)

(31) *Government departments, employers and unions should devote more attention to preventive health through work organization, conditions and amenities, and in other ways.* (Chapter 9, pp. 195–96)

(32) *Local authority spending on housing improvements under the 1974 Housing Act should be substantially increased.* (Chapter 9, p. 197)

(33) *Local authorities should increasingly be encouraged to widen their responsibilities to provide for all types of housing need which arise in their localities.* (Chapter 9, p. 198)

(34) *Policies directed towards the public and private housing sectors need to be better co-ordinated.* (Chapter 9, p. 197)

(35) *Special funding, on the lines of joint funding, for health and local authorities should be developed by the government to encourage better planning and management of housing, including adaptations and provision of necessary facilities and services for disabled people of all ages by social services and housing departments.* (Chapter 9, p. 199)

Our recommendations reflect the fact that reduction in health inequalities depends upon contributions from within many policy areas, and necessarily involves a number of government departments. Our objectives will be achieved *only* if each department makes its appropriate contribution. This in turn requires a greater degree of coordination than exists at present.

(36) *Greater co-ordination between government departments in the administration of health-related policies is required, by establishing inter-departmental machinery in the Cabinet Office under a Cabinet sub-committee along the lines of that established under the Joint Approach to Social Policy (JASP), with the Central Policy Review Staff also involved. Local counterparts of national co-ordinating bodies also need to be established.* (Chapter 9, p. 201)

(37) *A Health Development Council should be established with an independent membership to play a key advisory and planning role in relation to a collaborative national policy to reduce inequalities in health.* (Chapter 9, p. 201)

30. Within such co-ordinating machinery major initiatory responsibility will be vested in the Department of Health and Social Security, and we recommend that the Cabinet

Committees we have proposed be chaired by a Minister, and by a senior DHSS official respectively, having major responsibility for health and prevention. Similarly it will be an important obligation upon the DHSS to ensure the effective operation of the Health Development Council.

The Debate

'Equalities and inequalities in health', British Medical Journal, Volume 281, 20 September 1980

The recent report by Sir Douglas Black and his colleagues on *Inequalities in Health*, so grudgingly made available by the DHSS, presents much detail rather selectively culled from a bibliography. The recommendations have a certain detachment from reality which explains, though it does not justify, Patrick Jenkin's dismissive foreword. It may be true that the Government cannot at present provide the money for an ideal policy within the overall budget on health and welfare. That is no reason, however, for the Secretary of State failing to look at the pattern of services which could be developed even within present resource limitations. [. . .]

Some of its comments seem a little facile. All those concerned with 'acute hospital services' must be growing tired of being told that they must cut back to allow some of the money saved to be spent outside the hospitals. [. . .]

High-technology medicine is the usual target for those who demand a larger share of NHS resources for community services and prevention. This latest report is even more emphatic than others and equally vague about the elements to be cut. [. . .] Too little attention has been paid in this and other reports to the misery entailed for some patients or families by long waiting times for surgical treatment or admission for long-term care.

Sir Douglas Black's group has done a valuable service in bringing out the importance of social welfare, housing and education services, and social security payments in maintaining health. [. . .]

The emphasis in the report on prevention is welcome but a little vague. [. . .]

'Equalities and inequalities in health', Letters, British Medical Journal, Volume 281, 11 October 1980

Sir,—The Secretary of State's dismissal of the report of our working group[1] has attracted much attention from the press. Moreover, only 260 copies were printed, its main purpose—to stimulate serious discussion of a critical health issue—thus being frustrated. Even major health authorities were not provided with a copy. Your return to the subject (20 September, p. 762) is therefore very welcome.

I could cavil at several statements in the leading article. We do not endorse the suggestion 'that savings should be made in the maternity services': 'We regard improvement of the quality of maternity care as crucial; there can be no scope for savings here' (p. 234). Nor did we join in the attack on 'acute hospital services'. Alternatives are presented, one involving a small cut in the Government's plans for a (slight) increase, and the other no cut at all (p. 244). And so on.

My object in writing, however, is to point out that, while commenting that the emphasis on prevention is 'a little vague', your leader, centred as it is on the NHS, gives no picture of the report's principal thrust on prevention, its principal diagnosis and recommendation for action. Social inequalities in health, we concluded quite conventionally, arise to a large extent out of the socioeconomic structure; and one of the main factors in the poor health record of the lower social classes is their poverty and the multiple disadvantages inherent in this. The realistic and, one hopes, preventive way to attack this is in childhood and, in the light of massive research, the first years of life. Hence 'We consider that the abolition of child poverty should be adopted as a national goal for the 1980s. We recognise that this requires a redistribution of financial resources far beyond anything achieved by past programmes, and is likely to be very costly. Recommendations are presented as a modest first step which might be taken towards this objective' (p. 366)— increase in child benefits, a new infant care allowance, higher maternity grants, expansion in day-care facilities for the under-5s and free school meals. These together, if fully implemented at once (which, of course, does not follow), would cost about £1,500m, three-quarters of the £2,000m a year considered by the Secretary of State to be 'quite unrealistic in present or any foreseeable economic circumstances'. The corresponding total budget on social service, it may be mentioned, is £45,000m.

This is old-fashioned social medicine indeed. 'How far the poor can be made less poor. . . . In the whole range of questions concerning Public Health, there is not, in my opinion, any one to be deemed more important. . . . '[2] Subsistence poverty is abolished now—there is no hunger, no bare feet—but serious residual poverty remains to blight the lives of sizable sections of the population. Late in the twentieth century we are still beset by nineteenth-century-type problems of deprivation. If we are to be rid of social inequalities in health, these will have to be resolved at the same time as more focused education and health-service measures are instituted and the incentives provided for changes in life style, diet and exercise, and smoking and drinking behaviour.

The Opposition will, of course, be raising the whole issue of the report and its treatment when Parliament reassembles. But should not medicine seek to prevent this national issue from becoming merely a party one? Will the Faculty of Community Medicine give a lead (27 September, p. 826)? As your leading article concludes, the report 'could be modified to become a long-term development plan for health and social services', something we shall require more than ever in the difficult days ahead.

J. N. Morris

Departments of Human Nutrition and Community Health,
London School of Hygiene and Tropical Medicine,
London WC1E 7HT

'*Commentary from Westminster: Mr Jenkin on the Black Report*', Rodney Deitch, *The Lancet*, 28 March 1981
The Black Report on Inequalities in Health in Britain has become something of a bible for the Opposition in the Commons. [. . .] Mr Jenkin, for his part, has kept virtual silence on the subjects for six months. However, speaking at a meeting in Cardiff recently, he took the offensive. He accepted that inequalities in people's health had been little reduced. But the Black report did not explain any of the fundamental causes for this. [. . .]

A separate question from differences in health between the social classes, he went on, was differences in health-care provision. Do the poor have less access to the NHS than the better-off? Black said 'yes'. But the DHSS, Mr Jenkin added, had looked at a lot more evidence. They found that poorer people tend to receive proportionately more services than the average for the population as a whole. [. . .]

Mr Jenkin was waiting for the fruits of the Department's research and then for an opportunity to publicise it. The DHSS effort was along the lines of, and confirmed, work

---

[1] Department of Health and Social Security. *Inequalities in health*. Report of a research working group (chairman Sir Douglas Black). London DHSS, 1980.
[2] Simon, J. *English sanitary institutions*. London: Cassell, 1890, 444.

done by Rudolph Klein and Elizabeth Collins at Bath University. [. . .] Research showing results more in line with Black's conclusions, Klein and Collins believe, is based on inadequate statistics. 'We can confidently conclude,' they say, 'that Britain's primary health care system does not speak with an upper-class accent.' This is in strong contrast to Black's assertion that severe under-utilisation of health facilities by the working classes is a complex result of under-provision in working class areas and of costs (financial and psychological) of attendance. [. . .]

If there is equal access to the NHS, Mr Jenkin nevertheless accepts that it is access to facilities which differ in quality and quantity from one area of the country to another. [. . .] However, Mr Jenkin doubts if extra spending is the answer to the problems identified by Black. Firstly, it is often possible to increase the service given by the NHS without spending more. But his doubts about the cheque-book solution go deeper. 'It may be that there is a correlation between socioeconomic group and state of health. But Black has not been able to identify causes which indicate specific treatment. They went for a high programme of spending with absolutely no evidence that it will have any effect. On the other hand, it does appear there is a very definite correlation between education and better health. Smoking habits show that especially well. [. . .] We have been spending money in ever-increasing amounts on the NHS for 30 years and it has not actually had much effect on increasing people's health. If it is just a question of spending more money, then why do we still have all the "diseases of affluence"?'

'The Black Report and Causality', Letters, *The Lancet*, 6 June 1981

Sir, [. . .] Mr Patrick Jenkin's view seems to be that Black and his colleagues have failed to explain any of the fundamental causes of inequality in health. No doubt this view will be shared by others, and I suggest that the debate on the Black report should now include discussion of what is meant by 'causality'—a concept which is used frequently, often with little attention paid to its precise meaning. [. . .]

The debate on the causal factors associated with diseases, such as smoking with lung cancer and diet and exercise with heart disease, tends to be focused at the 'micro' level, scientific progress taking the form of successive clarification of causal associations between observable phenomena and the mechanisms involved. Although it makes extensive reference to studies of this kind, the Black report focuses on the 'macro' level and seeks an explanation of social inequalities in health, in social structural terms. This means the study of social and economic relationships and other complex social phenomena which, although real enough to us as social beings, are not so readily observable, in the sense of being accessible to the senses, as the causal factors considered at the 'micro' level. This, however, should not render them any the less powerful as explanations. The report devotes an entire chapter to the need for further research on these questions. [. . .]

Medical historians such as Prof. T. McKeown have described past improvements in health in terms of better socioeconomic environments, so the approach is hardly novel. As Sir Douglas Black has commented, his report did not exactly explain how poverty caused ill health but my point is—do we really have to elucidate mechanisms at the micro level, relating ill-health to poverty, before taking action to abolish poverty, bad housing, and poor working and living conditions? [. . .]

Medical Department,
Grampian Health Board,
Aberdeen AB9 8QP
                                                                    Keith Paterson

'*Commentary from Westminster: The Debate on the Black Report*', Rodney Deitch, *The Lancet*, 18 July 1981

The Government clearly does not think it has yet won the ideological debate which has raged around its health policy. [. . .] This is demonstrated in the extensive research now taking place, under DHSS aegis, into the theses of the Black report on Inequalities in Health and into the relationship between unemployment and ill-health. [. . .]

There have been accusations from the Labour benches that the Government has deliberately suppressed work which does not support its ideology, followed by indignant denials from DHSS Ministers. A case in point is a study (commissioned by the DHSS) of unemployment and health in families by Dr Leonard Fagin. This series of case studies suggested that unemployment can indeed have powerful effects on the health of the unemployed person and his family. Why had no effort been made to publicise the report, asked Labour spokesman, Mr Gwynneth Dunwoody, in the Commons? Retorted the Under-Secretary Sir George Young: 'That is untrue.' The DHSS had made the report available to the press, who took little interest in it, he said. (Health correspondents will confirm, nevertheless, that the Fagin study was scarcely publicised by the Department, in striking contrast to its attitude to the work of Klein and Collins.)

There is much further research being done for the DHSS at the moment. [. . .]

But what does Mr Jenkin hope for from all this work? Is he simply a searcher after truth, as he is happy to dub himself? If the balance of the research suggests that the health of the worse-off can only be improved by massive extra funding of health projects, will Mr Jenkin then campaign in the Cabinet for extra spending?

Extracts from the Introduction to the Pelican Edition of The Black Report*

The government's reaction

Mr Patrick Jenkin, then Secretary of State for Social Services, received the report early in April 1980. The Secretary of State's dismissal was brief. [. . .]

[In] the spring of 1981 the Secretary of State drew attention to what he considered to be the report's three principal shortcomings. First, he claimed it did not adequately explain the causes of inequalities in health, and 'its enormously expensive' programme of recommendations could not therefore be accepted. Second, Mr Jenkin argued that new evidence disproved the thesis that the working class suffered poorer access to the health services. [. . .] Third, Mr Jenkin argued that there was no evidence that more money would make any difference (so missing the main point of the report). [. . .] All three objections raised by government ministers—explanations, access and money—have been strongly contested by the members of the Working Group.

In the late 1970s the class differences in infant mortality diminished, but there tend to be fluctuations in such rates from year to year and it will be a few years before this welcome trend can be confirmed. So far as we are aware, no other substantial evidence of any qualifications that may be attached to the conclusions about class have emerged. On the contrary, later evidence would seem to confirm the greater part of the analysis in the report. [. . .]

The Secretary of State also drew on selected studies to cast doubts on the voluminous evidence marshalled by the Working Group showing that on the whole the richer occupational classes make more use of the National Health Service than do poorer occupational groups. [. . .]

* Edited by Peter Townsend and Nick Davidson, and published in 1982.

The study quoted by the Secretary of State (Collins and Klein, 1980) is based on material from the General Household Survey *for only one year*. Because of the wide fluctuations reported by class in utilization of services the Working Group, with full support from DHSS statisticians, had deliberately analysed such material for a succession of years. Second, the paper by Collins and Klein was based on the *numbers* of users of primary care, and not on the *frequency* of use. Third, the data considered were not related to *severity* of need as measured by days of illness or seriousness of condition. Fourth, even the restricted data discussed in the paper were not re-examined in relation to the much higher percentage of partly skilled and unskilled manual workers who were in the categories of '*chronic sick*'. And, finally, no data are given on *children*, among whom there is the greatest inequality of access. [. . .]

Lack of resources is the third, and superficially the most conclusive, of the three arguments of government Ministers against the Black Report. Are there resources available to commit to new positive health strategies? First, other countries which are at a comparable stage of economic development are spending more of their GNP on health services. The figures quoted as the cost of the Black Report's recommendations represent an addition of only 4½ per cent of total public expenditure on the social services (social security, health and personal social services, education and housing), or less than 3 per cent of total public expenditure. Second, the Working Group made clear that the recommendations deserve to be phased, with priorities, and that the full cost need not be met all at once. The Working Group take a modest view. As many as twenty-three of their thirty-seven recommendations would not be expensive to implement and the remaining recommendations could be implemented by stages. Third, while it was no part of the Working Group's terms of reference to go into detail about methods of financing the proposed changes, illustrations were given of three possible strategies for reducing the total cost. Fourth, there were all kinds of indirect benefits from developing a more efficient social policy in the interests of a healthy workforce and population. There were implications for production by reducing mortality and morbidity among adults of economically active age but also the long-term contribution to morale and vitality from a reduction in pain, discomfort and stress and the enhancement of a sense of security.

7.5

Reforming US Health Care: the Consumer Choice Health Plan

Alain Enthoven

The US health care financing system is a mixture of public and private enterprise, 42 per cent paid for by the public sector.

The two largest public health care financing programs are Medicare and Medicaid. Medicare is a federal program that pays for hospital and physician services for 29 million aged and disabled persons. Medicare spending doubled every four years through the 1970s and reached $37 billion in 1980. Medicaid is a joint federal–state program to pay for care for 22 million people with low incomes. In 1980, Medicaid spending reached $27 billion, nearly twice its 1975 level.

Most other Americans obtain health insurance through employment. Because employer expenditures on the health care of employees are a tax deductible business expense for employers, but are free of income and payroll taxes on employees, the federal government is, in effect, paying about 40 per cent of the cost of employer-paid health insurance. This has acted as a powerful incentive for employers to offer employees very comprehensive insurance.

Health care spending in the United States has grown rapidly, from $27 billion and 5.3 per cent of GNP in 1960 to $249 billion and 9.5 per cent of GNP in 1980. Real per capita spending nearly tripled between 1960 and 1980 and reached $1,075 in 1980.

While many factors contribute to this rapid growth of spending, I believe the main explanation is the combination of several factors:

1. Nearly universal comprehensive insurance with free choice of doctor blocks economic competition among physicians and does not provide incentives to be cost-conscious. Since the bills are mostly paid by third-party intermediaries, especially when people are seriously ill, patients have no reason to choose economical styles of care, and physicians have no incentive to be economical.

2. Fee-for-service payment of physicians rewards them with more income for providing more, and more costly, services, whether or not more are necessary or beneficial to the

patient. In the presence of much uncertainty, this is an incentive to resolve all doubts in favor of more care.

3. In effect, hospitals have been paid on the basis of cost reimbursement. The third party intermediaries have had little or no authority to question hospital charges or the need for services.

4. A great proliferation of new medical technologies has given physicians an almost limitless supply of services they can offer their patients.

5. Solo practice, the dominant form of medical practice, is likely to mean an absence of professional restraints. An increasing supply of physicians leads to 'physician induced demand' for services.

Are we paying more than is necessary for health care? I believe that there is a great deal of care that yields little or no benefit to patients. If our total health care delivery system performed with the efficiency of some of our more economical health care delivery organizations, we could obtain essentially all the benefits we now receive for roughly 25 per cent less cost.

Health Maintenance Organizations Cost Less

While our traditional and dominant health care financing and delivery system has no cost consciousness, it is not the only system in operation in the United States. We now have about 13 million people who voluntarily choose to receive their care through Health Maintenance Organizations (HMOs). Some of these organizations have been in operation since the 1940s. By their nature HMOs, in contrast to the traditional fee-for-service system, are competitors with built-in incentives for economy. Four principles that illustrate this point are discussed below.

First, in the insured fee-for-service system, premiums or taxes are paid to a financial intermediary. After care has been provided, the patient or the provider sends the bill to the intermediary who usually has little choice but to pay it. In an HMO, premiums are paid directly to an organization that accepts responsibility for providing comprehensive care. The payment is set in advance on the basis of a fixed amount per person per month. Thus, more services do not mean more revenue for the providers. The provider organization has a fixed budget within which to deliver the care.

Second, in an HMO, the provider organization is responsible for a voluntarily enrolled population. It can plan resource use to match the needs of this population. Preventing medical problems or treating them in less costly ways is rewarded. In the insured fee-for-service system, there are no defined populations to whom provider organizations are responsible. There is no basis for planning resource use. And less costly treatment is not rewarded.

Third, in the insured fee-for-service system, the patient has free choice of doctor, and, as I explained earlier, the system precludes economic competition among physicians. In an HMO, the patient voluntarily accepts a limited choice of doctors, including only those participating in that particular system, in exchange for what he perceives to be better care or lower costs. The premium charged by the HMO reflects the cost generating behavior of the providers within that system. Patients may be able to pay lower premiums for comprehensive care by signing up with economical providers. In such a system, economical providers may be able to attract more patients.

Fourth, the HMO organizes, provides or arranges the services. Thus, it can exercise management controls over quality, cost and appropriateness of care. In the insured fee-for-service solo practice system, such controls generally do not exist.

There are several types of HMO, and a considerable variety within each type. The most successful is the prepaid group practice (PGP). The essential principles of prepaid group practice are that an organized group of physicians, working together full time, agree to provide comprehensive health care services for a periodic *per capita* payment fixed in advance to a defined population of voluntarily enrolled members. There are many variations on the theme. For example, some own their own hospitals, while others do not.

Studies comparing costs of care under traditional insured fee-for-service with the costs for similar people, usually in the same employee group, cared for in prepaid group practices found that the total *per capita* costs in the prepaid group practices were some 10 to 40 per cent lower. Most of the difference could be ascribed to a 25 to 45 per cent reduction in hospital use. HMOs cut cost without cutting the quality of care in several ways.

Cutting Cost Without Cutting the Quality of Care

In the fee-for-service sector, physicians earn more per unit of time caring for hospitalized patients than for patients in their offices, and they earn more for doing surgery and other procedures than for taking histories and giving advice. In prepaid group practices physicians are salaried and do not face powerful economic incentives to hospitalize or to do procedures.

Other things equal, 10 per cent more surgeons *per capita* are associated with 3 per cent more surgery. A health care organization can be economical by retaining the right number of surgeons to keep them fully occupied. They are not under economic pressure to recommend surgery in doubtful cases. The same point applies to all specialities and to facilities such as hospital beds, clinical laboratories, and CT scanners.

In 1975, about 15,000 open heart surgery operations were done in 91 hospitals in California; the annual volume in 48 of the hospitals was less than 100. About 24 per cent of the cost could have been saved if all that surgery had been concentrated in 30 hospitals each doing 500 operations. Hospitals having high annual volumes have much lower surgical mortality rates than low volume hospitals. This suggests that appropriate regional concentration can lead to better care at less cost.

A great deal of medical care provided today is of no benefit to patients: unnecessary operations, prolonged hospital stays, frequent diagnostic tests, etc. Prepaid group practices generally curtail such useless care.

Prepaid group practices make extensive use of organized home nursing care and surgery on an outpatient basis as alternatives to costly inpatient care. These developments have been impeded by the irrational structure of health insurance that often pays for costly in-hospital care but not for less costly alternatives.

New technologies are frequently developed and applied very widely without a careful determination of which indications are appropriate for their use. Coronary artery bypass graft surgery is a case in point. Important economies are achieved in prepaid group practices by a more selective use of new technologies and by more systematic controlled evaluations to determine more precisely the circumstances in which they would be beneficial.

Finally, there is a great deal of room for simple cost consciousness that doesn't exist today. For example, duplication of diagnostic tests, often done when patients are admitted to a hospital, should be avoided by use of a single shared comprehensive medical record for each patient used by all physicians seeing the patient.

An examination of what efficient organizations actually do provides convincing evidence that they do cut cost substantially without cutting the quality of care. I would suggest 25 per cent as a good average figure. The achievement is all the more impressive when one recognizes that they have done this in a market in which price competition, if it exists at all, is greatly attenuated. One cannot but wonder what they might achieve if they faced serious competition from similar organizations in which most consumers were price sensitive.

One should avoid confusing spending on health care services with the total social cost of illness and its treatment. Some forms of limiting spending are not cost reduction; they merely represent a shift of cost from government or some other payer to patients. A reduction in government spending achieved at the cost of increased waiting times for surgery may be no cost reduction at all. The increased cost in discomfort or suffering of patients, though difficult to measure and perhaps invisible to much of the population, may far exceed the reduction in government spending.

The appropriate goal is to create a system in which physicians and managers are constantly seeking to find new and better ways to reduce the cost of illness and its treatment, ways to cut cost while improving the quality of care. Prepaid group practices and similar Health Maintenance Organizations with built-in incentives for quality and economy are now delivering medical care to millions of people at a cost substantially below the cost for similar people cared for under insured fee-for-service. I propose now to describe how this successful experience might eventually be made available to the whole population.

Principles of Fair Economic Competition

Analysis of successful experiences reveals principles that would describe a system of fair economic competition of alternative health care financing and delivery systems, a set of market conditions that would be favorable to the growth of economical organized systems of care that served their members well.

The first principle is *consumer choice*. Each consumer must be offered an annual choice of any of several comprehensive health care financing and delivery plans serving his area of residence.

The second principle is *cost conscious choice through fixed-dollar subsidies*. Everyone must receive a fixed-dollar subsidy usable only as a premium contribution toward the health plan of his choice. Whatever financial assistance people get must not be in the form of an open-ended entitlement as predominates today. Those persons who choose more costly health plans must pay the extra cost themselves.

The third principle is more complex: *equal rules must be applied to all competitors*. Rules governing premium setting, enrollment practices, benefits covered, and other aspects of operation are needed to make the system workable and fair. An especially important rule is community rating by actuarial class. Each health plan may set its own premiums in the light of competitive market conditions, but it must charge the same premium for the same benefits to all persons in the same actuarial rating category. It may not charge higher premiums to individuals within a category who have greater medical needs. Community rating assures high risk people of financial access to affordable health insurance.

Rules are needed to prevent healthy consumers from taking a 'free ride' by going without health insurance, pocketing the premium savings and then trying to insure or be cared for at public expense when they get sick. Rules are needed to curb deceptive and inadequate coverages and to prevent marketing strategies that make it difficult for consumers to make price comparisons. I believe the system must be designed in the frank recognition that the details of health insurance policies are difficult for people to understand. We should require all plans to cover at least a uniform package of comprehensive health care services.

The fourth principle is *physicians in competing economic units*. In a system of effective competition, everyone must be offered a choice so that people who choose economical providers can realize for themselves the savings in the form of lower premiums. *The choice being proposed is one among different provider organizations, not among different levels of insurance.*

Consumer Choice Health Plan

In 1977, while serving as a consultant to the Secretary of Health, Education and Welfare, I developed a proposal for universal health insurance based on these principles, called Consumer Choice Health Plan. In that proposal, everybody would receive a fixed-dollar subsidy usable only as a premium contribution toward membership in the qualified health care plan of his choice. The subsidy would be related to actuarial risk category and average costs in each geographic area. For people who are not poor, it would equal 60 per cent of the average per capita cost of covered services. This would replace the subsidy to employer-paid health insurance through the tax system. People with low incomes would receive additional help. Poor people would receive subsidies large enough to pay for an average comprehensive plan. Qualified health plans, eligible to receive subsidized premium contributions would have to comply with a system of rules along the lines of those I just outlined. They would have to participate in an annual open enrollment in which any eligible person could enroll in the plan of his choice, practice community rating by actuarial class, and limit aggregate out-of-pocket expenses for covered services.

The Carter Administration did not accept my proposal. By the time I delivered it, they were already irrevocably committed to their unsuccessful campaign for federal spending controls on hospitals. However, Consumer Choice Health Plan did generate a great deal of discussion.

I believe that Consumer Choice Health Plan would reconcile universal comprehensive health insurance and the need for cost conscious purchasers. Providers of care, those best qualified to make the key decisions, would be under economic pressure to organize care efficiently. Consumers would choose what they perceived to be in their best interest, and the total health care system would be transformed gradually and voluntarily into one made up of efficient organized systems that give consumers a good value for their money.

Let me mention and comment on some of the issues that have been raised.

First, what about the poor and residents of rural underserved areas? Would Consumer Choice Health Plan induce doctors to go where they are needed? People on our political left quickly equate any notion of market system with disadvantage for the poor. I reply that our present tax and Social Security laws create a subsidized open-ended demand for doctors in attractive areas where upper income people live. Consumer Choice Health Plan would put a limit on the subsidies to upper income groups and would put adequate stable medical purchasing power into the hands of the poor and residents of rural areas. One can separate questions of income distribution from the form of economic organization used to provide the services.

Another point of concern is the time it would take to transform the delivery system. Politicians and their staffs usually have extremely short time horizons. They want to know whether the proposal would do any good by the next election. I reply that Consumer Choice Health Plan must be seen as a long-term solution. It will take years to develop the management and the capital required to carry out this transformation. Under the most favorable conditions, it would take a decade or more for half the population to be covered by HMOs or other cost conscious delivery systems. But Consumer Choice Health Plan must be judged realistically against real alternatives. I do not believe there is any feasible way of transforming the health care delivery system quickly.

Prospects for the Future

What are the prospects for Consumer Choice Health Plan or any version of the incentives reform strategy now? Prediction is especially difficult at this time.

The federal budget deficit will persist, and health care spending will make an increasing contribution to it. There will be a continuing search for ways of reducing spending and increasing revenues.

The process of cutting Medicare and Medicaid without reforming the health care system will continue for a time, but it will run into increased opposition as the hardships inflicted on the poor and the aged become more apparent. However, the growth in real spending per beneficiary in Medicare of about 8 per cent per year cannot be sustained.

I think one of the biggest unknowns in the public policy arena lies in the conflict between short-term incentives for politicians and the need for long-term fundamental structural reform. Can we ever get an Administration and a Congress to support and enact long-term solutions even if that involves serious short-term political costs? If we can, then the Consumer Choice strategy for health services reform remains the option that would be most feasible for the federal government to administer, and the option most compatible with American pluralism and values.

Conclusion

Consumer Choice Health Plan is a proposal to assure universal comprehensive health insurance coverage—a traditional but elusive goal of the left—in a manner that should be acceptable to the taxpayers who would have to pay for it. It would offer conservatives a private market system with the least restraints on individual freedom consistent with universal access to good quality care. Upper income people would retain or gain the right to choose their health care plan, but they would have to pay the extra cost of a more costly plan out of their own net-after-tax incomes. Publicly supported care for the poor would be relatively economical.

These ideas are not terribly complicated. But their acceptance will require greater sophistication on the part of the body politic and its political leaders that we have seen so far. Will they be willing to think beyond traditional categories? I hope so. Because the evidence is quite clear that neither traditional socialist concepts nor a free market nor the traditional fee-for-service solo practice model offers a satisfactory solution. We ought to be ready for something new.

Alain Enthoven is an American health economist, and is the Marriner S. Eccles Professor of Public and Private Management at the Graduate School of Business, Stanford University. This article has not previously been published in English.

7.6

Alternative Medicine: Prospects and Speculations

Ruth West

Alternative medicine is witnessing a scene that a few years ago it would not have dreamed of. It has the favour of the media, the public voting for it with its feet and the medical profession taking note of its existence. It is even gaining enough of a voice to begin asking questions about taking up its rightful place within the country's health care system. However, for those practitioners who remember the earlier years, when they were all-but back street operators and the mention of their names was anathema to doctors, this new-found acceptance is regarded warily. The sight of the British Medical Association's juggernaut hurtling after them lurks in their mind's eye.

It was only in the sixties that the practice of alternative medicine was labelled 'fringe medicine'. Meant in a kindly way by those who coined the term—it was around the time of the Edinburgh Fringe—the association with 'lunatic fringe' was perhaps a little too close for comfort. And so a more fashionable, though challenging, title was substituted—that of 'alternative medicine', after 'alternative London' and 'alternative life-styles'. Since then two other labels have been invented, both of which seek a more comfortable place alongside orthodox medicine. The World Health Organisation has adopted the title 'traditional medicine'. This has worked well in developing countries, where the traditional healers and medicine men represent the indigenous non-Western medicine. But in 'developed' countries it has proved to be confusing as people have associated traditional with orthodox Western medicine and so wondered what all the fuss was about. The most recent title to be introduced is 'complementary medicine'. This has found currency with those who wish to make it clear that they are not doctor-bashers, but are wanting to achieve a partnership with orthodox medicine, each recognising the need for the other.

What is 'alternative medicine'?

If the choice of a title raises problems, then decisions as to what the title is meant to cover compounds them. There are two main options on offer. The first is to follow the World Health Organisation and include all forms of health care provision that 'usually lie outside the official health sector' including formalised traditional systems of medicine such as Ayurveda, Unani and traditional Chinese medicine; the practice of traditional healers, such as traditional birth attendants and medicine men; and the practice of biofeedback, chiropractic, naturopathy, osteopathy, homeopathy, 'and even Christian Science'.[1]

In the UK, such a categorisation would mean the inclusion of about sixty therapies, which may be divided as follows. First the physical therapies: these include naturopathy, herbal medicine, manipulative therapies (osteopathy, chiropractic, the Alexander technique, rolfing and reflexology), oriental therapies (shiatsu, acupressure), systems of medicine (acupuncture, homeopathy, anthroposophical medicine), exercise/movement therapies (T'ai chi, yoga, dance) and sensory therapies (music, art, colour). Second, the psychological therapies: psychotherapy (analysis, hypnotherapy), humanistic psychology (gestalt, transactional analysis, primal work, rebirthing, encounter. . . to name but a few), and transpersonal psychology. And lastly, paranormal therapies: healing (hand healing, exorcism, radionics and the like) and paranormal diagnosis (palmistry, astrology, iridology).

A possible objection to this option is that it treats the alternatives rather like the contents of a dustbin, some of which are of value and may with luck be rescued, but the majority of which belong in the dustbin and should remain there. A second possibility is to divide the alternatives into two basic types: those that require a high degree of professional training and skill and those that are at heart variations on first aid, do-it-yourself, and self-care techniques. Osteopathy, chiropractic, medical herbalism, homeopathy, naturopathy and acupuncture would fit under the first category; and everything else, barring a few psychotherapies, under the second. Assuming for the moment that their efficacy and safety could all be established, the first category could take its place alongside the medical profession, whilst the second category could join the ranks of the professions supplementary to medicine.

Professional and public attitudes to alternative medicine

Judging from articles in the medical and scientific journals, attitudes within the medical profession are not changing. Their pages from time to time deride alternative medicine as 'the flight from science'; they have been known to compare chiropractic which goes beyond the 'treatment of bone and joint abnormalities' with the 'occult business of divination of the future by examination of a bird's entrails'[2] and to put much of the survival of alternative medicine down to the 'needs of desperate patients for whom orthodox medicine has not succeeded'. Small wonder that the recent action of the medical trade union, the British Medical Association (BMA), raised such alarm and suspicion among alternative therapists. The association seemed to be responding to the criticisms levelled at it by their President, Prince Charles, during his term of office;

> I would suggest that the whole imposing edifice of modern medicine, for all its breath-taking success is, like the celebrated Tower of Pisa, slightly off balance . . .

> Don't overestimate the 'sophisticated' approach to medicine. Please don't underestimate the importance of an awareness of what lies beneath the surface of the visible world and of those ancient unconscious forces which still shape the psychological attitudes of modern man . . . When it comes to helping people it seems to me that account has to be taken of those sometimes long-neglected complementary methods of medicine . . .

It was shortly after this second message that the BMA announced that it had set up a committee to investigate alternative therapies. The alternatives have good reason to worry about the outcome of this committee's work. They know all too well the sceptics' reaction to the success of their treatment. It can all be put down to a good bedside manner and/or the strength of the placebo effect: if you think something is going to work, no matter how hocus-pocus it is, then there is a 40 per cent chance it will. Of the former, Dr Tony Smith, writing in the *British Medical Journal*, has this to say:[3]

> The patients are given time, courtesy and individual attention . . . which may relieve many of the symptoms of a chronic or terminal disease, but do nothing to arrest the disease process.

Two alternative systems often cited as mere placebo are homeopathy, in which any real effect is challenged on the grounds that it mostly uses medicines diluted to the extent that not one molecule of the original substance remains; and osteopathy, in which the effective treatment of anything except back pain is ridiculed on the grounds that manipulating the spine could not conceivably cure such problems as headache. Moreover, scoff the sceptics, 'if patients are resorting to practices based upon the obsolescent relics of the prehistory of modern medicine', then 'this requires urgent attention'.

But this habit of linking orthodox medicine with modern, scientific ways of thinking and alternative medicine with prescientific thinking; of equating scientific with good, effective medicine, and anything else with irrational quackery, has been described as nothing more than an example of a doctor's trained incapacity to accept any medicine as legitimate beyond his own, so dominant has the modern medical profession become in the health care system of most societies. It belongs naturally with those who hold a monopoly position: and as Lowell Levin warns:[4]

> there may be . . . sinister reasons for professional neglect of the lay resource in health. Bluntly stated, there may be some protecting of professional (for which, in many areas, read 'financial') power preserves.

While the pundits cling to their placebo theories, or argue the ethics of using or recommending the use of potentially dangerous treatments for their patients, a growing proportion of their customers, it seems, are expressing doubts and criticisms regarding the value of *orthodox* medical care. Taylor Nelson Medical is a marketing research company that has been monitoring changes in attitude to doctors, medicine and health over the past ten years. In 1978, 52 per cent of the population said that they trusted the doctor to know what they needed; this fell to 39 per cent in 1980, when 22 per cent also confessed to having less faith in doctors than they used to. General practice consultations have also been declining since 1978.

The rise of alternative medicine

A survey carried out in 1980 on behalf of the Threshold Foundation found that the number of alternative medicine consultations was increasing at the rate of 10–15 per cent per year; and the estimates for the numbers of practitioners and consultations showed that alternative medicine is growing five times as rapidly as orthodox medicine.[5]

The reasons for these changes can, in the main, only be guessed at. A survey, carried out by *Which?* in 1981, revealed that two-thirds of those who had received alternative medicine treatment during the last five years said that they had been having treatment with conventional medicine, but that it was not helping or they did not like it—because of side-effects, for example.[6] The increasing hazards to health of taking modern drugs must be contributing significantly to the trend away from conventional medicine. It has been estimated that two out of every five patients taking prescribed drugs are likely to suffer from side-effects of the drug; some drugs also produce dependence; and then there are the problems created by interactions between the drugs a patient may be taking. It is also becoming evident that there is a serious mismatch between health care provisions and real needs. Modern medicine is hospital-based, yet the vast majority of medical problems do not require hospital care. In any one month, a recent study has shown, out of 1,000 adults, 750 will develop a symptom of some kind; 250 of these will go to their general practitioner; 10 will be referred to hospital; and only 1 will be admitted. The World Health Organisation (Europe) is in fact now suggesting that the centralised notion of medical care, based on the large, expensive, industry-modelled, high technology hospital, 'providing leadership, controlling other levels and generally exercising the main responsibility for the entire spectrum of patient care' is misconceived. Perhaps what is needed are 'services . . . [to be] provided using the lowest necessary level of care, as close to the community as possible. In this perspective, the starting point for health services is the people themselves and their families, with primary health care personnel providing the necessary professional care.'[7]

While the medical world awaits its reorganisation, alternative medicine takes up the slack—as is witnessed by the growing transfer of allegiance from the doctor's surgery to the alternative medicine clinic and practitioner.

Reports such as they are on the outcome of treatment are favourable. Government Commissions of Enquiry, and Consumer Association surveys, all provide evidence in support of the alternatives: New Zealand (on chiropractic), Australia and the Netherlands (on a range of alternatives in practice) have all reported favourably; the consumer magazine *Which?* found that 9 out of every 10 people surveyed said that they would use again the form of alternative they had tried and only 10 per cent felt that the treatment had been useless. The pattern seems to be that people's first use of alternative medicine is as a last resort; but then they stay and use it again, but this time as a first choice if there is a recurrence of the problem; then gradually begin to substitute it for orthodox medicine to supply their primary health care needs—their osteopath or acupuncturist, for example, taking the place of their general practitioner. One per cent of the UK population, Taylor Nelson Medical finds, now say that they use an acupuncturist; 2 per cent go to homeopathic physicians; and, in terms of self-care, 3 per cent are practising meditation, 7 per cent use natural medicine, and 16 per cent buy health foods.

The future

Increasingly, alternative practitioners are worrying that such progress is not enough. Although the majority feel that it would injure their practice to be brought into the National Health Service (because of constraints on time and freedom to practise as they see fit, unsupervised by doctors), there is a growing sense of urgency to secure some formal recognition by Act of Parliament. But just how, and for whom, is difficult to sort out.

For many reasons, it might be best to leave things as they are: everyone practising what they want, providing that they do not claim to be a doctor or to treat certain diseases. But there is a threat from orthodoxy. Already the medical acupuncturists are pressing to be the only group able to practise acupuncture, and if the trend by young doctors to learn an alternative therapy continues, then the worry is that the alternatives that appeal to the doctors will be medicalised. They will be learnt as extra techniques on weekend courses, the monopoly will thus reassert itself, and all lay practitioners will be outlawed. The emergence, in September 1983, of a new association for doctors, the British Holistic Medical Association, which includes in its statement of principles that the holistic practitioner will be 'willing to use . . . an expanded range of interventions' to include 'acupuncture, counselling, dietary advice, exercise, osteopathy and meditative techniques' has certainly added to this concern.

If one looks for encouragement to other countries to see how they are legislating for alternative health care, then the situation is fairly bleak. There are only two countries which have managed to truly integrate Western orthodox medicine with other systems; these are China and Nepal. Certain other developing countries (mainly in South Asia) have legalised alternative medicine to the extent that it is allowed to co-exist with orthodox medicine. But the rest of the world, on the whole, legislates only for the practice of orthodox medicine. And this, alternative medicine's detractors would argue, is right and proper. Alternative medicine should only receive official recognition if it is able to gain its laurels in the same way as any orthodox branch of medicine—by laboratory work with *in vitro* or animal experiments, followed by a double-blind, controlled trial (to eliminate any possible placebo effect).

Alternative medicine feels caught in a cleft stick. In order to survive, it needs research to demonstrate its efficacy. But many practitioners object to animal experimentation and all are adamant that the above methods are not suited to them. Those therapies, for example, that involve touching the patient claim that technique and therapist, like the song and the singer, cannot be separated. So a blind, controlled trial of osteopathy would mean that one person simulates the manipulation in order to compare manipulation with no manipulation for a particular disorder. The fact that the osteopaths say you cannot pull the wool over people's eyes in this way, and that they have an alternative research design that they believe to be acceptable to both parties, leaves the funding bodies unconvinced. And so the research is not done. Similar problems are raised with acupuncture, in which the individual acupuncturist's taking of the patient's pulses and putting in the needles are essential parts of the treatment; and with reflexology, where the practitioner, rubbing the feet and talking to the patient, does not divide his technique from his art.

Left to orthodox research, the prospects for alternative medicine are exceedingly gloomy. Given the present state of affairs, the following is all that can be accepted as valid medicine: acupuncture analgesia (because it is now 'known' that it causes the brain to produce endorphins—natural morphine-like substances); certain medicines based on extractions from plants; certain vitamins for the treatment of specific deficiency diseases; and manipulation for back pain, if the criterion for success is a speedier return of the sufferer to work, i.e. it is more economical as a treatment than orthodox medicine. Yet there are some (small, vaguely perceptible) signs of change. For example, a research group at Harvard Medical School has established that there is a very real physiological response that is evoked in the body by relaxation techniques that encourages the body's own self-healing forces. This helps unravel the mechanisms of meditation, for example, and it may be a means of understanding the gift of healing that some people claim to possess.

In the meantime, whatever may be surmised about the success of the alternatives, in one particular respect they are being acknowledged as having the edge on orthodox medicine—in that they recognise that most diseases afflicting Western nations today are psychological, not organic, in origin, In fact, many alternative practitioners would say that the service they are providing, rather than covering the gaps left by orthodoxy's inadequacies, is a new, or rediscovered, holistic medicine. Instead of concentrating on illness, they look at the person who is ill and ask *why* they have become susceptible to disease. 'Organic illness is what we say we cure but don't', the maverick F. G. Crookshank wrote half a century ago. 'Functional disease is what the quacks cure and we wish we could.' Instead of looking for magical cures, alternative practitioners expect patients to collaborate in their treatment by making changes in their lifestyle. It is, after all, nearly a quarter of a century since René Dubos concluded that the improvements that had taken place in people's health had been brought about not, as we assumed, by medicine, but by improved standards of nutrition and sanitation. Furthermore, today's diseases, says Thomas McKeown, are the 'result of behavioural and environmental changes associated with industrialisation'. For McKeown the shape of things to come depends upon public action and modification of behaviour. In the present circumstances, any sensible foetus should take the following advice. He will:

> come about as near to immortality as human genes permit by electing to become the wife of a rural clergyman; well-to-do but living frugally; fertile but with few children; physically active but avoiding field sports, especially hunting; taking no drugs, alcohol or tobacco; and keeping to a diet low in salt, fat, sugar and meat, and so rich in fruit, vegetables and grains that the addition of bran would be an indulgence.[8]

Some alternative therapies have already established their usefulness within a society afflicted by 'psychosocial disease'. But whether alternative medicine will grow as a genuine alternative is difficult to say. At the moment, the amount of attention it is receiving is way out of proportion to its actual size. In the UK today, there are only 2,000 practitioners in some form of professional organisation compared with 30,000 general medical practitioners. It could just be that members of the public are clinging to any bit of driftwood for help as orthodoxy sinks—or whilst waiting for the official rescue party. This would fit in with the finding that, apart from the purchase of health foods, which is a middle-class preoccupation, the use of alternative medicine is spread evenly across the population.

A perhaps more appealing interpretation is one that sees its popularity as a sign of a wider social change that is taking place. The pendulum is swinging—away from dependence on experts and specialists, towards more consumer participation and self-reliance. Alternative medicine is just one way of exercising a belief in the importance of the democratisation of life as witnessed by the growth in self-help groups.

However, looking to the year 2000, there are three possible futures in which alternative medicine may have a place. In one, we continue much as we are. The economy survives; material well-being is maintained; and the health services are extended, modified and improved to cope with an increasing population that is weighted towards old age. In a second, disaster strikes, and we are in a life-boat economy. Alternative medicine takes up a 'barefoot doctor' role in the struggle to provide any kind of health care. In the third, society is transformed. People change from being 'outer-directed', looking for the achievement of material goals, to becoming self-explorers, seeing inner growth as the way forward. Alternative medicine takes its place as a resource for self-care, leading to health, wellbeing and personal development. Now this, according to the experts, is not such a far-fetched vision of the future.

References

1. Bannerman, R. H., Burton, J. and Wen-Chieh, Ch'en *Traditional Medicine and Health-care Coverage. A reader for health administrators and practitioners,* World Health Organisation, Geneva p. 292 (1983).
2. See, for example, 'The flight from science' in the *British Medical Journal* (5 January 1980); 'Alternative medicine is no alternative' in *The Lancet* (1 October 1983, p. 773); 'Homeopathy, fact or fiction?' in *New Scientist* (22 March 1984, p. 46).
3. 'Alternative medicine' in the *British Medical Journal* (30 July 1983, p. 307).
4. Levin, Lowell, S. 'Self-care in health: potentials and pitfalls' in *World Health Forum,* **2**(2), 177–84 (1981).
5. Fulder, Stephen and Monro, Robin 'The status of complementary medicine in the United Kingdom', Threshold Foundation Bureau, London (1981).

6. 'Alternative medicine' in *Which?* (August 1981).
7. From a document submitted for discussion by the World Health Organisation Regional Committee for Europe at its 33rd session in Madrid in September 1983.
8. McKeown, Thomas, 'A basis for health strategies: a classification of disease' in *British Medical Journal*, 287 (27 August 1983).

Ruth West is director of the Koestler Foundation in London, which was formed to promote research into unorthodox areas of science. She is co-author (with Brian Inglis) of *The Alternative Health Guide* (published in 1983 by Michael Joseph), author of a forthcoming book on parapsychological experiences and is currently compiling a bibliography of alternative medicine. This article has not appeared in print before.

7.7

Cancer and Work: Guidelines for Workers Taking Collective Action over Health Hazards

General, Municipal, Boilermakers and Allied Trades Union (GMBATU)

Hundreds of GMBATU members employed in making or handling town gas, dyestuffs, rubber goods, asbestos, radiation, water-purification agents, nickel, PVC, cadmium and other products have been killed by the chemicals and other harmful agents which they worked with. They suffered, then died, from cancer. In many cases, important clues to the cancer risks were ignored, sometimes for decades, by their employers and government departments responsible for their health.

Today, at least 1,400–11,000 cancer deaths a year are caused by harmful substances found at work. (Accidents at work kill about 1,000 workers a year.) Most of these cancer deaths are preventable. This pamphlet is part of the Union's campaign to prevent occupational cancer.

How can Occupational Cancer be prevented?

Cancer is caused by carcinogens—that is, cancer-causing agents—found in the environment in which we live and work. By preventing exposure to carcinogenic substances, we can prevent most cancer. Many carcinogens have not yet been identified, but some have.

Union policy is to demand prohibition or rigorous control of all probable and suspect carcinogens without waiting for dead workers to 'prove' that a substance is carcinogenic. Workers, not chemical substances, must be given the benefit of the doubt.

Start your cancer campaign by getting a *written* assurance that your employer does not use any of the substances in Appendices 1 and 2 (or any other suspected carcinogen) at work. If a likely carcinogen is being used, make sure:

* that substitute chemicals are considered and used, where possible;
* that likely carcinogens are handled in closed systems, with engineering controls that do not allow any exposures to workers;

* that continuous monitoring of the workplace makes sure that the engineering controls are containing the chemical; and that you get results of the monitoring;
* that workers are fully informed, in writing, of the risks, and trained in the precautions to be followed;
* that all sources are prominently labelled 'cancer hazard';
* that full personal protection for maintenance and other workers is provided;
* that effective medical and epidemiological (i.e. surveys of disease patterns among the workers) checks are provided; and
* that a 'no fault' compensation scheme is agreed with the employer which guarantees adequate protection for your dependents if you do get cancer—but don't sign anything without advice from the Union's Legal Department.

What Evidence is used to identify a Carcinogen?

This evidence comes from four main sources:

1. *Humans* (i.e. epidemiological studies). By studying the pattern and distribution of disease in groups of people epidemiologists can tell us whether there is too much cancer, and sometimes what is likely to be causing it. For example, studies of GMWU members making town gas found too many cases of lung and bladder cancer compared with the rest of the population. Workers often notice the first signs of human evidence—read on to find out how to follow up your suspicions.

The trouble with this source of evidence is that by the time we've got it, many workers will have died. Waiting for human evidence usually means experimenting with worker 'guinea-pigs'. As cancer can take a long time to appear (5–50 years), a lot of deaths can be in the pipeline before the human evidence is available.

2. *Animals*. Rats, mice and other animals can be used instead of workers. The animals are exposed to chemicals, and their cancer experience is compared with that of 'control' animals who haven't been exposed to the chemical. The experiment usually takes 2/3 years to complete. This is how all medicines and foodstuffs are tested *before* they can be marketed. Unfortunately, most of the 60,000 chemical substances in common use at work *haven't* been tested in this way.

Animal evidence can be used to predict cancer in humans if action is taken quickly enough. Here are some examples where it wasn't:

* in the 1920s GMWU gas workers complained of early deaths amongst their members; in the 1930s the tars and pitches they were exposed to caused cancer in rats; in the 1950s the epidemiologists showed excess lung and bladder cancer in gas workers;
* in the early 1930s GMWU dyestuffs and rubber workers complained of early deaths among their members; in 1938 a substance they were exposed to (betanapthylamine) was found to cause cancers in dogs (having failed to cause cancer in rats); and in the 1950s epidemiologists showed excess bladder cancer in UK dyestuffs and rubber workers (cancer found earlier in German and Swiss workers having been ignored by the UK chemical and rubber industries);
* in the 1970s the chemical VCM was found to cause cancer in animals, four years before epidemiologists discovered liver cancer in VCM workers.

Four other human carcinogens (mustard gas, 4-aminobiphenyl, melphalan and DES) have also been predicted by animal experiments, so that *positive animal evidence should* be taken as sufficient proof of cancer to justify handling substances as though they were carcinogenic for man.

Some people argue that it is cruel to use animals for cancer testing. It is, but until better methods are invented, it is better to use animals than humans.

3. *'Short-term' tests.* It is thought that most carcinogens cause cancer by changing the structure of genes in the body's cells. If substances can do this they are called 'mutagenic' substances, and are quite likely to cause cancer. Scientists have therefore devised experiments to test the mutagenicity of substances—the *Ames test* is the most famous of these. If a substance is positive in one, or several, of those tests, then it should be treated with great suspicion.

4. *Chemical structure and behaviour.* Chemicals which have a similar arrangement of atoms and molecules in their structures often behave in the same way, so that if one of them is found to be carcinogenic, then others with a similar structure should be treated with suspicion. For example, groups of chemicals such as 'aromatic amines' are known to be carcinogenic, so that any substance from these groups should be treated as a likely carcinogen.

How is the Evidence weighed up?

Before workers, or scientists, can decide whether a substance is carcinogenic or not, they have to answer two questions.

First, what *weight* will they put on the four kinds of evidence described above? For example, many experts will accept only human evidence, and will ignore the animal and other evidence, as they did with our gas workers. Other people, like the unions, the International Agency for Research on Cancer, and workers who are actually exposed to the substances being evaluated, put much more weight on animal and other non-human evidence.

Second, what *level of proof* will be used to say that substance X is a likely carcinogen? For example, scientists usually use a very high level of proof to say that 'A' causes 'B'. The level of proof they use is similar to that which we all demand from our *criminal* courts, where someone is proved to be guilty only after 'all reasonable doubt' about other suspects has been removed by the evidence. This high level of proof is used to protect us from getting our science wrong, and from convicting innocent people.

The *civil* courts, where people who have injured others are sued for damages, provide a lower level of proof. The judges in civil cases will award damages to the injured party if *'on the balance of probabilities'*, the evidence suggests that the person being sued did cause the injury. The injured party is given the benefit of the doubt.

In the trial of chemical substances suspected of being cancer killers, what level of proof should be used, and who should get the benefit of the doubt—workers or chemicals?

Many experts insist on the high level of proof ('beyond all reasonable doubt') before accepting that a substance is carcinogenic. Other experts and unions say that the lower level of proof ('balance of probabilities') is sufficient because it gives greater protection to workers.

What are the Costs of being Wrong?

If the unions are wrong, and a substance turns out *not* to have been carcinogenic after all, there will have been some unnecessary alarm and cleaning up of workplaces, and possibly some lost sales for that particular substance. But if the experts are wrong, and substances turn out to be carcinogenic, workers will have died needlessly. Which approach do you prefer?

What are the Clues about Cancer risks at Work?

The substances used are likely carcinogens. See the list in Appendices 1 and 2.

Epidemiological studies have shown 'excess' cancer. See the list of industries or occupations in Appendix 3. If you are in one of these industries, make sure exposures to all substances are kept as low as possible.

There are one or two 'rare' cancers among the workers. See Appendix 4. If there are two or more of these cancers in even large workforces (i.e. several thousands), there should be an immediate investigation. For example, a GMWU safety representative noticed several cases of skin cancer that turned out to be malignant melanoma—a rare cancer. An epidemiological investigation then revealed an excessive number of these cancers.

There are some young cancer deaths. For example, lung cancers in 30–45-year-olds, especially if any are non-smokers, are suspicious. For example, less than 5 per cent of all deaths among 35–44-year-olds should be from lung cancer, so if there is, say, three times that proportion among your members, ask for an investigation.

There seems to be too many cancer deaths among the members. Appendix 5 gives some idea of the proportion of cancer deaths in all deaths to expect. For example, if stomach cancer deaths are more than, say, 6 per cent of all deaths (instead of the 2.5 per cent you'd expect), then this should be investigated.

Gathering Further Evidence

If you want to follow-up any of the clues to cancer risks described above, you will need to collect evidence about:
(i)   the cancer deaths and other causes of death;
(ii) the numbers of workers who may have been exposed; and
(iii) the processes and substances used at work.

This work is not easy. It can take many months and you may be accused of scaremongering, of threatening jobs, or of being a militant. Try and avoid these problems by getting the support of the Shop Steward Committee, or Union Safety Committee, and by working without broadcasting what you are doing to everyone. If you can trust your employers, you may want to work together. If not, avoid antagonising them, or alerting them to what you are doing. *It will still be useful at an early stage to try and get written evidence that personnel and other records from many years ago still exist,* so that any further studies are not prevented by an absence of good records.

The Cancer Deaths and Causes of Death
The *minimum* information you need to be able to show that there might be a cancer problem in your workplace is:

* the total number of cancer deaths in a certain period;
* the type of cancers in that total
    AND
* the numbers of all other deaths amongst employees in the same period

OR
* the approximate numbers of employees from which the cancer cases came (the 'numbers at risk').

    With this information it may be possible to show that:

* the PROPORTION *of cancer deaths in all the deaths* is much higher than the national average (say, 40 per cent instead of 20 per cent)—this is called the *PROPORTIONAL MORTALITY RATIO or PMR*
OR
* the NUMBER *of cancer deaths you have observed in your group of employees is higher than you would expect* if they were similar to the national average—this is called the *STANDARDISED MORTALITY RATIO or SMR.*
    The PMR and the SMR are two basic tools of epidemiology that help to answer the important question 'Is there a cancer problem?'
    The evidence you collect will be used by the Union to see if your suspicions are confirmed by a preliminary investigation. But the most important part of any investigation is the collection of evidence, and safety reps are often in the best position to collect this.

Sources of Evidence on Deaths

There are at least seven sources of evidence that you should try.
    1. *Union members, relatives and friends.* Ask around, especially the older members, pensioners, ex-branch secretaries, wives, anyone involved in sick clubs, supervisors who came off the shopfloor years ago, etc. Try to persuade them to keep your investigation as confidential as possible so that any alarm is kept to a minimum.
    2. *Union records.* Ask branch secretaries, regional officials and area district regional finance or benefits officers. Many unions need to see a death certificate (see below) before they pay out funeral or death benefit, so they will know if someone has died, and maybe the cause of death, if benefit has been claimed. Dust off old boxes of records—you may find just what you need.
    3. *Obituary columns in the local newspaper.* This involves real detective work, but you often find that some people look at these columns regularly. Ask them to look at the last five years in the local library to see if they recognise anyone, making a note of the name, age, address and next of kin if they do. You may be able to help them with a list of employees so that they don't have to rely on recognising someone they know.
    4. *Death certificates.* These are *public documents,* available to anyone. They are not confidential. And they are the best source of evidence on deaths. For everyone who dies in Britain there must be a death certificate stating the cause of death. Several causes may be mentioned, recording the chain of events that led to death. For example, if lung cancer led to respiratory failure and then cardiac arrest (or heart failure), each of these would be mentioned (see the specimen copy in Appendix 6). Most analyses of deaths are based on the *underlying cause of death* and there are strict rules for deciding which is the underlying cause, so that everyone interprets or 'reads' a death certificate in the same way.
    In general, if CANCER is mentioned in Part I of the death certificate, it is considered to be the underlying cause, but not if it is mentioned in Part II. If two types of cancers are mentioned in Part I, e.g. 'brain' and 'lung', the second one is considered to be the underlying cause of death. You will need to know some of the jargon that doctors

use if you are not to miss some cancers, and common jargon is explained in Appendix 7. If in doubt, ask your GP or a medical student, or consult a medical dictionary in your local library (see 'Sources of Information' in Appendix 11).

Death certificates may not always be accurate, or complete. In general, studies have shown that only 60–80 per cent of death certificates are accurate when checked against the best evidence available from hospital records, post-mortems, etc. So *if you think a member has died from an occupational cause, and it's not too late, try and get a post-mortem and an inquest.*

In addition, some workers will get cancer yet not die from it, so other sources which identify cancer *cases* (called 'cancer *incidence*') instead of just cancer deaths (called 'cancer *mortality*') may need to be used when you're investigating cancers that can be successfully treated, e.g. skin or thyroid cancer. This booklet concentrates on cancer mortality, but if you come across live cancer cases in your searches keep a record of them as they may be useful later.

5. *Post-mortem and inquest reports.* Copies of post-mortem reports ordered by the coroners can be obtained from their local offices by any properly interested person such as a trade union representative or a close relative. *Coroners* will hold an inquest if they believe the death was 'unnatural' and *they have been instructed by the Home Office to take account of the wishes of relatives, trade union representatives and HSE Inspectors when deciding whether to hold an inquest.* If an inquest is held, then union representatives can attend, question witnesses and afterwards receive copies of the post-mortem report and notes of evidence.

6. *Company records.* Employers may have information about employees' deaths in their medical, pensions or personnel files, and if you are able to cooperate with your employer this can be the quickest and most comprehensive source of evidence. *There is nothing confidential about deaths—you are not asking for medical records—so if employers have this information they should share it with you.*

7. *National records.* Details of everyone's death in Britain are recorded and epidemiologists can obtain copies of these details for their investigations. This helps them to trace at least 95 per cent of the employees they look for.

How to Collect the Evidence

Use the sources of information described above to collect details of the deaths amongst current or ex-employees in the department/s or factory that you are concerned about. Choose at least a *five to ten year period*, and exclude those who worked for less than a year. Try and get copies of death certificates of the cancer deaths from relatives or other written proof of cause of death from them or your employer, but if that's impossible read Appendix 8, 'How to obtain copies of death certificates', and get them yourself. Make sure you have the correct name and approximate date of death before you start looking, as this will save you time. Remember, death certificates are public records. Use the 'Cancer case sheet' in Appendix 9 to fill in as many details as you can, but don't worry if you can only get the

* name
* approximate age at death
* date of death
* type of cancer
* approximate length of service in relevant dept or area
* usual job or department

because this will be enough to get a rough answer to 'Is there a problem?' *You only need this detail for the cancer deaths* because a simple PMR analysis can be done with just *the numbers (and preferably the ages) of other deaths* in the department or area.

Numbers of employees at risk

Employees at risk are those who have worked in the relevant department or factory. Usually the longer they have worked there, the more they are at risk, but some cancers have been caused in workers who have had only several months exposure. Epidemiologists will make detailed calculations on this but the *minimum* needed for our simple analysis is:

* the size of the workforce in the relevant department/s or factory during the period chosen for the deaths (i.e. the last 5–10 years);
* approximate turnover; and
* approximate ages of the employees in rough ten-year groups, e.g. 25—34, 35–44, etc., to 74 (a guess at this 'age distribution' will be better than nothing).

Substances or processes used by employees

If you can show that the cancer cases come mainly from particular departments or areas, then the evidence of any occupational link becomes stronger. Use the 'Department or factory information sheet' in Appendix 10 to summarise the information about the department/s or factory under suspicion, and another department (if there is one) that seems not to cause any cancers.

What *substances or processes* are used in the department/s or factory under suspicion? Main *sources* of this information are:

* labels—the chemical names of over 1,000 dangerous substances are now required by the 1978 and 1981 Labelling Regulations;
* the Substances Audit which employers should have for each department;
* the information from suppliers/importers/manufacturers of substances which has to be given to safety representatives, via employers, under Section 6 of the HSW Act and the Safety Representatives Regulations (see GMWU recommended Chemical Data Sheet and Checklist, available from the Regional Health and Safety Service);
* the supplies or stores department of your workplace;
* the Health and Safety Executive, who should ensure that employers tell employees what toxic substances they are working with;
* your employer's safety or occupational hygiene department, if there is one;
* reference books on production processes; or
* epidemiological or occupational hygiene studies of similar work processes that appear in scientific journals.

At a later stage the epidemiologists will be interested in *how much* of the substances workers have been exposed to, so find out now *if your employer or the HSE has ever monitored the working environment for dust or fume levels, etc.* As a safety representative, you have a legal right to these monitoring results. If there has not been any monitoring, crude but valuable measures of exposure can be obtained by asking workers and supervisors to estimate whether particular workers or jobs received 'high', 'medium' or 'low' exposure.

Using the Evidence

Use whatever evidence or clues you may have to get some further investigation by your employment medical advisory service doctor or sympathetic experts. Seek advice from your union's regional health and safety officer. Your suspicions may turn out to be misplaced, but if you are right, as several GMWU safety reps have been, you will have helped prevent some future deaths, and possibly helped to get compensation for families.

It will take time for any investigation to finish. Do not let the wait for results hold up any cleaning up of the plant, especially if toxic substances or suspected carcinogens are being handled.

Finally, ignore the charge of 'you're unreasonable'. As Bernard Shaw said, 'all progress depends on unreasonable men—and women'.

This is an edited extract from an occupational cancer prevention package produced by David Gee, National Health and Safety Officer of the General Municipal, Boilermakers and Allied Trades Union, one of the largest British trade unions for manual workers. The full package is available from the Union at: Thorne House, Ruxley Ridge, Claygate, Esher, Surrey KT10 0TL (UK).

7.8

Brave New World

Aldous Huxley

A squat grey building of only thirty-four storeys. Over the main entrance the words, CENTRAL LONDON HATCHERY AND CONDITIONING CENTRE, and, in a shield, the World State's motto, COMMUNITY, IDENTITY, STABILITY.

The enormous room on the ground floor faced towards the north. Cold for all the summer beyond the panes, for all the tropical heat of the room itself, a harsh thin light glared through the windows, hungrily seeking some draped lay figure, some pallid shape of academic goose-flesh, but finding only the glass and nickel and bleakly shining porcelain of a laboratory. Wintriness responded to wintriness. The overalls of the workers were white, their hands gloved with a pale corpse-coloured rubber. The light was frozen, dead, a ghost. Only from the yellow barrels of the microscopes did it borrow a certain rich and living substance, lying along the polished tubes like butter, streak after luscious streak in long recession down the work tables.

'And this', said the Director opening the door, 'is the Fertilizing Room.'

Bent over their instruments, three hundred Fertilizers were plunged, as the Director of Hatcheries and Conditioning entered the room, in the scarcely breathing silence, the absent-minded soliloquizing hum or whistle, of absorbed concentration. A troop of newly arrived students, very young, pink and callow, followed nervously, rather abjectly, at the Director's heels. Each of them carried a note-book, in which, whenever the great man spoke, he desperately scribbled. Straight from the horse's mouth. It was a rare privilege. The DHC for Central London always made a point of personally conducting his new students round the various departments.

'Just to give you a general idea,' he would explain to them. For of course some sort of general idea they must have, if they were to do their work intelligently—though as little of one, if they were to be good and happy members of society, as possible. For particulars, as everyone knows, make for virtue and happiness; generalities are intellectually necessary evils. Not philosophers, but fret-sawyers and stamp collectors compose the backbone of society.

'Tomorrow', he would add, smiling at them with a slightly menacing geniality, 'you will be settling down to serious work. You won't have time for generalities. Meanwhile...'

Meanwhile, it was a privilege. Straight from the horse's mouth into the note-book. The boys scribbled like mad.

Tall and rather thin but upright, the Director advanced into the room. He had a long chin and big, rather prominent teeth, just covered, when he was not talking, by his full, floridly curved lips. Old, young? Thirty? fifty? fifty-five? It was hard to say. And anyhow the question didn't arise; in this year of stability, AF 632, it didn't occur to you to ask it.

'I shall begin at the beginning,' said the DHC, and the more zealous students recorded his intention in their note-books: *Begin at the beginning.* 'These', he waved his hand, 'are the incubators.' And opening an insulated door he showed them racks upon racks of numbered test-tubes. 'The week's supply of ova. Kept', he explained, 'at blood heat; whereas the male gametes,' and here he opened another door, 'they have to be kept at thirty-five instead of thirty-seven. Full blood heat sterilizes.' Rams wrapped in thermogene beget no lambs.

Still leaning against the incubators he gave them, while the pencils scurried illegibly across the pages, a brief description of the modern fertilizing process; spoke first, of course, of its surgical introduction—'the operation undergone voluntarily for the good of Society, not to mention the fact that it carries a bonus amounting to six months' salary'; continued with some account of the technique for preserving the excised ovary alive and actively developing; passed on to a consideration of optimum temperature, salinity, viscosity; referred to the liquor in which the detached and ripened eggs were kept; and, leading his charges to the work tables, actually showed them how this liquor was drawn off from the test-tubes; how it was let out drop by drop on to the specially warmed slides of the microscopes; how the eggs which it contained were inspected for abnormalities, counted and transferred to a porous receptacle; how (and he now took them to watch the operation) this receptacle was immersed in a warm bouillon containing free-swimming spermatozoa—at a minimum concentration of one hundred thousand per cubic centimetre, he insisted; and how, after ten minutes, the container was lifted out of the liquor and its contents re-examined; how, if any of the eggs remained unfertilized, it was again immersed, and, if necessary, yet again; how the fertilized ova went back to the incubators; where the Alphas and Betas remained until definitely bottled; while the Gammas, Deltas and Epsilons were brought out again, after only thirty-six hours, to undergo Bokanovsky's Process.

'Bokanovsky's Process,' repeated the Director, and the students underlined the words in their little note-books.

One egg, one embryo, one adult—normality. But a bokanovskified egg will bud, will proliferate, will divide. From eight to ninety-six buds, and every bud will grow into a perfectly formed embryo, and every embryo into a full-sized adult. Making ninety-six human beings grow where only one grew before. Progress.

'Essentially', the DHC concluded, 'bokanovskification consists of a series of arrests of development. We check the normal growth and, paradoxically enough, the egg responds by budding.'

Responds by budding. The pencils were busy.

He pointed. On a very slowly moving band a rackful of test-tubes was entering a large metal box, another rackful was emerging. Machinery faintly purred. It took eight minutes for the tubes to go through, he told them. Eight minutes of hard X-rays being about as much as an egg can stand. A few died; of the rest, the least susceptible divided into two; most put out four buds; some eight; all were returned to the incubators, where the buds began to develop; then, after two days, were suddenly chilled, chilled and checked. Two, four, eight, the buds in their turn budded; and having budded were dosed almost to death with alcohol; consequently burgeoned again and having budded—bud out of bud out of bud—were thereafter—further arrest being generally fatal—left to develop in peace. By which time the original egg was in a fair way to becoming anything from eight to ninety-six embryos—a prodigious improvement, you will agree, on nature. Identical twins—but not in piddling twos and threes as in the old viviparous days, when an egg would sometimes accidentally divide; actually by dozens, by scores at a time.

'Scores,' the Director repeated and flung out his arms, as though he were distributing largesse. 'Scores.'

But one of the students was fool enough to ask where the advantage lay.

'My good boy!' The Director wheeled sharply round on him. 'Can't you see? Can't you *see*?' He raised a hand; his expression was solemn. 'Bokanovsky's Process is one of the major instruments of social stability!'

Major instruments of social stability.

Standard men and women; in uniform batches. The whole of a small factory staffed with the products of a single bokanovskified egg.

'Ninety-six identical twins working ninety-six identical machines!' The voice was almost tremulous with enthusiasm. 'You really know where you are. For the first time in history.' He quoted the planetary motto. 'Community, Identity, Stability.' Grand words. 'If we could bokanovskify indefinitely the whole problem would be solved.'

Solved by standard Gammas, unvarying Deltas, uniform Epsilons. Millions of identical twins. The principle of mass production at last applied to biology.

'But, alas', the Director shook his head, 'we *can't* bokanovskify indefinitely.'

Ninety-six seemed to be the limit; seventy-two a good average. From the same ovary and with gametes of the same male to manufacture as many batches of identical twins as possible—that was the best (sadly a second best) that they could do. And even that was difficult.

'For in nature it takes thirty years for two hundred eggs to reach maturity. But our business is to stabilize the population at this moment, here and now. Dribbling out twins over a quarter of a century—what would be the use of that?'

Obviously, no use at all. But Podsnap's Technique had immensely accelerated the process of ripening. They could make sure of at least a hundred and fifty mature eggs within two years. Fertilize and bokanovskify—in other words, multiply by seventy-two—and you get an average of nearly eleven thousand brothers and sisters in a hundred and fifty batches of identical twins, all within two years of the same age.

'And in exceptional cases we can make one ovary yield us over fifteen thousand adult individuals.'

Beckoning to a fair-haired, ruddy young man who happened to be passing at the moment, 'Mr Foster,' he called. The ruddy young man approached. 'Can you tell us the record for a single ovary, Mr Foster?'

'Sixteen thousand and twelve in this Centre,' Mr Foster replied without hesitation. He spoke very quickly, had a vivacious blue eye, and took an evident pleasure in quoting figures. 'Sixteen thousand and twelve; in one hundred and eighty-nine batches of identicals. But of course they've done much better', he rattled on, 'in some of the tropical Centres. Singapore has often produced over sixteen thousand five hundred; and Mombasa has actually touched the seventeen thousand mark. But then they have unfair advantages. You should see the way a Negro ovary responds to pituitary! It's quite astonishing, when you're used to working with European material. Still', he added, with a laugh (but the light of combat was in his eyes and the lift of his chin was challenging), 'still, we mean to beat them if we can. I'm working on a wonderful Delta-Minus ovary at this moment. Only just eighteen months old. Over twelve thousand seven hundred children already, either decanted or in embryo. And still going strong. We'll beat them yet.'

'That's the spirit I like!' cried the Director, and clapped Mr Foster on the shoulder. 'Come along with us and give these boys the benefit of your expert knowledge.'

Mr Foster smiled modestly. 'With pleasure.' They went.

In the Bottling Room all was harmonious bustle and ordered activity. Flaps of fresh sow's peritoneum ready to cut to the proper size came shooting up in little lifts from the Organ Store in the sub-basement. Whizz and then, click! the lift-hatches flew open; the

Bottle-Liner had only to reach out a hand, take the flap, insert, smooth-down, and before the lined bottle had had time to travel out of reach along the endless band, whizz, click! another flap of peritoneum had shot up from the depths, ready to be slipped into yet another bottle, the next of that slow interminable procession on the band.

Next to the Liners stood the Matriculators. The procession advanced; one by one the eggs were transferred from their test-tubes to the larger containers; deftly the peritoneal lining was slit, the morula dropped into place, the saline solution poured in . . . and already the bottle had passed, and it was the turn of the labellers. Heredity, date of fertilization, membership of Bokanovsky Group—details were transferred from test-tube to bottle. No longer anonymous, but named, identified, the procession marched slowly on; on through an opening in the wall, slowly on into the Social Predestination Room.

'Eighty-eight cubic metres of card-index,' said Mr Foster with relish, as they entered.

'Containing *all* the relevant information,' added the Director.

'Brought up to date every morning.'

'And coordinated every afternoon.'

'On the basis of which they make their calculations.'

'So many individuals, of such and such quality,' said Mr Foster.

'Distributed in such and such quantities.'

'The optimum Decanting Rate at any given moment.'

'Unforeseen wastages promptly made good.'

'Promptly,' repeated Mr Foster. 'If you knew the amount of overtime I had to put in after the last Japanese earthquake!' He laughed good-humouredly and shook his head.

'The Predestinators send in their figures to the Fertilizers.'

'Who give them the embryos they ask for.'

'And the bottles come in here to be predestined in detail.'

'After which they are sent down to the Embryo Store.'

'Where we now proceed ourselves.'

And opening a door Mr Foster led the way down a staircase into the basement.

The temperature was still tropical. They descended into a thickening twilight. Two doors and a passage with a double turn ensured the cellar against any possible infiltration of the day.

'Embryos are like photograph film,' said Mr Foster waggishly, as he pushed open the second door. 'They can only stand red light.'

And in effect the sultry darkness into which the students now followed him was visible and crimson, like the darkness of closed eyes on a summer's afternoon. The bulging flanks of row on receding row and tier above tier of bottles glinted with innumerable rubies, and among the rubies moved the dim red spectres of men and women with purple eyes and all the symptoms of lupus. The hum and rattle of machinery faintly stirred the air.

'Give them a few figures, Mr Foster,' said the Director, who was tired of talking.

Mr Foster was only too happy to give them a few figures.

Two hundred and twenty metres long, two hundred wide, ten high. He pointed upwards. Like chickens drinking, the students lifted their eyes towards the distant ceiling.

Three tiers of racks: ground-floor level, first gallery, second gallery.

The spidery steelwork of gallery above gallery faded away in all directions into the dark. Near them three red ghosts were busily unloading demijohns from a moving staircase.

The escalator from the Social Predestination Room.

Each bottle could be placed on one of fifteen racks, each rack, though you couldn't see it, was a conveyor travelling at the rate of thirty-three and a third centimetres an hour. Two hundred and sixty-seven days at eight metres a day. Two thousand one hundred and thirty-six metres in all. One circuit of the cellar at ground level, one on the first gallery, half on the second, and on the two hundred and sixty-seventh morning, daylight in the Decanting Room. Independent existence—so called.

'But in the interval', Mr Foster concluded, 'we've managed to do a lot to them. Oh, a very great deal.' His laugh was knowing and triumphant.

'That's the spirit I like,' said the Director once more. 'Let's walk round. You tell them everything, Mr Foster.'

Mr Foster duly told them.

Told them of the growing embryo on its bed of peritoneum. Made them taste the rich blood-surrogate on which it fed. Explained why it had to be stimulated with placentin and thyroxin. Told them of the *corpus luteum* extract. Showed them the jets through which at every twelfth metre from zero to 2040 it was automatically injected. Spoke of those gradually increasing doses of pituitary administered during the final ninety-six metres of their course. Described the artificial maternal circulation installed on every bottle at Metre 112, showed them the reservoir of blood-surrogate, the centrifugal pump that kept the liquid moving over the placenta and drove it through the synthetic lung and waste-product filter. Referred to the embryo's troublesome tendency to anaemia, to the massive doses of hog's stomach extract and foetal foal's liver with which, in consequence, it had to be supplied.

Showed them the simple mechanism by means of which, during the last two metres out of every eight, all the embryos were simultaneously shaken into familiarity with movement. Hinted at the gravity of the so-called 'trauma of decanting', and enumerated the precautions taken to minimize, by a suitable training of the bottled embryo, that dangerous shock. Told them of the tests for sex carried out in the neighbourhood of Metre 200. Explained the system of labelling—a T for the males, a circle for the females and for those who were destined to become freemartins a question mark, black on a white ground.

'For of course', said Mr Foster, 'in the vast majority of cases, fertility is merely a nuisance. One fertile ovary in twelve hundred—that would really be quite sufficient for our purposes. But we want to have a good choice. And of course one must always leave an enormous margin of safety. So we allow as many as thirty per cent of the female embryos to develop normally. The others get a dose of male sex-hormone every twenty-four metres for the rest of the course. Result: they're decanted as freemartins—structurally quite normal (except', he had to admit, 'that they *do* have just the slightest tendency to grow beards), but sterile. Guaranteed sterile. Which brings us at last', continued Mr Foster, 'out of the realm of mere slavish imitation of nature into the much more interesting world of human invention.'

He rubbed his hands. For, of course, they didn't content themselves with merely hatching out embryos: any cow could do that.

'We also predestine and condition. We decant our babies as socialized human beings, as Alphas or Epsilons, as future sewage workers or future. . . .' He was going to say 'future World Controllers', but correcting himself, said 'future Directors of Hatcheries' instead.

The DHC acknowledged the compliment with a smile.

They were passing Metre 320 on Rack 11. A young Beta-Minus mechanic was busy with screw-driver and spanner on the blood-surrogate pump of a passing bottle. The hum of the electric motor deepened by fractions of a tone as he turned the nuts. Down, down. . . . A final twist, a glance at the revolution counter, and he was done. He moved two paces down the line and began the same process on the next pump.

'Reducing the number of revolutions per minute,' Mr Foster explained. 'The surrogate goes round slower; therefore passes through the lung at longer intervals; therefore gives the embryo less oxygen. Nothing like oxygen-shortage for keeping an embryo below par.' Again he rubbed his hands.

'But why do you want to keep the embryo below par?' asked an ingenuous student.

'Ass!' said the Director, breaking a long silence. 'Hasn't it occurred to you that an Epsilon embryo must have an Epsilon environment as well as an Epsilon heredity?'

It evidently hadn't occurred to him. He was covered with confusion.

'The lower the caste', said Mr Foster, 'the shorter the oxygen.' The first organ affected was the brain. After that the skeleton. At seventy per cent of normal oxygen you got dwarfs. At less than seventy, eyeless monsters.

'Who are no use at all,' concluded Mr Foster.

Whereas (his voice became confidential and eager), if they could discover a technique for shortening the period of maturation, what a triumph, what a benefaction to Society!

'Consider the horse.'

They considered it.

Mature at six; the elephant at ten. While at thirteen a man is not yet sexually mature; and is only fully grown at twenty. Hence, of course, that fruit of delayed development, the human intelligence.

'But in Epsilons', said Mr Foster very justly, 'we don't need human intelligence.'

Didn't need and didn't get it. But though the Epsilon mind was mature at ten, the Epsilon body was not fit to work till eighteen. Long years of superfluous and wasted immaturity. If the physical development could be speeded up till it was as quick, say, as a cow's what an enormous saving to the Community!

'Enormous!' murmured the students. Mr Foster's enthusiasm was infectious.

He became rather technical; spoke of the abnormal endocrine coordination which made men grow so slowly; postulated a germinal mutation to account for it. Could the effects of this germinal mutation be undone? Could the individual Epsilon embryo be made to revert, by a suitable technique, to the normality of dogs and cows? That was the problem. And it was all but solved.

Pilkington, at Mombasa, had produced individuals who were sexually mature at four and full grown at six and a half. A scientific triumph. But socially useless. Six-year-old men and women were too stupid to do even Epsilon work. And the process was an all-or-nothing one; either you failed to modify at all, or else you modified the whole way. They were still trying to find the ideal compromise between adults of twenty and adults of six. So far without success. Mr Foster sighed and shook his head.

Their wanderings through the crimson twilight had brought them to the neighbourhood of Metre 170 on Rack 9. From this point onwards Rack 9 was enclosed and the bottles performed the remainder of their journey in a kind of tunnel, interrupted here and there by openings two or three metres wide.

'Heat conditioning,' said Mr Foster.

Hot tunnels alternated with cool tunnels. Coolness was wedded to discomfort in the form of hard X-rays. By the time they were decanted the embryos had a horror of cold. They were predestined to emigrate to the tropics, to be miners and acetate-silk spinners and steel workers. Later on their minds would be made to endorse the judgement of their bodies. 'We condition them to thrive on heat,' concluded Mr Foster. 'Our colleagues upstairs will teach them to love it.'

'And that', put in the Director sententiously, 'that is the secret of happiness and virtue—liking what you've *got* to do. All conditioning aims at that: making people like their unescapable social destiny.'

In a gap between two tunnels, a nurse was delicately probing with a long fine syringe into the gelatinous contents of a passing bottle. The students and their guides stood watching her for a few moments in silence.

Aldous Huxley (1894–1963) was a member of a famous family including Thomas Huxley and the scientist Julian Huxley. He wrote in a wide range of genres: the short story, travel books, historical studies and essays.

Brave New World was first published by Chatto and Windus in 1932, and has been reprinted many times. The extract included here comprises the opening pages of the book.

Index